Video Atlas of Hypospadias Surgery

Springer Nature More Media App

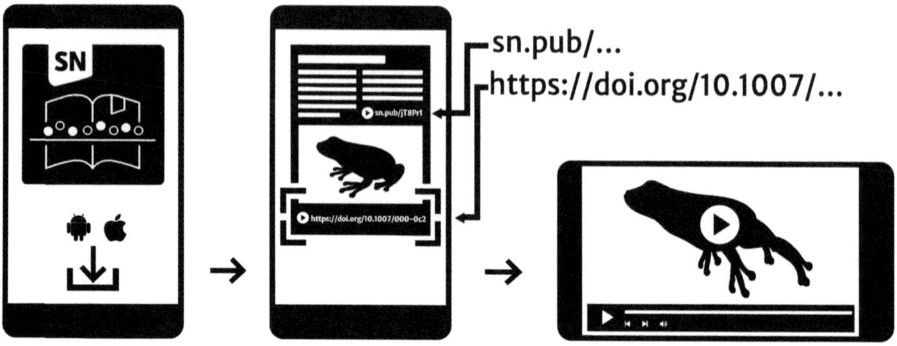

1. Download → 2. Scan Link → 3. Enjoy Video

Tariq O. Abbas
Editor

Video Atlas of Hypospadias Surgery

Springer

Editor
Tariq O. Abbas
Weil-Cornell Medical College-Qatar
Sidra Medicine
Doha, Qatar

ISBN 978-981-99-0794-6 ISBN 978-981-99-0795-3 (eBook)
https://doi.org/10.1007/978-981-99-0795-3

This Springer imprint is published by the registered company Springer Nature Singapore Pte Ltd.
The registered company address is: 152 Beach Road, #21-01/04 Gateway East, Singapore 189721, Singapore

Preface

With profound appreciation and modesty, I introduce this comprehensive video atlas of hypospadias surgery. The successful completion of this venture rested on the steady encouragement and support of my valued family, who stood by my side at each phase. I am deeply indebted to my wife, whose constant support of my aspirations has been a tremendous source of motivation, as well as to my children, whose tolerance and support have sustained me throughout challenging periods of my academic journey.

Furthermore, my gratitude extends to the diligent and knowledgeable contributors of the chapters, whose contributions have enhanced the quality of this atlas and rendered it an indispensable asset for practicing surgeons and trainees. Their eagerness to impart their expertise and perceptions will undeniably prove advantageous to a variety of individuals dealing with the complexities of hypospadias reconstruction.

As we traverse the intricacies of surgical practice, may this atlas function as an illuminating light and source of motivation and knowledge, enabling us to deliver hypospadias patients the utmost quality of care.

Sincere regards,

Doha, Qatar | Tariq O. Abbas

Contents

Part III Procedures for the Repair of Proximal Hypospadias

Part IV Procedures to Correct Penile Curvature

Part I

Introduction

Training and Knowledge Transfer in Hypospadias Reconstruction

1

Tariq O. Abbas

Abstract

Hypospadias presents with a wide range of patient phenotypes and severity levels, resulting in the development of several hundred different procedures for corrective surgery. Over the past 20 years, advances in optical magnification, finer suture materials, and new methods for inducing artificial erection have led both surgeons and patients to expect improved aesthetic and functional outcomes. Hypospadias surgery is complex and requires a level of precision and specialization that surpasses many routine urology procedures. Consequently, appropriate training, expert mentoring, and relevant experience exert major influences on post-operative results. Following technical advances including global internet connectivity and access to portable electronic devices, online educational materials are now an integral part of the surgical educational arsenal. While platforms such as YouTube have contributed to the widespread availability of surgical videos, these typically lack careful explanation of pre-, intra-, and post-operative details that are considered crucial for surgical trainees. Related information such as anatomical variables, key indications, patient selection criteria, and complications are also routinely overlooked. Production of high-quality, peer-reviewed videos that can be integrated into online repositories should therefore be a high priority for future educational efforts in this field, which is the main goal of this *Video Atlas of Hypospadias Surgery*.

Keywords

Hypospadias · Urethroplasty · Video · Learning, skills · e-book · Residents · Specialists · Surgery · Urology · Video-based learning

T. O. Abbas (✉)
Pediatric Urology Section, Sidra Medicine, Doha, Qatar
e-mail: tabbas@sidra.org

T. O. Abbas (ed.), *Video Atlas of Hypospadias Surgery*,
https://doi.org/10.1007/978-981-99-0795-3_1

1.1 Introduction

Hypospadias incidence and clinical experience with this condition vary significantly between regions. North America has the highest current rate of hypospadias, at 34.2 cases per 10,000 live births, whereas Asia has the lowest prevalence at just 0.6–69 cases per 10,000 newborns [1, 2]. The penile curvature (PC) associated with this defect can cause problems during sexual activity, spraying of the urine stream, inability to urinate while standing, infertility due to poor sperm deposition, and dissatisfaction with genital appearance [3–6]. The primary objective of hypospadias correction is therefore to restore normal appearance and function of the penis, for which multiple different techniques have been developed over time. The anatomy of the penis and urethra is intricate, hence surgical correction of hypospadias requires a detailed understanding of these complex structures [7]. However, since hypospadias correction is a very delicate procedure, surgeons often have limited exposure to these cases during surgical skills training, which is a major barrier to improving patient outcomes [8]. Surgeons must be familiar with the diverse surgical techniques used to correct hypospadias and select the most appropriate method for each patient [9]. Indeed, since hypospadias presents in various forms and degrees of severity, it is extremely challenging to achieve a standardized correction strategy. Hypospadias surgery is also technically difficult and requires a high level of precision, hence surgeons must be capable of suturing and handling delicate tissues without causing injury and triggering associated complications (including urethral fistula/strictures and glans dehiscence). To mitigate negative impact on patients, surgeons must also be trained to identify and manage these complications promptly. To address these numerous obstacles, specialized training programs in hypospadias surgery have been developed to equip surgeons with the skills and experience necessary in this field. Typically, these programs combine didactic lectures, hands-on surgical training, and mentorship from seasoned surgeons.

1.2 Need to Improve and Standardize Training in Hypospadias Repair

There are over 250 different methods of hypospadias correction, the effectiveness of which largely depends on surgical expertise and the availability of tissues suitable for repair [10]. The majority of prior research has been in the form of observational studies, and yet common techniques for hypospadias correction remain unstandardized, partly due to the lack of uniform definitions for patient phenotype and result assessment [11, 12]. As a result, ~40% of patients who undergo surgery for proximal hypospadias later report voiding problems including hesitation and spraying [13, 14].

After comprehensive, systematic assessment of numerous hypospadias repair methods, no single urethroplasty approach is demonstrably superior to the others. In addition, lack of consistency in reporting makes it difficult to compare series in the scientific literature, thus hindering the formation of general recommendations

[15–18]. Hypospadias repair procedures require dedicated surgical skills to overcome specific technical challenges. According to Manzoni, a surgeon should ideally perform 40–50 hypospadias repairs annually, and still higher numbers would be appropriate for challenging redo cases [19]. The current paradigm for training surgeons is mainly based on Halstedian frameworks, [20] in which students learn by observing experienced doctors perform relevant surgical procedures. This provides the opportunity to gain knowledge, technical abilities, and critical judgment necessary to perform safe and effective procedures on patients. Surgical knowledge is essential to healthcare, but educating competent surgeons is difficult due to factors including work time directives, [21] and limited opportunities to practice fundamental procedures [22, 23].

Hypospadias reconstruction is one of the most frequently performed specialist operations in pediatric urology, but a recent online poll of fellowship graduates indicated a need for extra training in repair surgery [24]. Younger faculty members are likely to employ web- and video-based teaching techniques more than textbooks, surgical atlases, and periodicals, but current learning resources for distal hypospadias repair are scant. The Computer Enhanced Visual Learning (CEVL) method [25] is currently the only online program that teaches the fundamentals of hypospadias surgery, by presenting static graphics of the procedure's most important phases. Prior research has revealed that learners typically prefer YouTube videos owing to their accessibility [26], but these often lack sufficient high-quality content to be recommended for training purposes. In a recent investigation, Haslam et al. found that YouTube videos of pediatric robotic pyeloplasty frequently omitted essential surgical procedures [27].

While there may be more than one "correct" method for completing a given surgical task, standardization is nonetheless the starting point for optimizing patient outcomes. Implementing and maintaining regular methods of operation as well as accurate databases of personal outcomes is a crucial first step for individual practitioners. If findings are to be published, care must be taken to detail every procedure in full.

It is critical to enhance and standardize training in hypospadias repair for several rationales:

1. Surgeons with adequate specialist training/standardized approaches to hypospadias repair are more likely to perform effective procedures and avoid complications.
2. Correction of hypospadias is associated with high incidence of urethral fistula/strictures and glans dehiscence. Improved training should lead to decreased complication rates, thereby reducing morbidity and lowering healthcare costs.
3. Hypospadias repair is a complex surgical procedure requiring technical skills and experience. Better access to high-quality training will increase the number of qualified surgeons available to perform these procedures, thereby enhancing patient access to care.
4. Standardized training will lead to greater consistency of surgical technique, thereby improving post-operative results and decreasing risk of complications.

5. Surgeons who receive continuous training and education are more likely to remain updated with new surgical techniques and best practices, resulting in better patient outcomes.

1.3 Video-Based Surgical Learning vs. Conventional Methods

Conventional training consists of observing surgeries, assisting in operations, and eventually conducting procedures under the close supervision of experienced surgeons. However, many trainees have limited exposure to specific surgical procedures, including repair of relatively uncommon and complex congenital anomalies such as hypospadias. Due to the need to balance patient safety with learning opportunities, conventional surgical training can limit a trainees' experience and scope to master key techniques. Conventional surgical education also lacks standardized teaching materials and protocols, leading to variable training quality and patient outcomes. Traditional approaches are poorly suited to ongoing education and training, whereas exposure to new surgical techniques and updated practices could improve post-operative results. New methods to support surgical skills, such as simulation-based training and online programs, provide trainees with more opportunities to gain hands-on experience, obtain immediate feedback, and benefit from standardized training.

Video-recorded surgical training (VRST) offers immediate low-cost benefits, including the provision of a more comprehensive learning environment for students. Trainees can view procedures multiple times and from different perspectives to fully grasp the intricacies of each surgical method. VRST also provides instant feedback to students, who can use this information to pinpoint weaknesses and refine their own technique. In addition, VRST can be used to standardize both training content and delivery methods, so that every trainee on an instruction course has access to the same materials. Trainees can learn at their own pace with VRST, which can support lifelong learning as new surgical methods are being developed, including by observing footage of other surgeons at work. According to a recent meta-analysis, use of video-based teaching methods resulted in better surgical skills/trainee satisfaction in 17/22 trials. Key benefits highlighted included the ability to control replay speed and navigate to specific portions requiring emphasis, [28] outlining of distinct anatomical structures, overlay with informative graphics, and the use of audio/text narrations [29]. Video editing also allows focus to be narrowed to the most crucial components needed for instruction via elimination of irrelevant material, [30] resulting in a deeper grasp of the key points being presented. This is consistent with the principles of distributed cognition, in which learning is enhanced when there is less mental work required to process information.

Using videos to educate students and professionals in a healthcare setting allows for standardization of instructional materials, serving as a uniform basis for future clinical trials, while also ensuring consistent delivery of high-quality content. Learning surgical techniques has historically relied heavily on workshop-based teaching and the apprenticeship model. However, recent studies point to significant benefits of augmenting surgical skills training with educational videos, [29] including the ability to disseminate key information via the Internet, study remotely, and control multiple aspects of material review [31]. Indeed, previous studies have indicated that a person recalls just 10% of what they read, 20% of what they hear, and 30% of what they see, but this figure rises to 40–50% when audio and video materials are combined together [32].

1.4 The Importance of Hypospadias Surgical Skills Maintenance and Self-Evaluation

Maintaining skills in hypospadias surgery is essential to ensure that surgeons can perform procedures safely and effectively. This is crucial to optimizing surgical outcomes, achieving high levels of patient satisfaction, and supporting ongoing professional development. Centralizing patient cases in specific centers can help provide surgeons with more opportunities to perform complex procedures, while also ensuring that patients are cared for by highly experienced surgeons. In 2011, Kogan et al. reported that pediatric urologists in the United States perform an average of just two proximal hypospadias repairs per year [33]. This figure highlights the fact that physicians are often performing very few procedures on patients with the most severe form of hypospadias [34]. Given this steep learning curve, surgeons typically face significant complication rates while seeking to gain adequate experience. It is therefore possible to enhance the treatment of children with complicated hypospadias by restricting the number of surgeons who manage these patients, thereby facilitating more rapid acquisition of relevant skills (particularly in re-operative scenarios).

1.5 How to Use This Surgical Video Atlas?

Large systematic reviews have shown that no one urethroplasty approach is superior to other methods of hypospadias correction. Indeed, it is hard to compare published series that use different reporting methods, hence it remains extremely difficult to make general recommendations for patient management [15]. There is now increasing appreciation that genetic factors underpin various anatomical features of hypospadias, each of which can combine to generate a broad spectrum of phenotypes, and that patient profile has major implications for post-operative outcome. At present, much of this variability is described and analyzed using highly subjective methods, reflecting that the underlying pathology is still poorly understood (and partly explaining the existence of >250 different repair methods). The aim of the hypospadias ecosystem is to begin examining how key components of disease etiology interact with patient phenotypic profiles to determine complexity [35–37]. In addition to altering our understanding of hypospadias defects, this can help to guide choice of surgical procedure and more objectively record patient outcomes (Fig. 1.1).

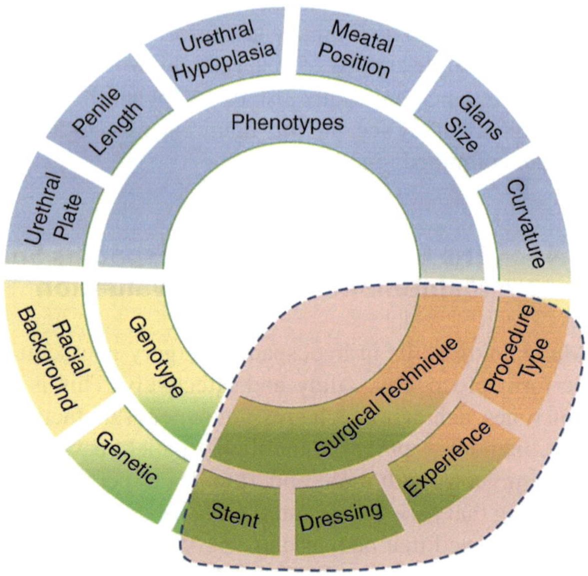

Fig. 1.1 Hypospadias ecosystem variables that influence repair outcome. This video atlas focuses on technical aspects of hypospadias repair by presenting peer review-quality videos prepared by experts in the field

The surgical video atlas aims to support high-quality education and instruction in hypospadias repair. Key steps for effective use include:

1. *Select procedure*: the video atlas covers a variety of hypospadias repair procedures, allowing you to select the most pertinent to your requirements.
2. *Watch attentively*: pay close attention to each step, the instruments used, and surgical technique, from the beginning to the end of each video.
3. *Take notes*: write down key aspects of each procedure, note important landmarks, and record any advice the surgeon offers.
4. *Repeat view*: watch the video more than once and focus on different aspects of the procedure each time (surgical instruments used, suturing technique employed, management of complications, etc.).
5. *Practice procedures*: after watching the video use a surgical simulator or practice the technique under supervision of an experienced mentor.
6. *Review methods*: re-watch videos after practicing the procedure in order to reinforce knowledge and abilities. These videos can also be played back during procedures to ensure that you are following the correct steps and techniques.

The surgical video atlas is intended to serve as a learning and training resource for hypospadias repair. By observing videos closely, taking notes, and practicing procedures, it will be possible to enhance surgical skills and knowledge leading to safer, more effective patient care.

References

1. Springer A, van den Heijkant M, Baumann S. Worldwide prevalence of hypospadias. J Pediatr Urol [Internet]. 12(3):152.e1–7.
2. Abbas T, McCarthy L. Foreskin and penile problems in childhood. Surg [Internet]. 2016;34(5):221–5.
3. Riedmiller H, Androulakakis P, Beurton D, Kocvara R, Gerharz E. European Association of Urology. EAU guidelines on paediatric urology. Eur Urol [Internet]. 2001;40(5):589–99.
4. Spinoit A-F, Waterschoot M, Sinatti C, Abbas T, Callens N, Cools M, et al. Fertility and sexuality issues in congenital lifelong urology patients: male aspects. World J Urol [Internet]. 2020.
5. Abbas TO. Evaluation of penile curvature in patients with hypospadias; gaps in the current practice and future perspectives. J Pediatr Urol [Internet]. 2021.
6. Beaudoin S, Delaage P-HH, Bargy F. No Title. 2000;22(3–4).
7. Baaklini GT, Abbas T, Hofer MD. Urethral anatomy, physiology, and regeneration. In: Abbas TO, editor. Hypospadiology [Internet]; 2023. p. 25–35.
8. Abbas T, Vallasciani S. Toward an ecosystem model of hypospadiology. In: Abbas TO, editor. Hypospadiology [Internet]; 2023. p. 1–23.
9. Abbas TO editor. Hypospadiology: current challenges and future perspectives. 2023. 190 p.
10. Abbas TO. Racial and demographic impacts on hypospadias phenotypical patterns and management approaches. J Pediatr Urol [Internet]. 2021;17(5):675–6.
11. Braga LH, Lorenzo AJ, Bagli DJ, Pippi Salle JL, Caldamone A. Application of the STROBE statement to the hypospadias literature: report of the international pediatric urology task force on hypospadias. J Pediatr Urol [Internet]. 2016;12(6):367–80.
12. Abbas TO. An objective hypospadias classification system. J Pediatr Urol [Internet]. 2022;18(4):481.e1–8.
13. Rynja SP, de Jong TP, Bosch JL, de Kort LM. Functional, cosmetic and psychosexual results in adult men who underwent hypospadias correction in childhood. J Pediatr Urol [Internet]. 2011;7(5):504.
14. Bethell GS, Chhabra S, Shalaby MS, Corbett H, Kenny SE. BAPS NOAH Contributors. Parental decisional satisfaction after hypospadias repair in the United Kingdom. J Pediatr Urol [Internet]. 2020;16(2):164.e1–7.
15. Castagnetti M, El-Ghoneimi A. Surgical management of primary severe hypospadias in children: systematic 20-year review. J Urol [Internet]. 2010;184(4):1469–75.
16. Snodgrass W. Hypospadias reporting – how good is the literature? J Urol [Internet]. 2010;184(4):1255–6.
17. Wilkinson DJ, Farrelly P, Kenny SE. Outcomes in distal hypospadias: a systematic review of the Mathieu and tubularized incised plate repairs. J Pediatr Urol [Internet]. 2012;8(3):307–12.
18. Abbas TO, Elawad A, Kareem A, Pullattayil SAK, Ali M, Alnaimi A. Preclinical experiments for hypospadias surgery: systematic review and quality assessment. Front Pediatr [Internet]. 2021;9:718647.
19. Manzoni G. Hypospadias repair failures: lessons learned. Eur Urol [Internet]. 2006;49(5):772–3.
20. Cameron JL, Halsted WS. Our surgical heritage. Ann Surg [Internet]. 1997;225(5):445–58.
21. McIntyre HF, Winfield S, Sen TH, Crook D. Implementation of the European Working Time Directive in an NHS trust: impact on patient care and junior doctor welfare. Clin Med [Internet]. 2010;10(2):134–7.
22. Cooper L, Din AH, O'Connor EF, Rose V, Roblin P, Mughal M. Trainee and trainer experiences and recommendations for plastic surgery training: a qualitative pilot study. JPRAS open [Internet]. 2022;31:76–91.
23. Parsons BA, Blencowe NS, Hollowood AD, Grant JR. Surgical training: the impact of changes in curriculum and experience. J Surg Educ [Internet]. 2011;68(1):44–51.
24. Wang M-H, Chen B, Kern D, Gearhart S. Pediatric urology fellowship training: are we teaching what they need to learn? J Pediatr Urol [Internet]. 2013;9(3):318–21; discussion 322

25. Hubert K, Johnson E, Estrada C, Diamond D, Maizels M. CEVL training for coronal/distal shaft hypospadias repair: a guide for attendings, residents, and OR staff. J Pediatr Urol [Internet]. 2015;11(1):3–4.
26. Celentano V, Smart N, Cahill RA, McGrath JS, Gupta S, Griffith JP, et al. Use of laparoscopic videos amongst surgical trainees in the United Kingdom. Surgeon [Internet]. 2019;17(6):334–9.
27. Haslam RE, Seideman CA. Educational value of YouTube surgical videos of pediatric robot-assisted laparoscopic pyeloplasty: a qualitative assessment. J Endourol [Internet]. 2020;34(11):1129–33.
28. Lwin AT, Lwin T, Naing P, Oo Y, Kidd D, Cerullo M, et al. Self-directed interactive video-based instruction versus instructor-led teaching for Myanmar house surgeons: a randomized, noninferiority trial. J Surg Educ [Internet]. 2018;75(1):238–46.
29. Saun TJ, Odorizzi S, Yeung C, Johnson M, Bandiera G, Dev SP. A peer-reviewed instructional video is as effective as a standard recorded didactic lecture in medical trainees performing chest tube insertion: a randomized control trial. J Surg Educ [Internet]. 2017;74(3):437–42.
30. Zhang D, Zhou L, Briggs RO, Nunamaker JF. Instructional video in e-learning: assessing the impact of interactive video on learning effectiveness. Inf Manag [Internet]. 2006;43(1):15–27.
31. Green JL, Suresh V, Bittar P, Ledbetter L, Mithani SK, Allori A. The utilization of video technology in surgical education: a systematic review. J Surg Res [Internet]. 2019;235:171–80.
32. Prinz A, Bolz M, Findl O. Advantage of three dimensional animated teaching over traditional surgical videos for teaching ophthalmic surgery: a randomised study. Br J Ophthalmol [Internet]. 2005;89(11):1495–9.
33. Kogan BA, Feustel PJ. What can we learn from pediatric urology certification logs? Urology [Internet]. 2011;78(1):147–52.
34. Hisamatsu E, Sugita Y, Haruna A, Shibata R, Yoshino K. The learning curve in proximal hypospadias repair. J Pediatr Urol [Internet]. 2021;17(3):330.e1–6.
35. Abbas TO, Vallasciani S, Elawad A, Elifranji M, Leslie B, Elkadhi A, et al. Plate Objective Scoring Tool (POST); An objective methodology for the assessment of urethral plate in distal hypospadias. J Pediatr Urol [Internet]. 2020;16(5):675–82.
36. Abbas TO, Braga LH, Spinoit AF, Salle JP. Urethral plate quality assessment and its impact on hypospadias repair outcomes: a systematic review and quality assessment. J Pediatr Urol [Internet]. 2021.
37. Abbas TO, AbdelMoniem M, Khalil I, Hossain MSA, Chowdhury MEH. Deep learning based automatic quantification of urethral plate quality using the Plate Objective Scoring Tool (POST). 2022.

Ergonomics of Hypospadias Surgery

2

Tariq O. Abbas

Abstract

During hypospadias surgery, increased technical complexity and sometimes inadequately adapted instruments have contributed to a rise in the incidence of complications and the distress of surgeon fatigue. Ergonomic integration and the proper instruments and operating asset environment for hypospadias surgery are essential for enhancing the efficiency, safety, and comfort of the operating team. This chapter discusses the primary ergonomic pillars of hypospadias surgery.

Keywords

Hypospadias surgery · Ergonomics · Instruments · Teamwork

2.1 Introduction

During hypospadias surgery, the increased technical complexity and sometimes inadequately adapted instruments have led to an increase in the incidence of complications and the discomfort of surgeon fatigue. Ergonomic integration and appropriate hypospadias surgery instruments and operating asset environment are crucial for enhancing the effectiveness, security, and comfort of the operating team. Complex hypospadias procedures necessitate a high level of concentration and skill. Consequently, it has been observed that the operating surgeon adopts a more immobile stance during hypospadias procedures compared to the open approach of the past. It has been demonstrated that these static postures are more disabling and detrimental than dynamic postures, as muscles and tendons accumulate lactic acid and toxins when held for extended periods in the same positions [1]. Using surface

T. O. Abbas (✉)
Pediatric Urology Section, Sidra Medicine, Doha, Qatar
e-mail: tabbas@sidra.org

T. O. Abbas (ed.), *Video Atlas of Hypospadias Surgery*,
https://doi.org/10.1007/978-981-99-0795-3_2

electromyography, investigators examined the muscle activation levels of surgeons and surgical assistants and found that the surgical assistants were associated with the same or even higher levels of muscle activity [2]. Consequently, it is essential for all surgeons performing hypospadias surgery as well as novices who have yet to be initiated into this field to comprehend the applications of ergonomics. This chapter aims to provide a foundational comprehension of the ergonomic challenges hypospadias surgeons face, as well as some simple modifications that can go a long way toward enhancing their operative practice. As a surgical skill requiring human dexterity and coordination, hypospadias reconstruction can unquestionably benefit from ergonomic gear.

2.2 What Is "Ergonomics"?

The term ergonomics is derived from the Greek words "ergon" which means work and "nomos" which means a natural order or arrangement. Ergonomics is "the scientific study of workers in terms of the design of equipment, layout at work, the working environment, safety, productivity, and training." Ergonomics is founded on the integration of anatomy, physiology, psychology, and engineering within a systems perspective. The significance of ergonomics cannot be emphasized enough. Studies have shown that ergonomics can reduce the time required for laparoscopic suturing [3].

2.3 Execution of Ergonomics Concepts in Hypospadias Surgery

Execution of surgical ergonomics in hypospadias reconstruction may be divided into three sections: (1) Pre-operative preparation issues, (2) Intraoperative Ergonomic concepts, and (3) contemporary concepts in team oversight, deliberate execution, and evaluation (Fig. 2.1).

2.3.1 Pre-operative Preparation Issues

2.3.1.1 Timing and Mental Preparation

Surgery is a motor exercise that requires practice, and there is a saying in the field that if you are away from the operating table for one week, you will notice it, after two weeks, your assistant will notice it, and after three weeks, your patient will notice it. The published evidence regarding the association among sleep deprivation/fatigue and performance is substantial. A recent meta-analysis found that insomniacs perform inadequately on tasks requiring working memory and problem-solving skills [4]. It is not unusual for a surgeon to visualize and rehearse the steps of a complex operation before performing it. Many have conscious or unconscious rituals that help them achieve peak performance. Visualization and ritual are

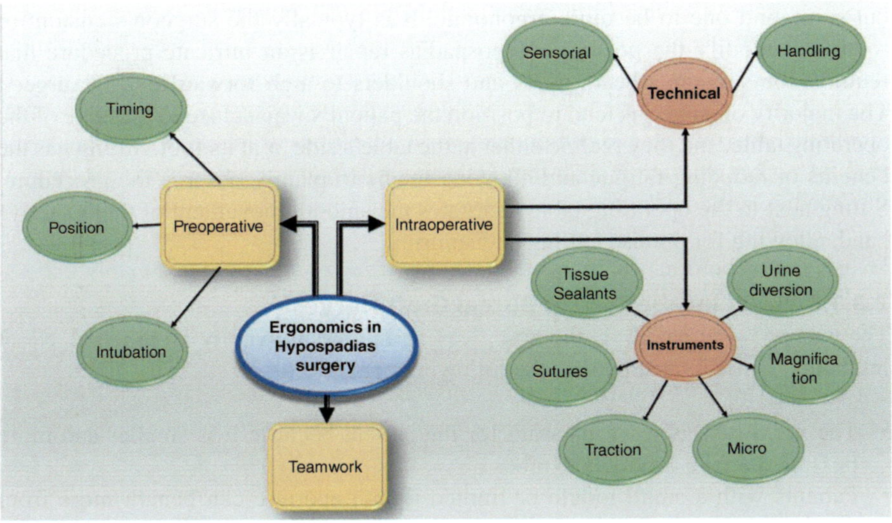

Fig. 2.1 Illustration of the key ergonomic concepts of hypospadias surgery discussed in this chapter

well-established techniques for increasing motivation and improving concentration and focus. Frequently, trainees will retain their breath in a futile attempt to achieve stability and eliminate tremor. Typically, this is counterproductive. A trainee's capacity to answer a question can be used to determine whether or not they can breathe and relax. Initial responses consist of groans. The familiarity with the procedure and ergonomics permits "yes" and "no" responses and brief sentences. A surgeon who is at ease will be able to carry on a lengthy conversation that is frequently extraneous to the procedure, also known as surgical banter. One may perceive the surgeon to be "in the zone." A recent study on the technical differences between expert and novice plastic surgeons used video-based motion analysis to quantify skills. Experts used their non-dominant hand more than trainees did and this resulted in a smoother, faster completion of relevant tasks [5]. Numerous activities requiring attention to detail and manual dexterity, such as athletics and surgical procedures, have been shown to be affected by the performer's "state of mind." Interestingly, Storm et al. recently showed that a significant increase in the rate of post-hypospadias repair complication was noted with morning vs afternoon cases for the group overall [6].

2.3.1.2 Operation Theatre Position

It is essential that the surgeon realizes and utilizes the operation table's function. The table's height complements the posture, and its inclination influences the angles. The accuracy of the final movement, such as the rotation of the needle, is ensured by judicious and punctual adjustments made throughout the operation, in conjunction with a shifting body position. The surgeon can perform hypospadias surgery in two distinct positions (sitting or standing). Both positions are practical, but some find one to be more ergonomic. It is typically the surgeon's custom or routine to modify the position. Hypospadias repair is an intricate procedure that requires the surgeon's head, neck, and shoulders to arch forward during surgery. The majority of surgeons tend to position the patient's waist close to the edge of the operating table, and they recline either at the table's side or at its foot. Sitting has the benefits of reducing fatigue and allowing others to plainly observe the procedure. Sitting next to the operating table facilitates the smooth movement of the operative hand, allowing for precise cutting and suturing.

2.3.1.3 Nasal Intubation for Buccal Graft Harvest

The patient is intubated via the nose, leaving the mouth wholly unimpeded. Nasal intubation is not a must but has the following benefits:

- The nasal tube is more pleasant for the patient because it is smaller and more flexible than the orotracheal tube.
- Patients with a small mouth or limited mouth aperture can benefit more from nasal intubation.
- At the outset of learning curve, nasal intubation is more useful.
- Patients requiring double graft harvestings benefit most from nasal intubation.

2.3.2 Intraoperative Ergonomic Concepts

2.3.2.1 Technical Skills and Handling

Sensorial Ergonomics

Sensorial ergonomics (manipulations and visualization) increase accuracy, dexterity, and confidence, whereas physical ergonomics convey surgeon comfort. These two elements of ergonomics increased safety, improved outcomes, and decreased tension [7]. As residents, we were taught to "see" with our hands as well as our eyes while acquiring the skills necessary to perform open surgical procedures. In an effort to attain the required level of dexterity for this dual task, we train our hands to develop the necessary dexterity. This is the tactile feedback that is conspicuously absent when one's arm rests without support.

Tissue Handling and Suturing Techniques

By using stay sutures, skin hooks, microsurgical instruments, and dissecting tissues in the proper plane, tissue trauma can be minimized. Furthermore, maintaining the proper vascularity of the flap for neo-urethra and skin is crucial for preventing ischemic complications. A subcuticular continuous suture with a fine needle is highly recommended for urethroplasty to attempt to keep both epithelial edges in contact and prevent edge eversion [8]. Eversion of the suture line increases periurethral reaction, which can lead to urinary leakage and the formation of fistulas or diverticula. A delicate balance must be reached between urine-tight anastomosis and the worse threat of tissue ischemia. Prior to stitching, the needle angle can be demonstrated, analogous to aligning the body with a golf club for a golf stroke. Once this alignment has occurred, the surgeon is in the ideal position to perform a flawless needle rotation.

2.3.2.2 Surgical Instruments

Magnification

The efficacy of hypospadias surgery hinges on precise dissection and tissue apposition. Therefore, magnification becomes a vital instrument in the surgical treatment of hypospadias in young children. High-powered spectacles, loupes, and an operating microscope are examples of different magnification instruments. The selection rests on the availability and familiarity with the magnification. Drawbacks of traditional magnifying loupes include poor neck posture and frequent head movement to refocus the view, in addition to the inability to share the magnified visual field with surgical residents and assistants. Magnification aids in avoiding breaching the epithelial lining of the neourethra during tubularization and decreases the likelihood of fistula formation [9]. In addition, the use of optical magnification in hypospadias surgery (2–5× magnification) was linked to a low cumulative complication rate [10]. Video Telescopic Operating Microscope (VITOM) provides excellent visualization of pediatric operations with improved surgeon comfort and may serve as a substitute for loupes. The VITOM exoscope provides images of superior quality, 2–16 times magnification zoom, and excellent illumination, which are displayed on large-format HD flat screens for the surgeon, assistants, and operating room staff to observe. Interestingly, VITOM imaging had a positive effect on the surgical technicians, who all found it simpler to track the progression of operations and believed that it enhanced the efficiency of the procedures [11] (Fig. 2.2).

Microsurgical Instruments

Key instruments are required for hypospadias surgery, and they must be extremely thin and delicate, and the scissors must be extremely sharp. Fine scissors, a fine needle holder (for 6/0 and 7/0 sutures), fine-toothed tissue forceps, and curved mosquito forceps to retain the stay sutures are required. Figure 2.3 depicts an example of a set of fine instruments that can be added to a standard pediatric set and are incredibly useful for hypospadias surgery (Table 2.1).

Traction Tools

The first part of the procedure involves applying traction and stabilizing the penis. This is accomplished by inserting a fine nonabsorbable material (5-0 nylon or silk on a small, rounded needle) traction suture in the glans penis. The Joshi-Kulkarni retractor (Fig. 2.4) provides stable, bloodless operative exposure by compressing tissue at the root of the penis without causing trauma. This retractor's self-retaining design also enhances ergonomics, thereby reducing surgeon fatigue [12]. In case such surgical retractors are not available, simple techniques can be used to apply traction on the penis during the surgery as shown in Fig. 2.5. By securing a stay

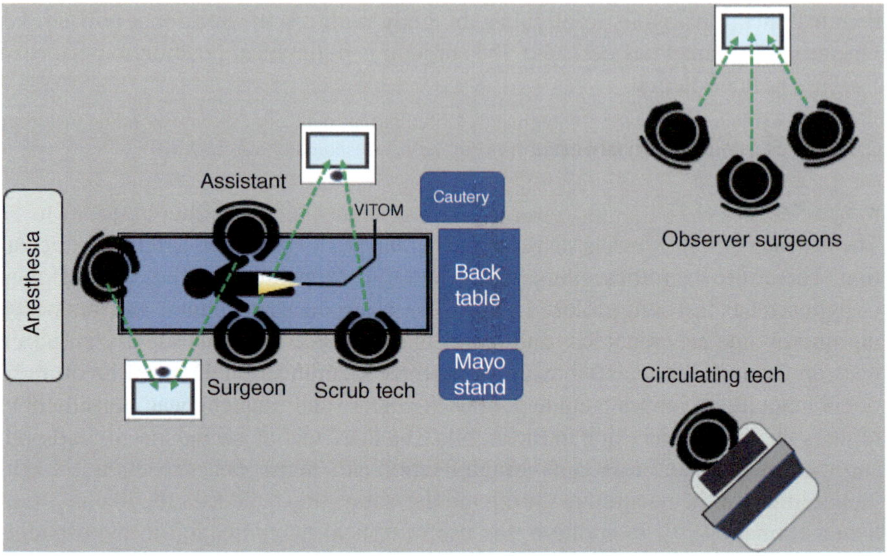

Fig. 2.2 Operation room (OR) ergonomics at the author's practice

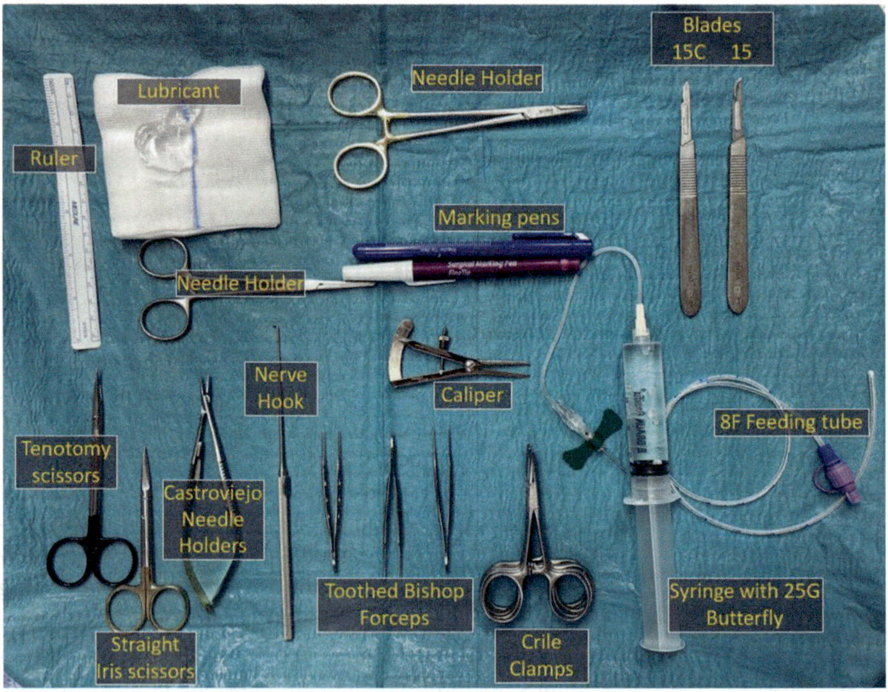

Fig. 2.3 An example set of surgical instruments to be used for hypospadias reconstruction surgery

Table 2.1 Peculiar uses relevant to hypospadias reconstruction for selected examples of surgical instruments

Instrument	Uses
Calipers	For measurements of glans anthropometrics and urethral plate anatomical features and flap dimensions
Spring needle holder	To help in urethroplasty
Tenotomy scissors	Useful for creating glanular wings, degloving, preparing dartos flaps for neourethral coverage and preputial flaps for Onlay reconstruction
Micro-toothed forceps	To provide firm yet atraumatic grip for glans and urethral tissues
Straight Iris scissors	For cutting delicate sutures
Nerve hooks	To help retract and expose very delicate narrow areas as at the area of the hypospadias meatus
Straight artery clips	For holding stay sutures of glanular wings
Adson toothed forceps	For handling preputial skin
Micro-mosquito forceps	To catch fine sutures and tissue flaps

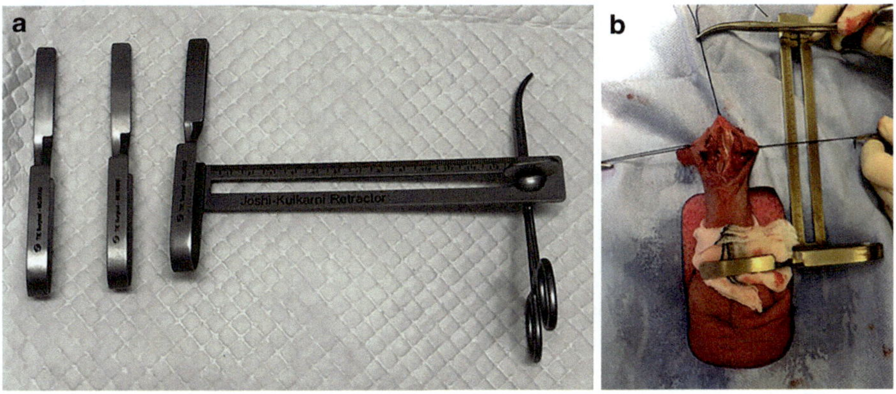

Fig. 2.4 (**a**) Components of the Joshi-Kulkarni retractor. (**b**) Use of retractor in dorsal inlay BMG penile urethroplasty. (Copyright © 2022, John Wiley and Sons reused with permission)

suture to surgical drape folds that have been purposefully made, traction is imparted to the penis.

Suture Material

The nature of suture material and the approach used for suture placing may have a substantial effect on the outcome of hypospadias surgery. The choice of suture in hypospadias surgery is influenced by a number of significant variables, including the required length of suture with the greatest tensile strength, suture retention at the

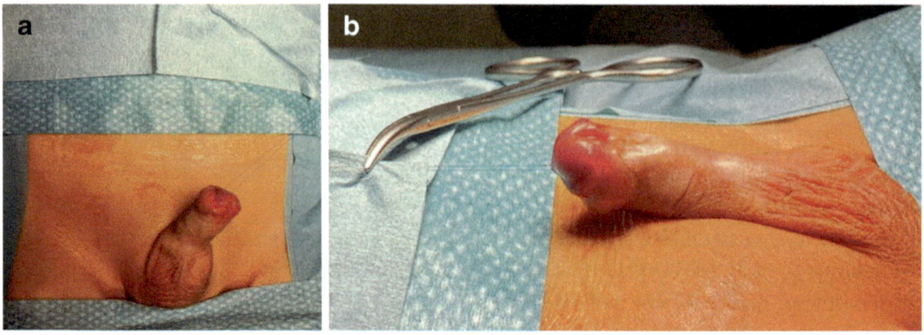

Fig. 2.5 Traction on the penis is applied by attaching a stay suture to purposely created folds in the surgical drapes (**a**) that can be then fixed to by a stay suture attached to the glans (**b**)

urethral level, the number of knots for each suture type, suture degradation time and products, as well as needle types. Due to the potential for stone formation, it is generally recognized that nonabsorbable sutures should be kept out of urothelial contact. In addition, the genitourinary tissues regain their tensile strength swiftly, eliminating the need for a prolonged suture.

Ulman and colleagues observed a significantly lower fistula rate (4.95% vs. 16.6%) in subcuticular repair compared to full thickness through-and-through technique [13], whereas others believe that the type of suture used, whether subcuticular or through-and-through, has no effect on the outcome as long as polyglactin suture is used [14]. Small fistulae may be caused by absorbable sutures left in place too long. Typically, polyglactin absorbable sutures are utilized for the closure of the innermost layer following epithelial inversion, whereas polyglyconate sutures are utilized for the closure of other layers [15].

Urinary Diversion
The most common nonsurgical form of intubated diversion is the self-retaining Foley urethral catheter. Ease of placement, plus the fact that it serves as a stent for the repair, represents a significant advantage for this form of diversion.

Tissue Sealants
Both natural and synthetic tissue sealants have been utilized in hypospadias surgery to reduce the incidence of urethrocutaneous fistulas after application like a thin layer of butyl cyanoacrylate over the suture line that was described in a recent systematic review [16]. Tissue sealants can be applied to the suture line, skin margins, and fistula site.

2.3.3 Contemporary Concepts in Team Oversight

Complex patient interventions must be performed by highly skilled operators backed by dependable teams to ensure patient safety. In structured micro-systems, operators must have a low tolerance for error and be supported by resilient, patient-centered teams [8]. Human errors in the operating room are rarely caused by a lack of technical performance alone, but rather by system malfunctions and non-technical errors by the operating team [17]. Therefore, team practice may have a greater impact on outcomes than individual warm-up. It is however constrained by significant resource, labor, and cost requirements [18].

References

1. Kant IJ, de Jong LC, van Rijssen-Moll M, Borm PJ. A survey of static and dynamic work postures of operating room staff. Int Arch Occup Environ Health [Internet]. 1992;63(6):423–8.
2. Zihni AM, Cavallo JA, Ray S, Ohu I, Cho S, Awad MM. Ergonomic analysis of primary and assistant surgical roles. J Surg Res [Internet]. 2016;203(2):301–5.
3. Joice P, Hanna GB, Cuschieri A. Ergonomic evaluation of laparoscopic bowel suturing. Am J Surg [Internet]. 1998;176(4):373–8.
4. Fortier-Brochu E, Beaulieu-Bonneau S, Ivers H, Morin CM. Insomnia and daytime cognitive performance: a meta-analysis. Sleep Med Rev [Internet]. 2012;16(1):83–94.
5. Glarner CE, Hu Y-Y, Chen C-H, Radwin RG, Zhao Q, Craven MW, et al. Quantifying technical skills during open operations using video-based motion analysis. Surgery [Internet]. 2014;156(3):729–34.
6. Storm DW, Lockwood GM, Bonnett MA, Cooper BJ, Harris LM, Cooper CS. The impact of perioperative and operative variables on early postoperative complications following primary hypospadias repair. Urology [Internet]. 2022;170:184–8.
7. Stylopoulos N, Rattner D. Robotics and ergonomics. Surg Clin North Am [Internet]. 2003;83(6):1321–37.
8. Manser T. Teamwork and patient safety in dynamic domains of healthcare: a review of the literature. Acta Anaesthesiol Scand [Internet]. 2009;53(2):143–51.
9. Rees MJW, Sinclair SW, Hiles RW, Smith PJB. A 10-year prospective study of hypospadias repair at Frenchay hospital. Br J Urol [Internet]. 1981;53(6):637–40.
10. Wacksman J. Results of early hypospadias surgery using optical magnification. J Urol [Internet]. 1984;131(3):516–7.
11. Frykman PK, Duel BP, Gangi A, Williams JA, Berci G, Freedman AL. Evaluation of a video telescopic operating microscope (VITOM) for pediatric surgery and urology: a preliminary report. J Laparoendosc Adv Surg Tech A [Internet]. 2013;23(7):639–43.
12. Flynn H, Joshi PM, Kulkarni SB, Desai D. How to do a penile urethroplasty using a novel self-retaining penile retractor. ANZ J Surg [Internet]. 2023;93(1–2):334–6.
13. Ulman I, Erikçi V, Avanoğlu A, Gökdemir A. The effect of suturing technique and material on complication rate following hypospadias repair. Eur J Pediatr Surg [Internet]. 1997;7(3):156–7.
14. Hakim S, Merguerian PA, Rabinowitz R, Shortliffe LD, McKenna PH. Outcome analysis of the modified Mathieu hypospadias repair: comparison of stented and unstented repairs. J Urol [Internet]. 1996;156(2 Pt 2):836.
15. Titley OG, Bracka A. A 5-year audit of trainees experience and outcomes with two-stage hypospadias surgery. Br J Plast Surg [Internet]. 1998;51(5):370–5.
16. Nurtamin T, Renaldo J, Kloping YP, Rahman IA, Hakim L. The use of tissue sealant in reducing urethrocutaneous fistula event following hypospadias repair: a systematic review and meta-analysis. Ann Med Surg [Internet]. 2022;78:103707.
17. Yule S, Flin R, Paterson-Brown S, Maran N. Non-technical skills for surgeons in the operating room: a review of the literature. Surgery [Internet]. 2006;139(2):140–9.
18. O'Leary JD, O'Sullivan O, Barach P, Shorten GD. Improving clinical performance using rehearsal or warm-up: an advanced literature review of randomized and observational studies. Acad Med [Internet]. 2014;89(10):1416–22.

Part II

Procedures for the Repair of Distal Hypospadias

Meatal Advancement and Glanduloplasty Incorporated (MAGPI)

3

Santiago Vallasciani

Abstract

The Meatal Advancement and Glandular Plasty Incorporated (MAGPI) technique, pioneered by Duckett in 1981, revolutionized the treatment of distal hypospadias. Durham Smith, in his 1997 historical review of hypospadias, recognized MAGPI as an evolutionary culmination of ideas originating from Duplay in 1874 and Beck in 1828. Duckett and Snyder later corroborated the efficacy of MAGPI through their extensive experience with over 1000 patients, boasting a low reoperation rate. However, criticisms emerged regarding potential abnormalities in the meatus resulting from dorsal advancement, leading to the exploration of alternative techniques and modifications. This video presentation elucidates the essential steps of the MAGPI procedure while showcasing the author's innovative modifications, addressing concerns and advancing the technique's efficacy in hypospadias repair.

Keywords

Hypospadias · Meatal advancement · Distal hypospadias · Glanuloplasty

Supplementary Information The online version contains supplementary material available at https://doi.org/10.1007/978-981-99-0795-3_3. The videos can be accessed individually by clicking the DOI link in the accompanying figure caption or by scanning this link with the SN More Media App.

S. Vallasciani (✉)
Division of Urology, Department of Surgery, Sidra Medicine, Doha, Qatar

Department of Urology, Weill Cornell Medical College Qatar, Doha, Qatar
e-mail: svallasciani@sidra.org

T. O. Abbas (ed.), *Video Atlas of Hypospadias Surgery*, https://doi.org/10.1007/978-981-99-0795-3_3

3.1 Introduction

The MAGPI technique was popularized by Duckett in 1981 [1] for the treatment of distal hypospadias. In his article on the history of hypospadias in 1997, Durham Smith [2] considered this technique to be the evolution of the initial ideas developed by Duplay in 1874 [3] and Beck in 1828 [4]. Duckett and Snyder published their experience with over 1000 patients ten years later, claiming a low reoperation rate [5]. Despite this, there were criticisms on where the dorsal advancement would result in an abnormal-looking meatus, and for this reason, other alternative techniques [6] or modifications to the original MAGPI were proposed [7–9]. In the present video, the critical steps of the MAGPI procedure are described together with the modifications developed by the author.

3.2 Indications/Case Selection

As we reported in 2007 [9], the presence of one or more of the following anatomical characteristics in a case should be considered as a relative contraindication for the use of this technique:

- Megameatus variant
- Hypospadiac meatus below the level of the glans wings
- Urethral hypoplasia

Any of them can result in increased tension in the ventral advancement of the urethra, which will result in retraction of the meatus in the long term. The technique can be abandoned and changed during the procedure for other surgical approaches such as Tubularized Incised Plate (TIP) with or without graft.

3.3 Video

https://1drv.ms/v/s!AnIDekwwlAN-gs1Y4LigZ5V14i-jVA?e=yOdfAF

3.4 Description of the Technique

1. After surgical field preparation and suture traction is placed on the glans, an initial intraoperative reassessment of the case is made for its suitability for the MAGPI technique. Keypoints as the position of the hypospadiac meatus within glandular wings and distal urethra elasticity are evaluated.
2. Degloving: it can be carried out by preserving the hooded prepuce for potential preputial reconstruction based on the preference of the patient/family and surgeon's experience (Fig. 3.1a, b).

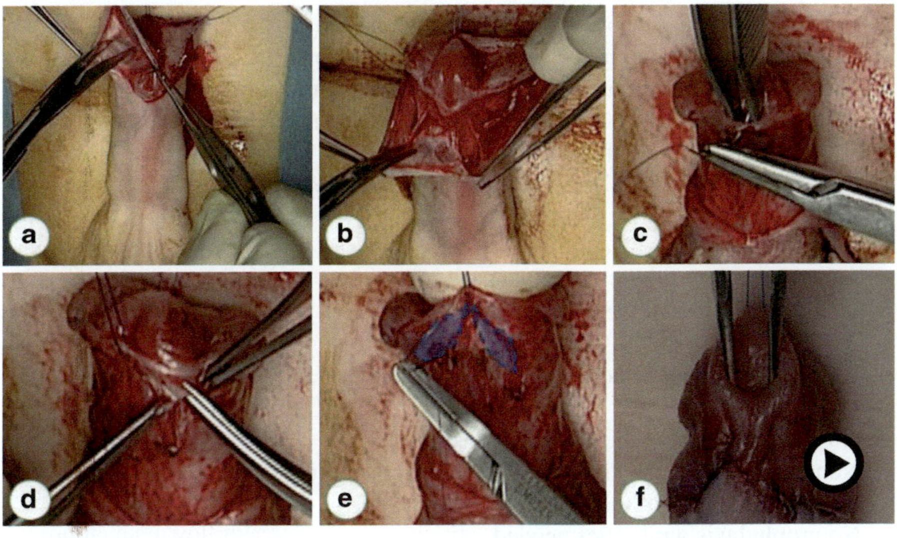

Fig. 3.1 Intraoperative images showing key steps of the procedure. Degloving (**a**, **b**) is followed by applying a traction suture at the ventral lip of the hypospadiac meatus (**c**) and the release of the glanular wings (**d**). Glanulopasty (**e**) is then performed by interrupted sutures in the glans tissue (blue shadow highlighted). Final appearance (**f**). MAGPI procedure (https://doi.org/10.1007/000-cmy)

3. A new assessment for the suitability of the case based on the previously mentioned anatomical characteristics.
4. Traction suture at the ventral lip of the hypospadiac meatus (Fig. 3.1c).
5. While the traction is kept cranially, the glandular wings are released (Fig. 3.1d) from the apex of the corpora to allow their rotation to the midline with no tension. This plane can be challenging to find due to particular glans configurations: in some cases, the thickness of the glans' wings can be reduced, and its vitality can be jeopardized during dissection. These issues can make it unable to place the sutures through robust glandular tissue to approximate the glandular wings to the midline.
6. The glans wings are sutured (Fig. 3.1e) to the midline with one to three tension-free interrupted subcuticular sutures in Polydioxanone or Polyglyconate 5 or 6/0 (the number of sutures will be subjectively determined depending on the glans configuration). The critical factors in the placement of these sutures are: (1) to be tension-free and (2) to have enough amount of tissue crossed by the suture. The surgeon can subjectively assess the former: if the needle is visualized in transparency through the tissue being crossed, the amount of tissue is insufficient.
7. Reconstruction of the mucosal collar is performed in three sub-steps:
   7.1 Dorsal midline incision of the mucosal collar allows ventrally healthy tissue transfer for its approximation without tension. This maneuver also allows the surgeon to remove any portion of the mucosal collar bearing areas of different colors or damage during the dissection for a better aesthetic result.
   7.2 One or two subcuticular interrupted Polydioxanone or Polyglyconate 6/0 to approximate mucosal collar to the midline.

7.3 Tailoring the mucosal collar ventrally and dorsally to a 3- or 4-mm length. The length of the mucosal collar is an additional factor that can negatively influence the mid and long-term outcome. This author's experience shows that an excessively long mucosal collar can lead to chronic edema providing the aspect of "mushroom" to the distal penis.

8. Resurfacing of the penile shaft (with or without the use of Byars' flaps according to the case) (Fig. 3.1f).

3.5 Postoperative Care

- Patient is discharged home the same day (unless another comorbidity requires otherwise).
- No catheter is left at the end of the procedure.
- Non-compressive dressing is left for 24 hours (the type is based on the availability and preference of the surgeon).
- No prophylaxis antibiotics needed.
- Any ointment cream for 1 or 2 weeks until the areas of the glans where the preputial adhesions were present are re-epithelialized.
- Follow-up visits at 1, 6, and 12 months and then based on parental or patient's request.

3.6 Conclusion

The MAGPI technique provides adequate aesthetic and functional results that are durable in time. Its use must be rigorously tailored to the patient's anatomy to achieve this. A further advantage of this approach is that at any time during the procedure, the surgical strategy can be changed to alternative and more invasive procedures (such as the TIP), not having tissues compromised by the previous dissections. This is particularly true when no dorsal advancement is performed as described in the original technique. In addition, not performing a dorsal incision as proposed by some authors [7–9] allows the surgeon to manage the case without needing a catheter in the postoperative period. A particular note has to be made on the neo-meatus aspect: while it presents with a slit-like aspect when exposed by retraction of the meatal lips, it is shown that it lies in the proximal aspect of it. This feature, however, does not compromise the functional and aesthetic results in the mid and long term.

References

1. Duckett JW. MAGPI (Meatoplasty and Glanuloplasty). A procedure for subcoronal hypospadias. Urol Clin North Am. 1981;8:513–9.
2. Durham SE. The history of hypospadias. Pediatr Surg Int. 1987;12:81–5.
3. Duplay S. De l'hypospadias perineo-scrotal et son traitement chirurgical. Arch Gen Med. 1874;133:513–657.

4. Beck C. A new operation for balanic hypospadias. New York Med J. 1898;67:147.
5. Duckett JW, Snyder H III. The MAGPI hypospadias repair in 1111 patients. Ann Surg. 1991;213:620–5.
6. Rodó Salas J, Perero Intriago M, Castañón García-Alix M. Changes in traditional techniques in anterior hypospadias. Cir Pediatr. 1985;8:164–6.
7. Taneli C, Genç A, Günsar C, Sencan A, Arslan OA, Daglar Z, Mir E. Modification of meatal advancement and glanuloplasty for correction of distal hypospadias. Scand J Urol Nephrol. 2004;38:122–4.
8. Baran CN, Sungur N, Kílínç H, Ozdemir R, Sensöz O. T-incision technique in distal hypospadias: a modification of meatal advancement and glanuloplasty. Plast Reconstr Surg. 2002;109:1018–24.
9. Vallasciani S, Spagnoli A, Borsellino A, Martini L, Ferro F. Simplifying the surgical approach to glandular and coronal hypospadias: longitudinal urethral incision and glanuloplasty. J Pediatr Urol. 2007;3:453–6.

Double Y Glanuloplasty (DYG) Procedure

4

Janu Ragunathan and Ahmed T. Hadidi

Abstract

Due to potential risks and possible unsatisfactory cosmetic outcome, glanular hypospadias were often not treated. However, in the last decades, the concern of parents about the future consequences of having an abnormal-looking penis has increased. Glanular forms of hypospadias with mobile meatus can now be corrected with a simple surgical technique, called double Y glanulomeatoplasty (DYG) described by Hadidi in 2010. It is a combination of advancement of the mobile meatus (the first Y) into a designed slit-like glans (second inverted Y). Proper selection of patients is mandatory. The technique is only suitable for patients with glanular hypospadias associated with mobile meatus. The operation results in excellent cosmetic and function result. The long-term success rate is 97%.

Keywords

Hypospadias · Distal · Glanular · Urethra · Meatus

Supplementary Information The online version contains supplementary material available at https://doi.org/10.1007/978-981-99-0795-3_4. The videos can be accessed individually by clicking the DOI link in the accompanying figure caption or by scanning this link with the SN More Media App.

J. Ragunathan · A. T. Hadidi (✉)
Hypospadias Center, Sana Klinikum Offenbach, Offenbach am Main, Germany
e-mail: janu.ragunathan@sana.de

T. O. Abbas (ed.), *Video Atlas of Hypospadias Surgery*,
https://doi.org/10.1007/978-981-99-0795-3_4

4.1 Introduction

Several procedures have been described for glanular hypospadias which have been developed based on the principle of urethral mobilization first described by Beck [1] and Hacker [2] in 1898, and the meatal advancement glanuloplasty incorporated (MAGPI) by Duckett [3], its modifications [4, 5], and by Ahmed T. Hadidi 2010 the double Y glanulomeatoplasty (DYG) technique [6]. The consequences of an unoperated hypospadias can be urinary, genital, or psychological [7].

DYG is a simple technique, suitable for patients with glanular hypospadias and a mobile meatus. This technique results in a terminal, slit-like meatus. The complication rate is minimal (2%). The principle of the technique is to make two (double) Y incisions: a Y incision along the lower part of the meatus and an inverted Y along the upper part of the meatus that extends to the tip of the glans. That is the reason why the technique is called double Y glanulomeatoplasty (DYG) [8].

4.2 Patients' Selection

- Primary hypospadias is classified into four grades: glanular (grade I), distal (grade II), proximal (grade III), and perineal (grade IV). Complicated, cicatricial hypospadias with inadequate skin and scarred tissue (inappropriately called crippled hypospadias) is classified as grade V hypospadias.
- As already described the DYG technique is only suitable for patients with glanular hypospadias and mobile meatus and without deep chordee. Usually, the patients have a small ridge distal to the meatus. This can be pulled with fine-toothed forceps to the tip of the glans. If this can be done without problems, the DYG technique is the ideal technique with minimal complications. The following table (Table 4.1) is the standard protocol for managment of hypospadias in the Hypospadias Center in Frankfurt:

Table 4.1 Techniques of hypospadias repair after chordee correction

Glanular (Grade I)	Distal (Grade II)	Proxima (Grade III)	Perineal (Grade IV)
DYG **D**ouble **Y** **G**lanuloplasty	SLAM **S**lit-**L**ike **A**djusted **M**athieu	LABO **L**ateral **B**ased **O**nlay	CEDU **C**hordee **E**xcision & **D**istal **U**rethroplasty

4.3 Video Demonstration

Factors	Findings
Age at surgery (month)	20 months
Gestational age (weeks)	39 weeks
Birth weight (g)	3020 g
Gestational risks	None
Family history	None
Testosterone (if yes, reason, and protocol used)	No
Any features of DSD	No

4.4 Operative Steps

1. An inverted Y incision is outlined on the glans. The center of the inverted Y is located at the tip of the meatus and the tip of the longitudinal limb is at the tip of the glans. The two oblique limbs embrace the meatus (Fig. 4.1).

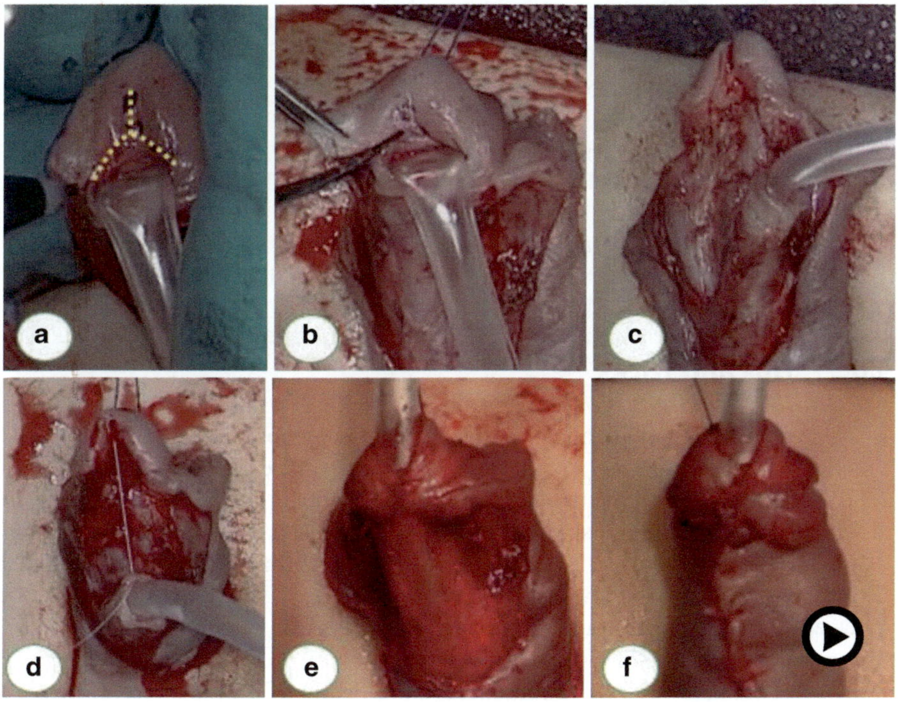

Fig. 4.1 (**a**) Inverted Y Incision. (**b**) The three flaps are elevated and proximally freeing the distal urethra (**c**). The apex of the meatus is sutured to the tip of the glans (**d**). The glanular wings are mobilized deep enough to wrap around the urethra and are approximated in the midline (**e**) where the 6 o'clock stitch is a 3-point stitch that brings the urethra and the two medial edges of the glanular wings together. (**f**) Final look with prepuce retained to prepare for foreskin reconstruction in a later session. (©Ahmed T. Hadidi 2021. All Rights Reserved). DYG procedure (https://doi.org/10.1007/000-cmz)

2. The three limbs are incised and deepened creating two glanular flaps laterally and the meatus and urethra downwards in the middle.
3. The meatus and urethra are mobilized, pulled upwards, and fixed to the tip of the glans.
4. The second Y is incised as shown in the figure to allow adequate mobilization of the urethra around a catheter size F12 whenever possible.
5. The glanular wings are sutured around the meatus in its new position.
6. The operative steps are illustrated in the figure.

4.5 Standard Postoperative Care After Hypospadias Surgery

(a) The catheter is removed in 1–2 days. Change of the dressing is not needed.
(b) The patient should receive second-generation cephalosporins antibiotics for 1 week (the wound is potentially contaminated with stools).
(c) Analgesia with Ibuprofen and/or Paracetamol.
(d) Oxybutynin is given in case of bladder spasms.
(e) The parents should use two diapers on top of each other for extra protection.
(f) The parents should keep the penis clean and dry. At the beginning the diapers should be changed every 2 hours.
(g) For 1 week they need to apply four times a day the gentamycin eye ointment on the wound.
(h) The patient is discharged home after he passes urine without the catheter and dressing.
(i) Our standard postoperative follow-up protocol includes examination after 3 months, 1 year, 3 years, and then every 5 years until the child is 15 years old.

4.6 Tips and Tricks

1. A tip is to start mobilization of the glanular wings proximally at the coronal sulcus, where the corpus spongiosum is better developed.
2. To avoid ischemia of the tissue the suture knots should not be tied too tight.
3. The use of a tourniquet is not necessary. We suggest a blood control by stretching the glans/penis fixed at the tip over the left index finger and exerting dorsal pressure. Like this it allows targeted hemostasis.
4. Deep glanular incision and mobilization of the glans wings are important for tension-free closure of the glans.
5. The use of catheter size F12 minimizes complications like meatus stenosis.
6. By compressing the penis against the abdominal wall with the dressing allows free mobility of the patient.
7. We suggest doing the surgery before the age of 3 years. The complications are more less, and the infants have quicker recovery.

4.7 Results and Conclusion

Since 2004 the DYG technique has become our standard technique for glanular hypospadias with mobile meatus. From 2004 to 2021 we used the technique on 546 patients. A slit-like meatus in a near normal-looking glans is considered as a satisfactory result. At the beginning we tried the DYG technique in coronal hypospadias. This resulted in meatal retraction in three patients. Furthermore, the use of catheter size F10 resulted in meatal stenosis in five patients. The use of catheter size F12 has helped to minimize this complication. Injury to the thin urethra occurs and should be repaired with Vicryl 7/0 and should be covered with a thin layer of preputial dartos fascia. The total complication rate is 3%. 97 patients have maintained 10-year follow-up with satisfactory results and meatus at the tip of the glans [8].

Because of the minimal complication rate and the simplicity of the technique and the good cosmetic and functional outcome, the DYG technique is ideal for glanular hypospadias with mobile meatus and no superficial chordee.

References

1. Beck C. A new operation for balanic hypospadias. New York Med J. 1898;67:147–8.
2. Hacker V. Zur operativen Behandlung der Hypospadia glandis. Bruns. Beitr Klin Chir. 1898:271–6.
3. Duckett JW. MAGPI (meatoplasty and glanuloplasty): a procedure for subcoronal hypospadias. Urol Clin North Am. 1981;8(3):513–9.
4. Decter RM. M inverted V glansplasty: a procedure for distal hypospadias. J Urol. 1991;146(2 (Pt 2)):641–3. https://doi.org/10.1016/S0022-5347(17)37881-3.
5. Arap S, Mitre AI, de Goes GM. Modified meatal advancement and glanuloplasty repair of distal hypospadias. J Urol. 1984;131(6):1140–1. https://doi.org/10.1016/s0022-5347(17)50846-0.
6. Hadidi AT. Double Y glanuloplasty for glanular hypospadias. J Pediatr Surg. 2010;45(3):655–60. https://doi.org/10.1016/j.jpedsurg.2009.11.019.
7. Mieusset R, Soulié M. Hypospadias: psychosocial, sexual, and reproductive consequences in adult life. J Androl. 2005;26(2):163–8.
8. Hadidi AT. Grade I: Glanular hypospadias; Double Y glanulomeatoplasty (DYG) technique. In: Hadidi AT, editor. Hypospadias surgery. Cham: Springer International Publishing; 2022. p. 361–9.

Tubularized Incised Plate (TIP) Urethroplasty

5

Amilal Bhat and Mahakshit Bhat

Abstract

Tubularized urethral plate urethroplasty is the commonest procedure done in distal hypospadias and done in selected cases of middle and proximal hypospadias. Usually, the circumcision is a part of the TIPU and dorsal dartos is used to cover the neourethra. The circumcision is less acceptable to both the parents/patients and the treating physician. Hence, prepucioplasty is more frequently demanded and done. Neourethra can be covered with ventral dartos and foreskin can be preserved for prepucioplasty. The basic principle in the management of hypospadias is to restore the normal or near normal anatomy. The tubularization of urethral plate, spongioplasty, and prepucioplasty reconstructs a near normal penis.

Supplementary Information The online version contains supplementary material available at https://doi.org/10.1007/978-981-99-0795-3_5. The videos can be accessed individually by clicking the DOI link in the accompanying figure caption or by scanning this link with the SN More Media App.

A. Bhat (✉)
Bhat's Hypospadias and Reconstructive Urology Hospital and Research Centre, Jaipur, Rajasthan, India

Dr S.N. Medical College Jodhpur, Jaipur, Rajasthan, India

Department of Urology, S.P. Medical College Bikaner, Bikaner, Rajasthan, India

P.G. Committee Medical Council of India New Delhi, New Delhi, India

Academic and Research Council of RUHS, Jaipur, Rajasthan, India

M. Bhat
Department of Urology, National Institute of Medical Sciences Medical College, Jaipur, India

T. O. Abbas (ed.), *Video Atlas of Hypospadias Surgery*,
https://doi.org/10.1007/978-981-99-0795-3_5

Keywords

Hypospadias · Tubularized urethral plate urethroplasty · Mobilization of urethral plate · Spongioplasty · Double Breasting Spongioplasty · Prepucioplasty · Foreskin reconstruction

5.1 Introduction

Hypospadias is the most common congenital anomaly of external genitalia. TIP is the choice of repair in distal hypospadias and is even feasible in selected cases of proximal hypospadias and is considered to be the most commonly done procedure for hypospadias repair. The basic principle in the management of any congenital anomaly is to restore the normal or near normal anatomy with the existing tissue or with supplementation of tissue. Ideal urethral replacement is only the urethra. The tubularization of urethral plate and spongioplasty reconstruct a near normal urethra. And adding the prepucioplasty reconstructs a near normal penis. Professor C. Thiersch (1869) first used the principle of tubularization of urethral plate in a child of epispadias and later, the same was used for hypospadias as the Thiersch-Duplay urethroplasty [1]. Even before Warren Snodgrass, King (1981) & Zaontz (1989) tubularized the urethral plate for distal hypospadias [2, 3]. Snodgrass (1994) added the dimension of relaxing incision in the urethral plate and deserves the credit of making it the most popular and commonly used technique world over [4].

5.2 Indications

1. Distal hypospadias with minimal or no chordee.
2. Middle and proximal hypospadias with no chordee, mild chordee corrected by penile degloving/single stitch dorsal plication, mobilization of urethral plate and spongiosum with well-developed urethral plate and spongiosum.
3. Augmented TIP in narrow urethral plate in distal and middle hypospadias.

5.3 Video Demonstration

Variable	Findings
Age at surgery (months)	24 months
Gestational age (weeks)	38 weeks
Birth weight	2900 g
Gestational risks	Nil
Family history	Not significant
Any features of DSD (e.g., undescended testes)	No
Testosterone	Not given
Clinical features	Sub-coronal hypospadias, Glans 12 mm urethral plate Stretched penile length 2.8 cm Urethral plate 8 mm Prepuce adequate

Video:

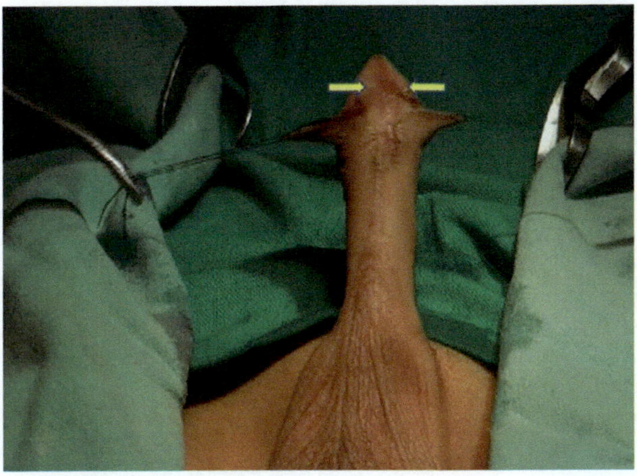

5.4 Steps of the Procedure [1]

- Partial penile degloving
- Mobilization of urethral plate and spongiosum
- Incising the urethral plate
- Tubularization of the urethral plate
- Spongioplasty modified Y-I, double breasting
- Glanuloplasty
- Frenuloplasty
- Dartosorraphy
- Prepucioplasty

5.4.1 Partial Penile Degloving [1]

Stay suture is applied in the glans and a Y-shaped incision is given encircling the urethral plate, starting from prepucial hood to meatus & then extended on to the penile shaft after injecting the I:1,000,000 adrenaline solution injected at the planned site of the incision and a urethral stent is inserted. The wings are extended up to the dorsal hood in patients having no chordee (Fig. 5.1a) and circumferential circum-coronal incision in cases with chordee. Skin and dartos are incised, and partial penile degloving is done (Fig. 5.1b). A complete penile degloving is done up to the root of the penis to correct chordee in cases with chordee keeping the level of dissection at Buck's fascia (Fig. 5.5a, b). Then, the chordee correction is evaluated by Gitte's test [1].

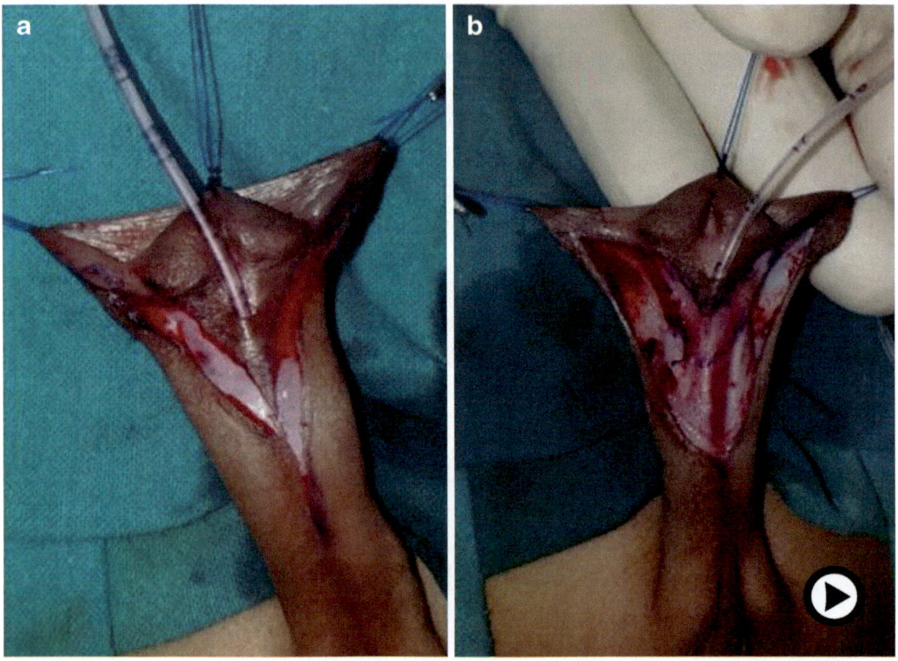

Fig. 5.1 Showing partial penile degloving. (**a**) Y shaped skin incision. (**b**) Mobilization of Dartos at the level of Buck's fascia. (With permission Bhat A.L. Reference [1] @ copyright Springer Nature Singapore). TIP procedure (https://doi.org/10.1007/000-cn0)

5.4.2 Mobilization of Urethral Plate [1]

There are varying views about mobilization of urethral plate and spongiosum. We feel tubularization of urethral plate and spongiosum can be done without tension on the suture line after mobilization. Another advantage is that mild curvature can also be corrected by it enlarging the scope of TIPU in patients with mild curvature and proximal hypospadias. Mobilization of the urethral plate and spongiosum is started creating a dissection plane at the tunica albuginea level proximal to the meatus. The mobilization is done proximal to distal and lateral to medial. Partial mobilization is sufficient in the patients of hypospadias having no chordee (Fig. 5.2a–d). The urethral plate and spongiosum is then dissected into the glans in the same plane of dissection beyond mid-glans up to the tip of the corpora to raise adequate glanular wings for glanuloplasty (Fig. 5.3a–d). Glanular wings are dissected adequately on both sides and deep up to the tip of corporal bodies, which will help get done the spongioplasty up to neo-meatus covering the sub-coronal area with spongiosum to prevent sub-coronal fistula. Deep and adequate mobilization of the glanular wings allows tension-free glanuloplasty even in cases of small glans [1].

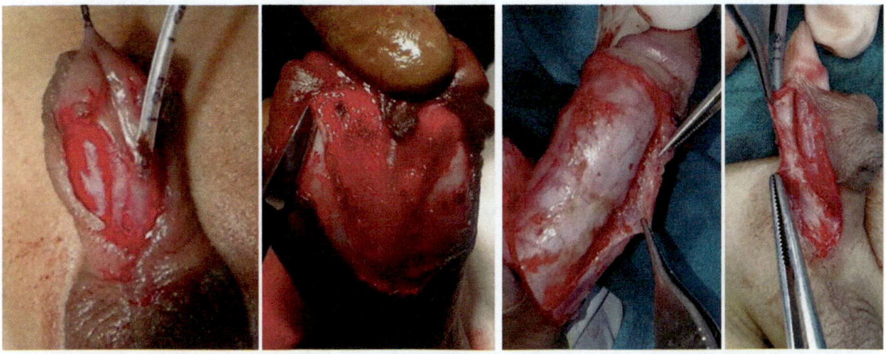

Fig. 5.2 Showing the mobilization of spongiosum and urethral plate

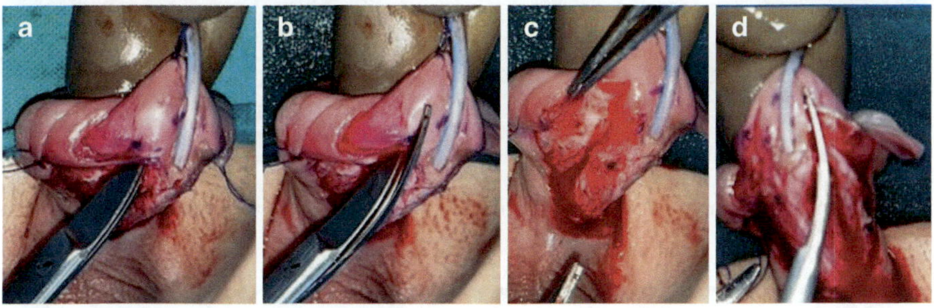

Fig. 5.3 Showing mobilization of urethral plate and spongiosum into glans: (**a**) Creating a plane at tunica albuginea. (**b**) Passing scissors in the same. (**c**, **d**) Incising the glans

5.4.3 Incising the Urethral Plate [1]

The incision in the urethral plate allows the tension-free tubularization of the urethral plate and the incision is started just inside the meatus with the knife extended up to mid-glans (Fig. 5.4a, b). While in cases with small glans it is extended up to tip of the glans margin and inlay graft is placed to prevent the meatal stenosis The incision depth is decided according to the urethral plate's width to tubularize the urethral plate with tension-free suturing. In case of the deep incisions and the narrow urethral plate we prefer to place the dorsal inlay graft in the urethral plate (Fig. 5.5a, b) [1].

5.4.4 Tubularization of the Urethral Plate [1]

Excessive skin on the margins of the urethral plate and meatus is excised and a suture is taken at the site of meatus to create a large meatus to prevent meatal stenosis. The bifurcation of the spongiosum and the urethral plate is well demarcated. Tubularization of urethral plate is stared about 1–2 centimetre proximal to the

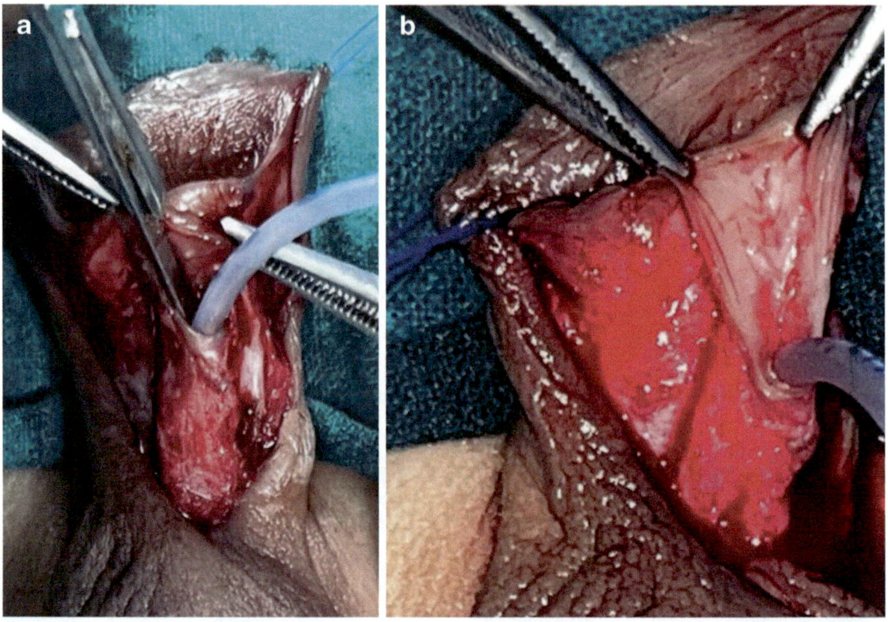

Fig. 5.4 Incising the urethral plate: (**a**) Starting just inside the meatus. (**b**) Incision up to mid-glans

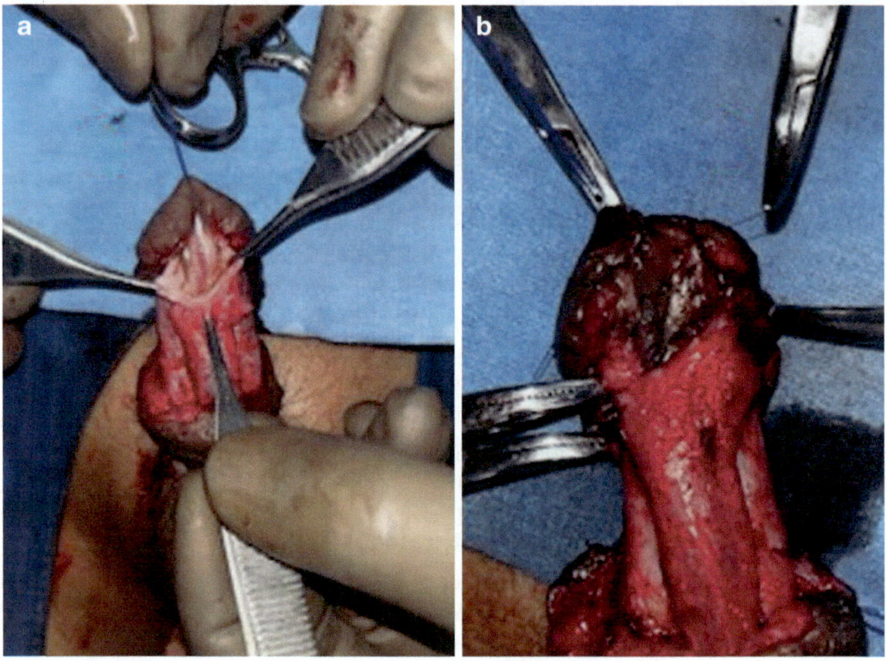

Fig. 5.5 Dorsal inlay graft: (**a**) incising the urethral plate. (**b**) fixed and quilted

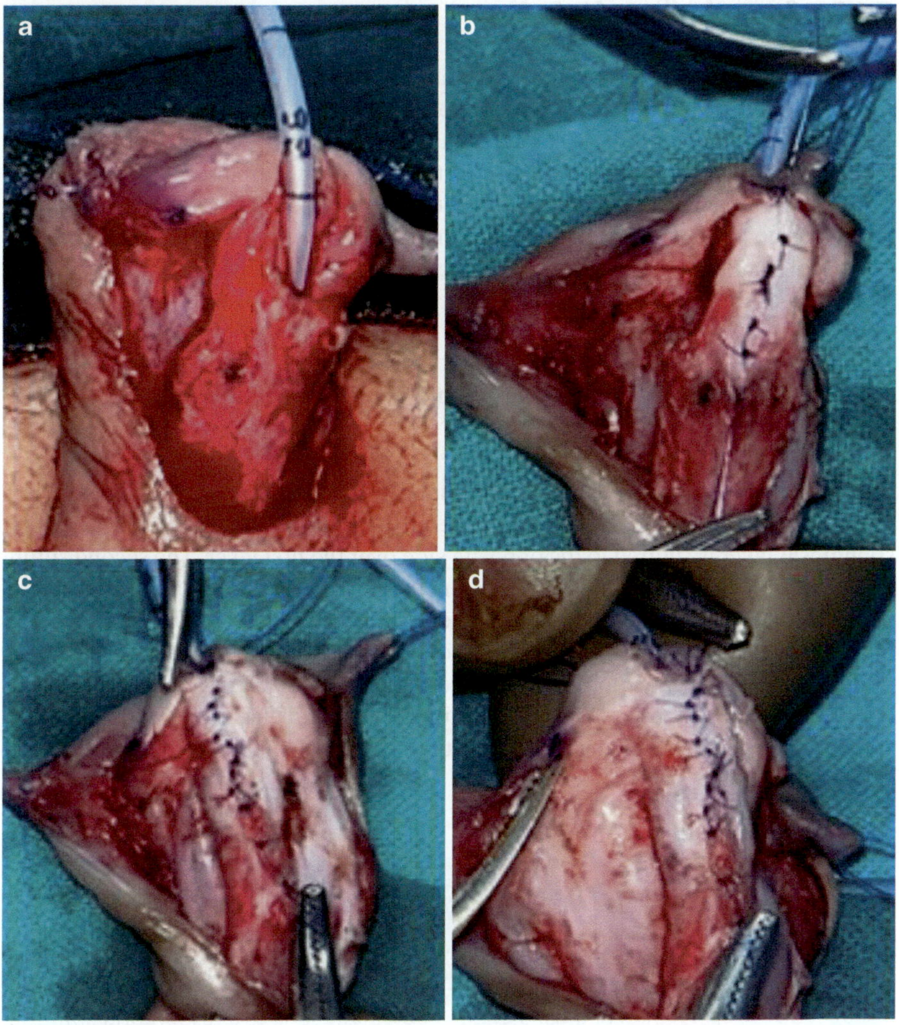

Fig. 5.6 Tubularization of the urethral plate and spongioplasty: (**a**) Mobilization of urethral plate and spongiosum. (**b**) Tubularization started 1 cm proximal to meatus and completed up to mid-glans. (**c**) Spongioplasty started 1 cm proximal to tubularized urethral plate. (**d**) Spongioplasty completed

meatus where the bifurcation of spongiosum starts. Tubularization of the urethral plate is done with 6/0–7/0 PDS inverting continuous or interrupted sub-epithelial sutures. Sutures through urethral plate margins should be avoided to prevent the micro fistulae [1]. We prefer to take subepithelial interrupted sutures to tubularize urethral plate (Fig. 5.6a, b).

5.4.5 Spongioplasty [1, 5, 6]

Covering the spongiosum over the tubularized urethral plate reconstructs a near normal urethra. Mobilization of spongiosum allows tension-free suturing of the spongiosum. Spongioplasty is started about a centimetre to the point of tubularization of urethral plate and done distally up to the tip of neourethra (Figs. 5.6c, b and 5.7a–c). Sutures can be either interrupted or continuous. Spongioplasty beyond mid-glans up to neo-meatus helps to prevent fistula at corona which is the commonest site of fistula. If the spongiosum is well developed and width is adequate then double breasting spongioplasty is feasible.

5.4.6 Double Breasting Spongioplasty (Figs. 5.8a–f and 5.9a–f) [5, 7]

The first layer of suturing of the spongiosum is done, keeping the suture line toward one side of the neo-urethral suture line laterally (Figs. 5.8c, d and 5.9b). The second spongiosal layer is sutured to the opposite side over the first layer. The second suture line toward the contralateral side buries the first layer's suture line with no overlapping of suture lines among all three layers (Figs. 5.8e, f and 5.9c, d). Thus, the neourethra is covered by two layers in a double breasting manner. The advantages of double breasting spongioplasty are covering neourethra by two layers of vascular tissue, avoid the superimposition of suture line of tubularization urethral plate, spongioplasty and skin closure, shape of the cylindrical, and preserve blood supply of urethral better.

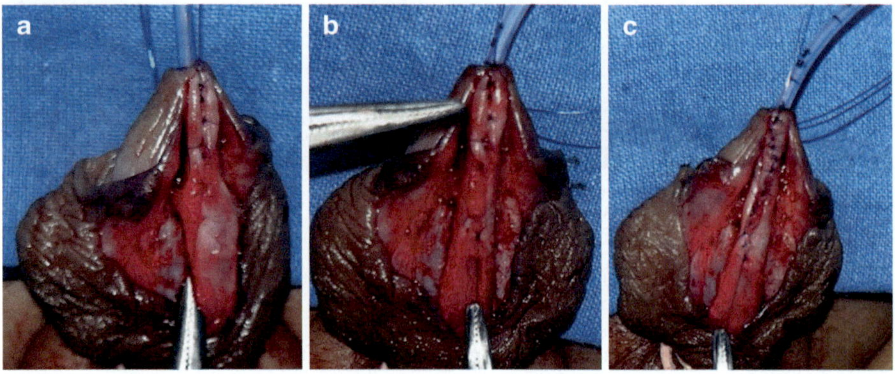

Fig. 5.7 Spongioplasty. (**a**) Tubularization started 1 cm proximal to meatus and completed up to mid-glans. (**b**) Spongioplasty started 1 cm proximal to tubularized urethral plate. (**c**) Spongioplasty completed

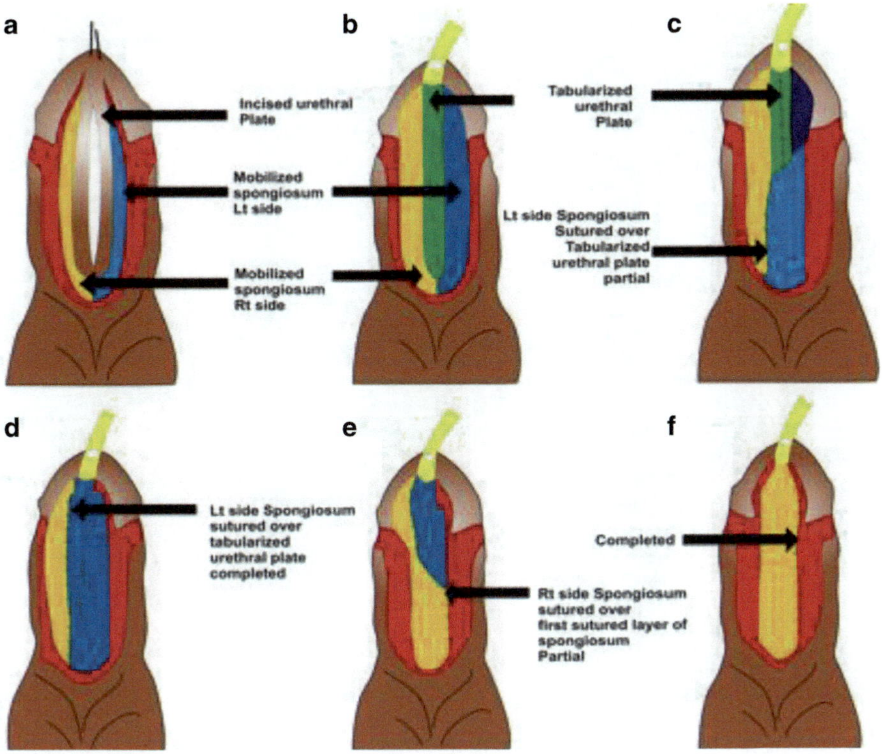

Fig. 5.8 Diagrammatic representation of double breasting. (**a**) Incised urethral plate, (**b**) Tubularized urethral plate, (**c**, **d**) Left side spongiosum sutured laterally to the suture line of tubularized urethral plate. (**e**, **f**). Right side spongiosum sutured to the lateral side as the second layer of double breasting. (With permission Bhat A.L. Reference [5] @ copyright Springer Nature Singapore)

5.4.7 Glansplasty [1]

Glansplasty brings the meatus and creates the conical normal looking glans. Adequate glanular wings are raised for tension-free suturing of the glans wings. Midline glanular wings are mobilized up to the tip of the corporal bodies (Fig. 5.10a) and laterally up to the mid of the shaft (Fig. 5.10b). Glansplasty is done in two layers keeping a space between the neo-urethra and sutured glanular wings (Fig. 5.11c). The second layer may preferably take subepithelial for cosmetically normal looking (Fig. 5.11a, b) but may be taken through the epithelium (Fig. 5.11c).

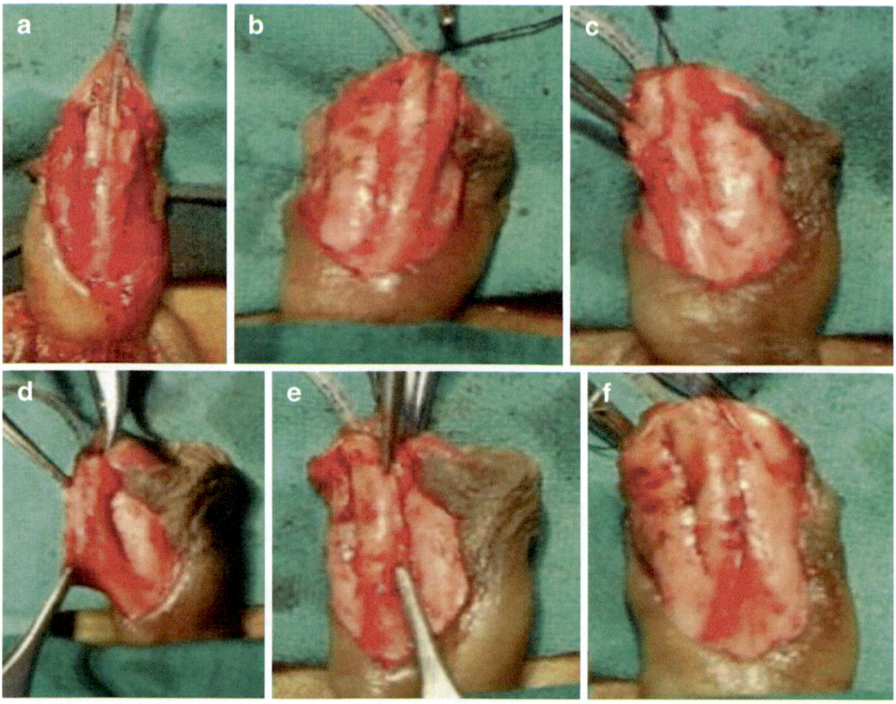

Fig. 5.9 Double breasting spongioplasty. (With permission Bhat A.L. Reference [5] @ copyright Springer Nature Singapore). (**a**) Mobilized urethral plate and spongiosum, (**b**) Tubularized urethral plate, (**c**, **d**) Suturing the left spongiosal pillar lateral to suture line of tubularized urethral plate. (**e**, **f**) Suturing the right spongiosal pillar over the sutured left spongiosal pillar covering the suture line

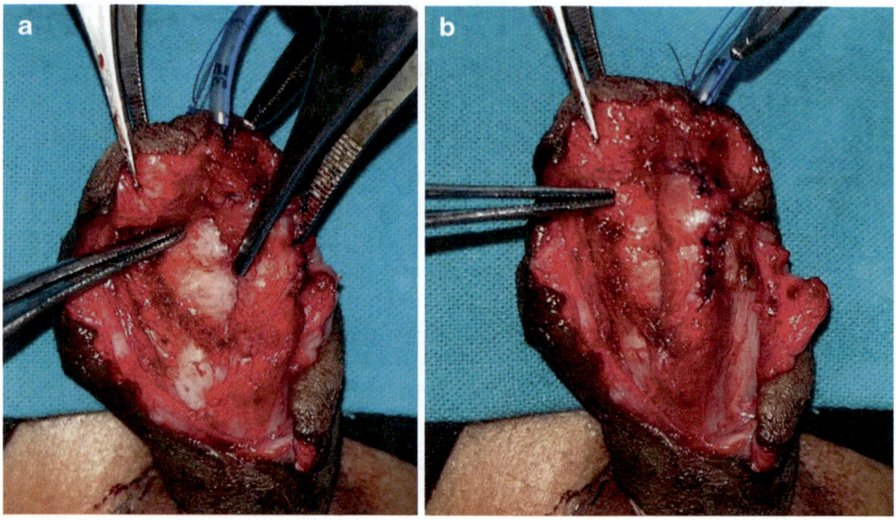

Fig. 5.10 Showing mobilization of glanular wing. (**a**) Medially up to the tip of the corporal body. (**b**) Laterally to the lateral border of corpora

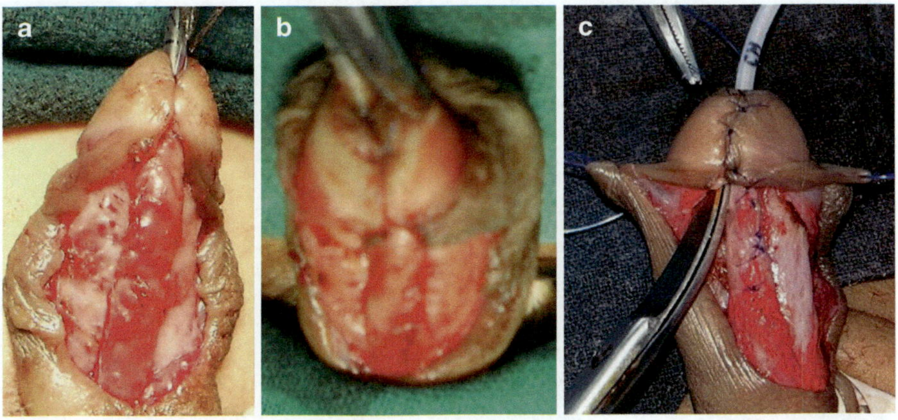

Fig. 5.11 Showing glansplasty. (**a**, **b**) Subcuticular sutures. (**b**) Showing adequate space between the neo-urethra and glansplasty. (**c**) Glansplasty completed

5.4.8 Frenuloplasty [1]

After competition of glansplasty para-glanular inner prepucial skin is sutured in midline to create a frenulum. Two to three sutures are taken to reconstruct the fraenulum of an adequate length. Reconstructing the frenulum is a part of prepucioplasty (Fig. 5.12a, b).

5.4.9 Dartosorraphy [1]

Conventionally, the dorsal dartos is brought ventrally after its mobilization which has a disadvantage of blood supply of superficial skin and skin necrosis. But in prepucial conservation repair the ventral dartos is utilized to cover the neo-urethra. It is necessary to dissect the dartos at the level of Buck's fascia and to have healthy dartos in partial penile degloving. A stay suture is applied at the prepucial skin and kept stretched to approximate the dartos up to prepuce (Fig. 5.13a, b). Dartos suturing is started from the proximal end of the incision and done distally to the prepucioplasty opening (Fig. 5.13a–c). Even in cases of complete penile degloving done at Buck's fascia level, the thick dartos is available to complete dartosorraphy (Fig. 5.14a, b). This thick layer of the dartos covers over the neourethra as a healthy interposing tissue layer to prevent fistula.

5.4.10 Prepucioplasty [1, 8–10]

A common goal to achieve normal or near-normal penile anatomy and good functional outcome, TIP (Tubularized Incised Plate) urethroplasty is the most common procedure. The dorsal hood is sacrificed in TIP to cover the tubularized urethral

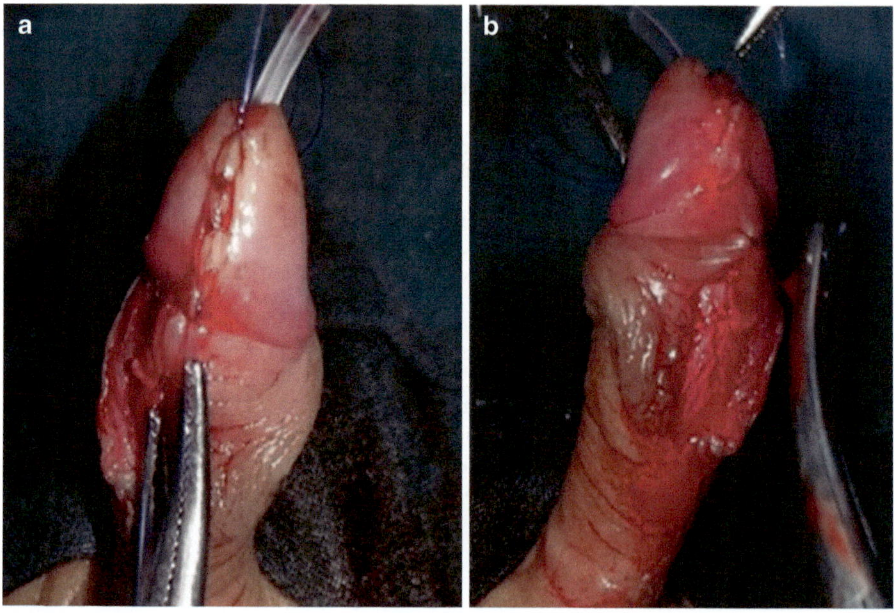

Fig. 5.12 (**a**, **b**) showing the frenuloplasty. (With permission Bhat A.L. Reference [1] @ copyright Springer Nature Singapore)

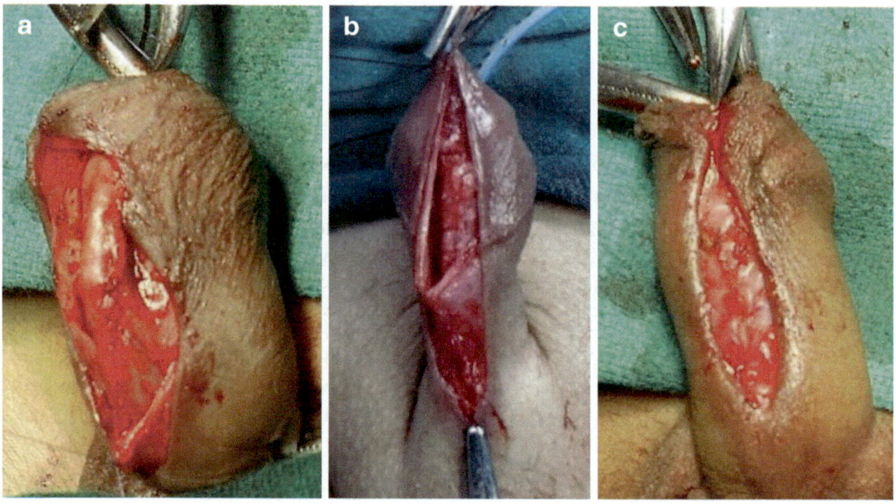

Fig. 5.13 Reconstitution of dartos "Dartosorraphy". (**a**, **b**) Dartos suturing started. (**b**) Half completed. (**c**) Dartos suturing completed. (With permission Bhat A.L. Reference [5] @ copyright Springer Nature Singapore)

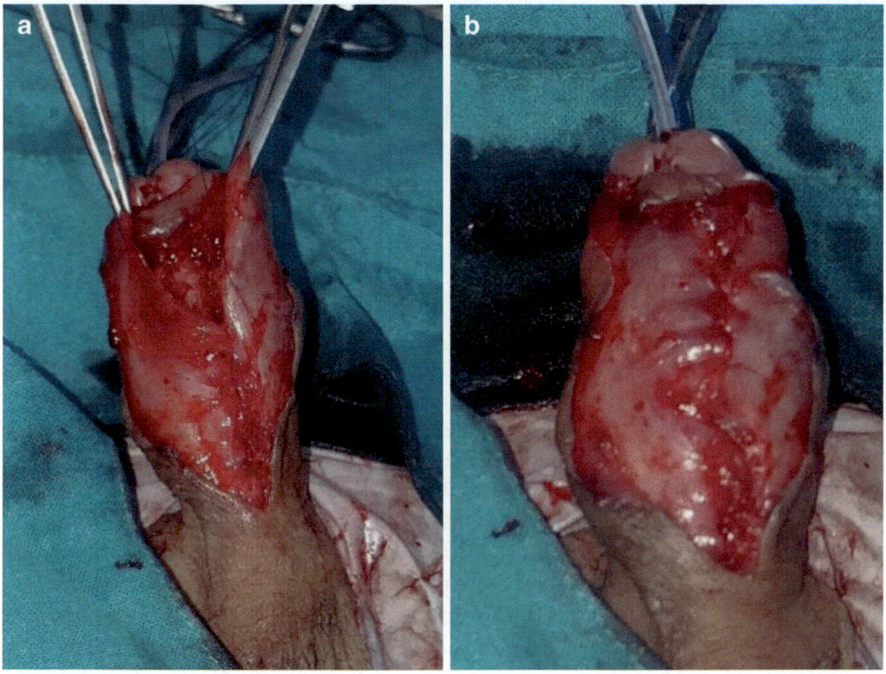

Fig. 5.14 Showing reconstitution of dartos "Dartosorraphy" in circumcision. (**a**) Dartos suturing Halfway down. (**b**) Dartos suturing completed. (With permission Bhat A.L. Reference [5] @ copyright Springer Nature Singapore)

plate as a dorsal dartos cover for waterproofing [8, 9]. But in recent times, circumcision has become less acceptable to both the parents/patients and the treating physician. Hence, prepucioplasty is done more frequently. The prepuce may easily be preserved for prepucioplasty by covering tubularized urethral plate with spongiosum and ventral/scrotal dartos or tunica vaginalis. Initially, prepucioplasty was done in distal hypospadias without chordee or mild chordee [8, 9]. With the advent of TIP repair, the number of patients undergoing prepucioplasty has increased significantly. It is now being done for both mid and proximal hypospadias with acceptable success. We had a well-formed retractable prepuce with 88.9% satisfactory results and better cosmesis in the proximal hypospadias patients. The incidence of complications was also similar to the complication rate (11.10%) in these cases without preputial reconstruction. The advantages of the prepucial reconstruction are the psychological benefit to the child of feeling equal to his colleagues for the shape of his penis, the preservation of the highly innervated and vascularized foreskin which plays a vital role in normal sexual intercourse [8]. Besides, a preserved prepuce can serve as a reserve of tissue if the hypospadias repair is unsuccessful. The preserved prepuce can be utilized in failed hypospadias as onlay flap urethroplasty, flap urethroplasty for stricture urethra, and healthy interposing tissue single or double dorsal dartos cover.

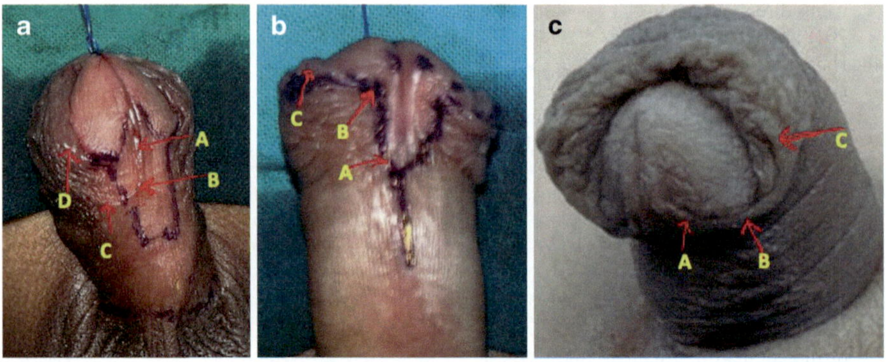

Fig. 5.15 (**a**–**c**) Showing surface marking for prepucioplasty. Arrow showing (**a**, **b**) Frenulum mark, (**b**, **c**) Prepucial skin flap mark

5.4.10.1 Measuring the Adequacy of Prepuce

Commonest complication of prepucioplasty is phimosis. So it is necessary to choose the right case for prepucioplasty. Reconstruction of the foreskin should be attempted in only those whose prepuce can be approximated in the midline without any tension at the coronal groove level. If the ventral defect is large, tension on suture line at corona or mid-glans reconstruction should be avoided. There are different techniques to measure the adequacy of the prepuce for prepucioplasty. Though marks for prepucial opening are marked in most of the cases (Fig. 5.15a–c). The methods to measure prepucial adequacy, are to measure the glans breadth at corona and mid-glans, and the prepuce's length and width with the Vernier callipers (Fig. 5.16a–d). Then compare these for adequacy of the skin. These dimensions will also help in the estimation of the distal limit of preputial reconstruction. Though we can measure the exact length, it is cumbersome to measure with the callipers in a child. Other methods of measuring are approximation of edges of the preputial hood with finger and thumb or forceps (Fig. 5.17a–d) and three stay sutures. These are easy methods and can be done on the table before proceeding for prepucioplasty. In the three-stay suture technique the three stay sutures are taken, one at the corona level, the distal end of prepucial hood at the junction of inner and outer prepucial skin and the penile shaft skin at the level of corona the maximum required width. The second suture preputial skin is pulled over the glans after fixing the inner prepucial skin at the corona by the first stay suture. Then the prepuce is retracted by the third stay suture. When the skin can be pulled over the glans and retracted easily, the prepucial hood is considered adequate (Fig. 5.18a–c).

5.4.10.2 Technique (Figs. 5.19a–f and 5.20a–e)

Apply two stay sutures on the prepuce at the margin of inner and outer prepucial skin (Fig. 5.17a, b). Prepucial incision should be eccentric to have a circular and large prepucial opening which helps in prevention of phimosis and is cosmetically normal looking (Fig. 5.19b). Prepucioplasty is done in three layers, first layer of inner prepucial skin, middle with dartos, and then third layer with outer prepucial

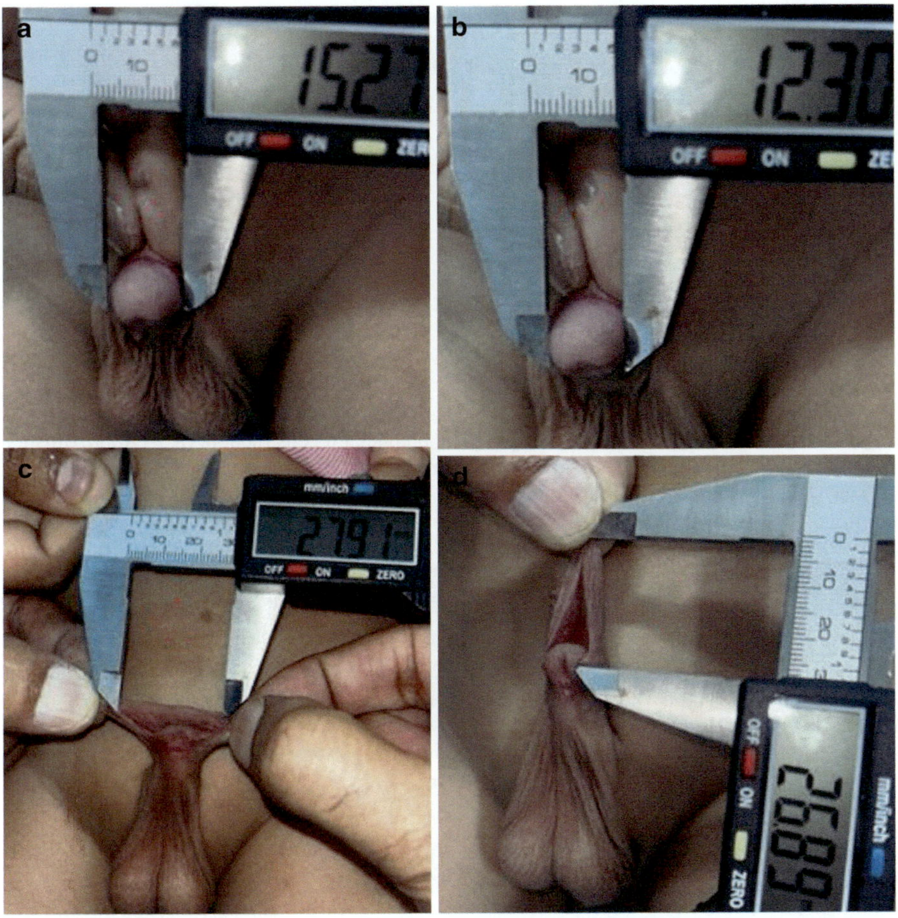

Fig. 5.16 Measurement of glans size and prepucial skin width and length. (**a**) Measuring glans at corona. (**b**) Measuring glans at mid-glans. (**c**) Measuring prepucial length, (**d**) Measuring prepucial width

skin. After reconstruction of frenulum the same is continued distally up to the marked distally for prepucial opening. A suture taken at the distal most limit of the prepucial closure and the inner layer is sutured with interrupted sutures. After completion of dartos closure up to corona the same is continued up distally keeping a traction with the suture applied at the distal limit. The closure of the dartos in prepuce completes the second layer of the prepucioplasty (Fig. 5.20b, c). The prepuce's outer layer is sutured to complete the prepucioplasty and skin closure done by subcuticular or through & through skin sutures (Figs. 5.19d–f and 5.20d, e). Application of traction is important to keep the alignment of all three layers in un-retracted prepuce (Fig. 5.20b, c). After completion of the prepucioplasty prepuce should be retracted back and the adequacy of the prepucial opening assessed. If it seems to be tight then dorsal prepucial vertical incision is given and sutured transversely to prevent phimosis.

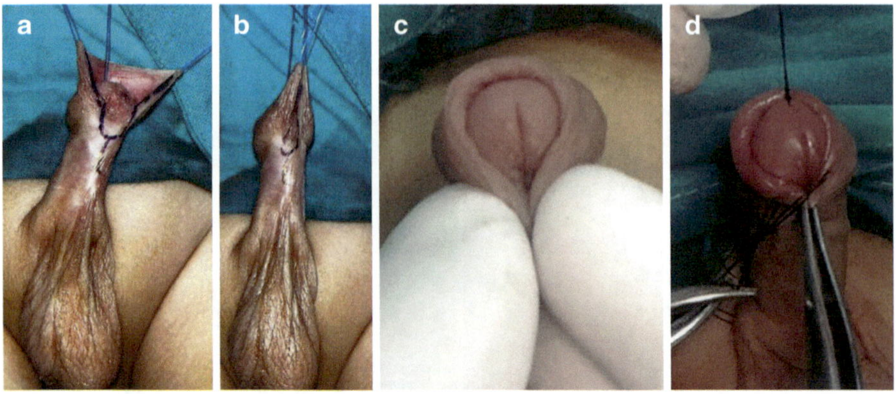

Fig. 5.17 Measurement of foreskin adequacy for prepucial reconstruction. (**a, b**) Approximation with stay suture. (**c**) Thumb and finger. (**d**) With forceps. (With permission Bhat A.L. Reference [8] @ copyright Springer Nature Singapore)

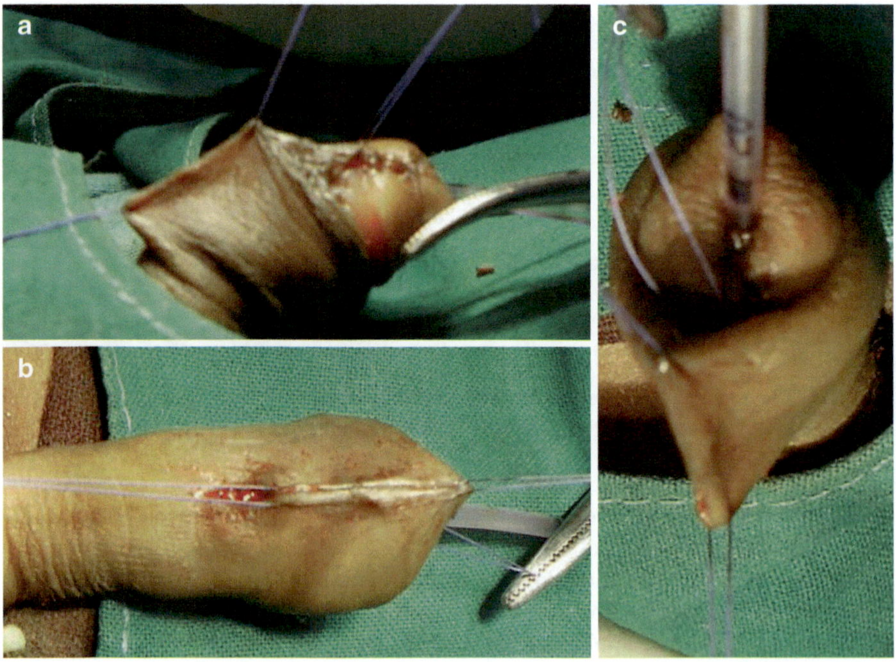

Fig. 5.18 Three stay sutures for adequacy of prepuce for prepucioplasty. (**a**) Photograph showing three sites of stay sutures. (**b**, **c**) Middle suture pulled up to see the adequacy of the prepuce. (With permission Bhat A.L. Reference [8] @ copyright Springer Nature Singapore)

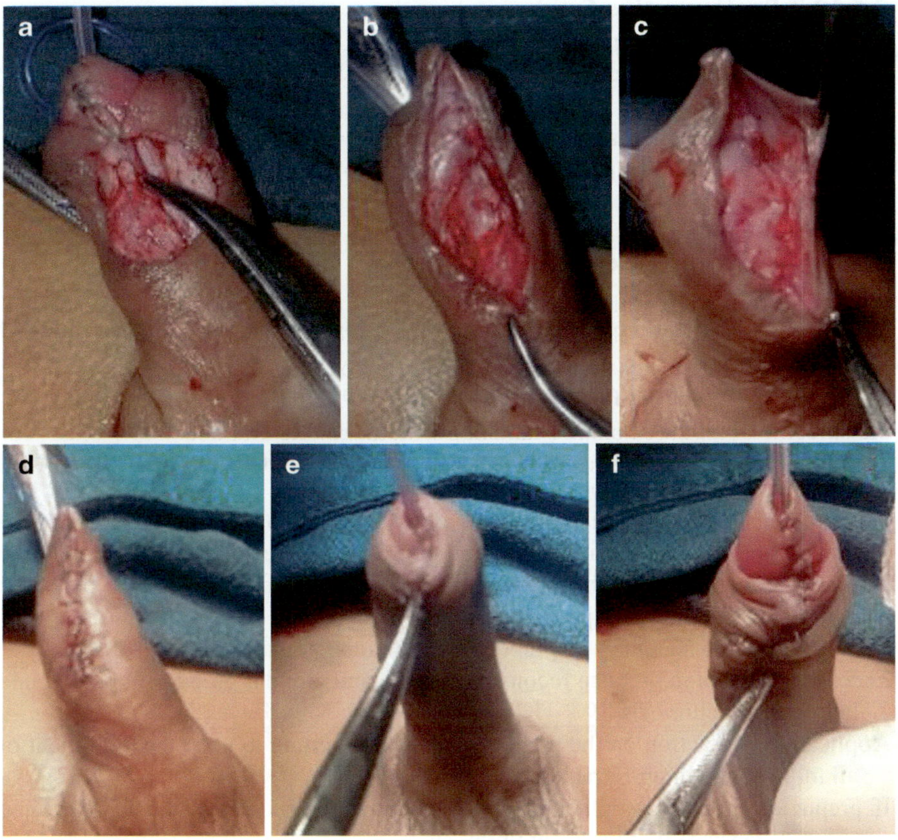

Fig. 5.19 Showing prepucioplasty in three layers. (**a**) Frenuloplasty. (**b**) Inner prepucial skin closure. (**c**) Dartos closure as second layer. (**d**) Outer layer skin closure (**e, f**) Retractable prepuce. (With permission Bhat A.L. Reference [8] @ copyright Springer Nature Singapore)

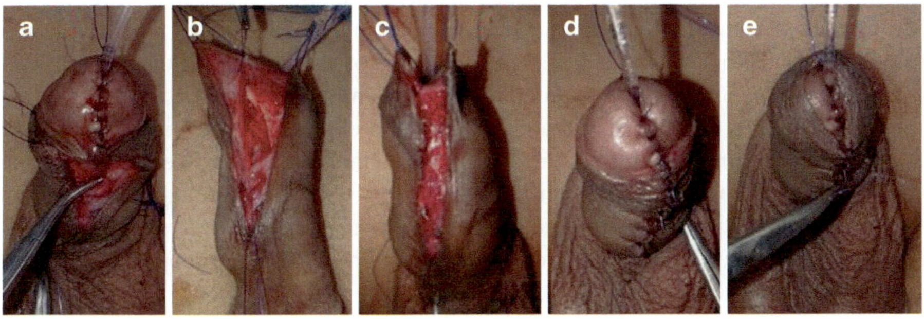

Fig. 5.20 Showing prepucioplasty in three layers. (**a**) Glansplasty and frenuloplasty. (**b**) Inner prepucial skin closure and dartos layer started. (**c**) Dartos closure as second layer completed. (**d**) Outer layer skin closure and retractable. (**e**) Well-formed prepucial opening

5.4.10.3 Postoperative Care

- Mild pressure dressing done to prevent oedema of prepucial skin.
- Stent/infant feeding tube is put to drain the bladder and kept in diaper for 7–9 days.
- Dressing and catheter are removed in 7 days.
- Antibiotics and anti-muscarinic are given for 7–10 days.

5.5 Tips and Tricks

Mobilization of urethral plate and spongiosum allows tension-free tubularization of urethral plate.

Mobilization of urethral plate with spongiosum into glans allows to add spongiosum up to neo-meatus, helps prevent coronal fistula.

Y-I spongioplasty or double breasting spongioplasty adds a locally available healthy tissue to cover tubularized urethral plate.

Double breasting spongioplasty has the advantage of two healthy layers over neo-urethra and avoids superimposition of suture line to prevent fistula.

Adding prepucioplasty with spongioplasty reconstructs normal looking penis for better satisfaction of the patients/parents.

Better to measure adequacy of prepuce before prepucioplasty.

Eccentric incision in prepuce reconstructs wide and circular prepucial opening and help prevent phimosis.

Application of traction on the prepucial skin is important to keep the alignment of all three layers in un-retracted prepuce.

If prepucial opening is tight then dorsal prepucial vertical incision is given and sutured transversely to prevent phimosis.

5.6 Results and Conclusions

Postoperative results are good: prepuce is normal looking, retractable (Fig. 5.21a–c), urinary stream is projectile and straight (Fig. 5.21d), and many a time it is not recognized whether the patient has been operated or not. The commonest complication is phimosis but can be prevented by better planning by eccentric incision of the prepucial hood & reconstructing a large prepucial opening, application of cortisone skin cream, and regular retraction of the prepucial skin after 8 weeks postoperatively. The phimosis after prepucioplasty needing circumcision and dehiscence of reconstructed prepuce was reported in 8% (10) but prepucioplasty itself does not increase the risk of urethroplasty complications, and the overall reoperation rate of hypospadias repair.

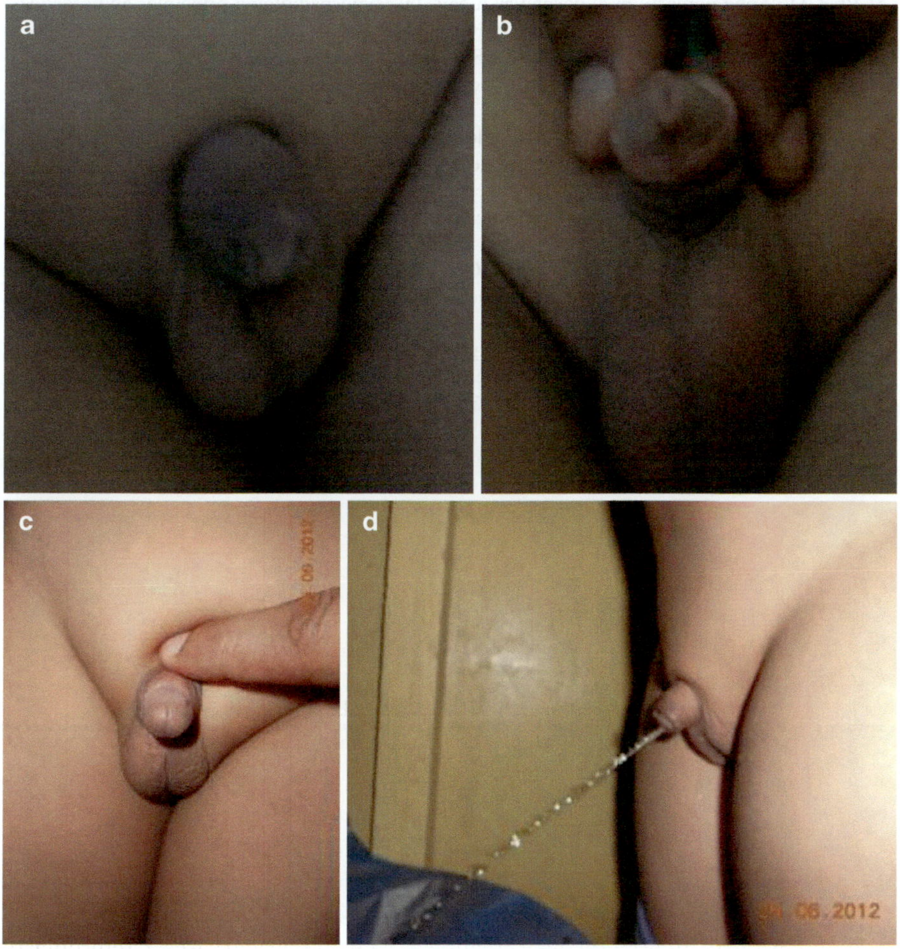

Fig. 5.21 Figure showing postoperative results. (**a**) Well-formed prepuce. (**b**, **c**) Almost normal appearing meatus and easily retractable prepuce. (**d**) Straight and projectile stream

References

1. Bhat AL. Modified tubularized incised urethral plate urethroplasty. In: Hypospadiology: principles and practices. Publishers Nature Springer Singapore Pte Ltd; 2022. p. 101–12.
2. King LR. Hypospadias—a one-stage repair with- out skin graft based on a new principle: chordee is sometimes produced by the skin alone. J Urol. 1970;103(5):660–2.
3. Zaontz MR. The GAP (glans approximation procedure) for glanular/coronal hypospadias. J Urol. 1989;141(2):359–61.
4. Snodgrass W. Tubularized, incised plate urethroplasty for distal hypospadias. J Urol. 1994;151(2):464–5.

5. Bhat AL. Spongioplasty in hypospadias repair. In: Hypospadiology: principles and practices. Publishers Nature Springer Singapore Pte Ltd; 2022. p. 101–12.
6. Bhat A, Sabharwal K, Bhat M, Saran R, Singla M, Kumar V. Outcome of tubularized incised plate urethroplasty with spongioplasty alone as additional tissue cover: a prospective study. Indian J Urol. 2014;30(4):392.
7. Bhat A, Bhat M, Kumar R, Bhat A. Double breasting spongioplasty in tubularized/tubularized incise plate urethroplasty: a new technique. Indian J Urol. 2017;33(1):58.
8. Bhat A, Bhat M, Khandelwal N. The prepuce and prepucioplasty in hypospadias repair. In: Hypospadiology: principles and practices. Publishers Nature Springer Singapore Pte Ltd; 2022. p. 101–12.
9. Bhat A, Gandhi A, Saxena G, Choudhary GR. Preputial reconstruction and tubularized incised plate urethroplasty in proximal hypospadias with ventral penile curvature. Indian J Urol. 2010;26(4):507.
10. Castagnetti M, Gnech M, Angelini L, Rigamonti W, Bagnara V, Esposito C. Does preputial reconstruction increase complication rate of hypospadias repair? 20-year systematic review and meta-analysis. Front Pediatr. 2016;4:41. https://doi.org/10.3389/fped.2016.00041. e Collection 2016.PMID: 27200322

6 Dorsal Inlay Tubularized Incised Plate (DTIP) Repair

Tariq O. Abbas

Abstract

It is recognized that multiple perioperative variables and anatomical components of the hypospadiac penis affect surgical prognosis. These characteristics are significant predictor variables that can aid in risk stratification and clinical decision-making. At the same time, the assessment of penile curvature is a crucial stage in the evaluation and management of hypospadias that can greatly influence the surgical technique chosen and long-term outcomes. Dorsal inlay tubularized incised plate is indicated whenever augmentation urethroplasty of the native urethral plate would lead to higher risk of complications "unfavorable" urethral plate.

Keywords

Hypospadias · Unfavorable · Urethral plate · Graft · Tubularized · Urethroplasty

6.1 Introduction

The tubularized incised urethroplasty (TIP), popularized by Warren Snodgrass in 1994, was rapidly adopted by surgeons around the world to treat distal and even proximal hypospadias [1]. Snodgrass and others assume that the dorsal surface of

---

Supplementary Information The online version contains supplementary material available at https://doi.org/10.1007/978-981-99-0795-3_6. The videos can be accessed individually by clicking the DOI link in the accompanying figure caption or by scanning this link with the SN More Media App.

T. O. Abbas (✉)
Pediatric Urology Section, Sidra Medicine, Doha, Qatar
e-mail: tabbas@sidra.org

T. O. Abbas (ed.), *Video Atlas of Hypospadias Surgery*,
https://doi.org/10.1007/978-981-99-0795-3_6

the incised urethral plate undergoes complete epithelialization [2, 3]. On the basis of studies showing tubularization of "narrow" urethral plates increases the prevalence of urethro-cutaneous fistulas and stenosis, some pediatric urologists have questioned the efficacy of this hypothesized healing process [4–6]. These data imply that at least a portion of the healing process involves fibrosis and retraction of the incised area, which leads to progressive strain and fistula formation [7–9]. To circumvent this "physiological" process, the placement of an inner preputial or oral mucosa graft (dorsal inlay graft) over the incised area has been suggested [10–13]. The proponents of dorsal inlay TIP (DTIP) claim that better healing occurs in the presence of the graft, resulting in a neourethra with a larger diameter, improved flow, and less stenosis [11, 14, 15].

6.2 Indications

(a) **Unfavorable urethral plate**

DTIP is recommended for unfavorable urethral plates, enhancing the healing of hypospadias without or with slight curvature [16, 17]. Based on this, we created an objective criterion to determine the properties of the urethral plate: The Plate Objective Scoring Tool (POST) score [18–21] (Fig. 6.1). Based on our findings, an AB/BC ratio of <1.2 indicates an unfavorable urethral plate, and in such cases, we advise a DTIP repair as opposed to a TIP repair [22, 23]. Future integration of artificial intelligence could further ease the use of this scoring system [24].

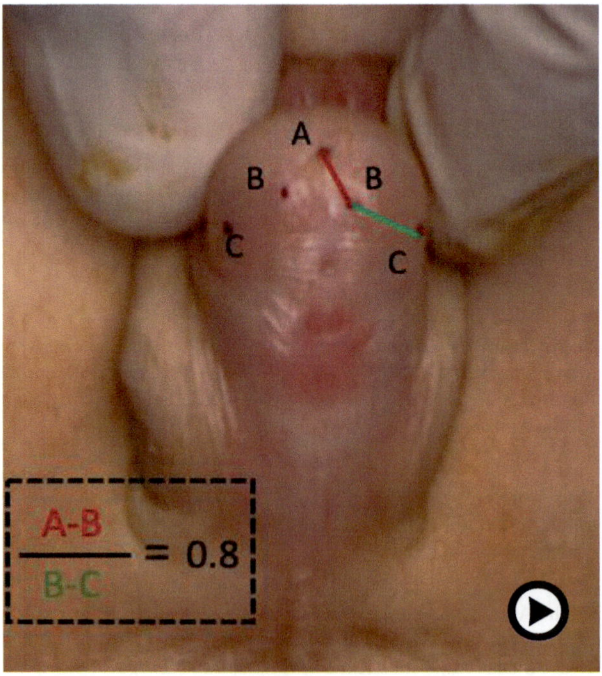

Fig. 6.1 Identification of anatomical landmarks for determination of POST score. A case of sub-coronal hypospadias, the borders of both the glans and urethral plate are identified followed by marking three distinct points: (**a**) distal extent of the urethral plate at the midline, (**b**) lateral border of the urethral plate where the knob of the glans is situated, and (**c**) where the coronal part of the glans commences and the glans edge diverges. Dorsal inlay TIP procedure (https://doi.org/10.1007/000-cn1)

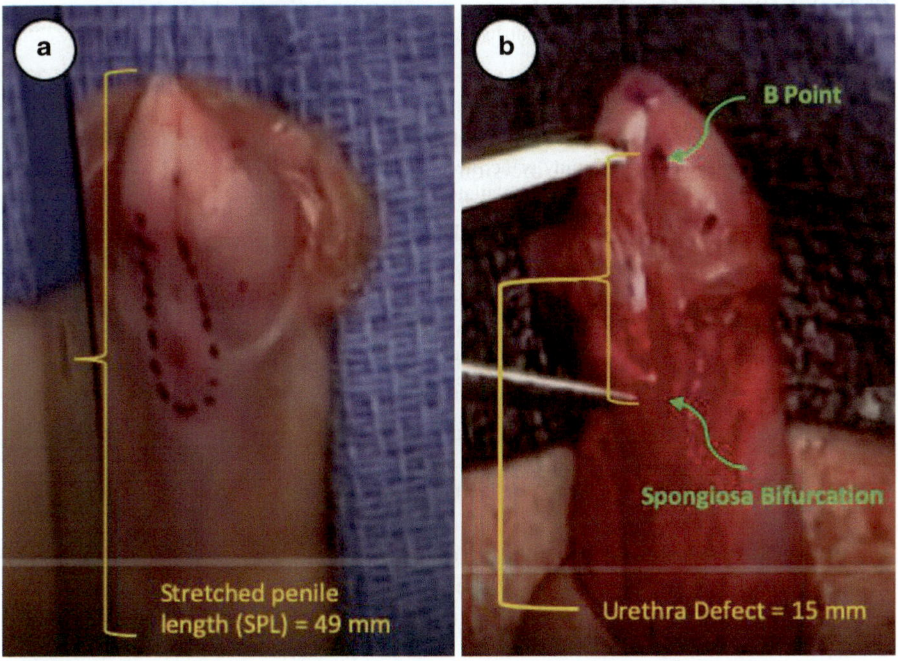

Fig. 6.2 A patient with sub-coronal hypospadias meatus. The precise quantification of the hypospadias severity is determined by the calculation of the urethral defect ratio (UDR) which is the result of urethral defect (UD) divided by the stretched penile length (SPL) (**a**); in this case, 15 ÷ 49 = 0.31 (i.e., Grade 1) (**b**)

(b) **Penile curvature <45°**
(c) **Hypospadias severity:** Grades 1 and 2 in urethral defect ratio classification [25] Fig. 6.2 (or distal to penoscrotal junction based on meatal position classification)

6.3 Video Demonstration

Factors	Findings
Age at surgery (months)	18
Gestational age (weeks)	37
Birth weight (g)	2850
Gestational risks (e.g., maternal co-morbidities, IVF, Twin)	None
Family history	None
Testosterone (if yes, reason, and protocol used)	Glans 11 mm, 2 mg/kg/dose 12, 8, and 4 weeks prior to surgery
Any features of DSD (e.g., undescended testes)	None

6.4 Steps of the Procedure

6.4.1 Penile Degloving

- A 5-0 polypropylene traction suture is placed in the dorsal midline of the glans
- Circumferential sub-coronal incision is done about 5–7 mm below the coronal sulcus and proximal to the hypospadiac meatus (Fig. 6.3)
- The penis is degloved just above the Buck's fascia
- An erection test is done without the use of a tourniquet by infusing normal saline with a large bore butterfly needle (21-gauge) [26] (Fig. 6.4)
- If chordee is present, it should be measured with a goniometer or by taking a lateral photograph and with a mobile device App (e.g., Angle Meter 360) in order to determine the exact degree of ventral curvature [16, 27, 28].

6.4.2 Preparation of Ventral Dartos Flap

- A ventral dartos flap is fashioned if a distal repair is anticipated. It should be dissected in the exact plane, just above the spongiosum and leaving with a wide base to maximize blood supply (Fig. 6.5).

6.4.3 Periurethral Plate Incision

- A U-shaped incision is made beginning at the glanular knobs (point B) and extending 1–2 mm proximal to the hypospadiac meatus (at a non-hypoplastic territory) (Fig. 6.6).

6.4.4 Chordee Correction

- If penile curvature is 20–45°, a midline dorsal plication is performed in situations with distal hypospadias where the erection test revealed a mild or moderate curvature with a normal-sized penis and excellent spongiosum all the way to the meatus (Chap. 20).
- A midline incision is made in the fascia of Bucks. The dorsal penile vein and any other structures in the midline are shifted laterally, revealing the tunica albuginea at 12 o'clock.
- Then, two parallel transverse incisions are made at the level of maximum curvature in the albuginea.
- Over the tiny incisions, 5-0 polypropylene inverted plication sutures are put to plicate the albuginea in that location.
- In situations with severe curvature (>45 degrees), poor spongiosum (long hypoplasia), or extremely small penis, the urethral plate is separated and a stepwise repair is planned, as detailed in another chapter of this book. Ventral lengthening

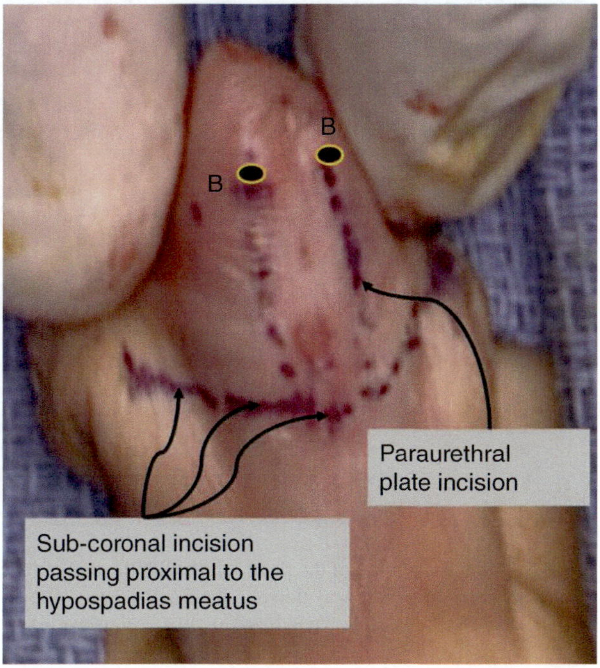

Fig. 6.3 Landmarks for the B points along with the paraurethral plate and sub-coronal incision that secure the preservation of the mucosal collar and the start of the penile degloving

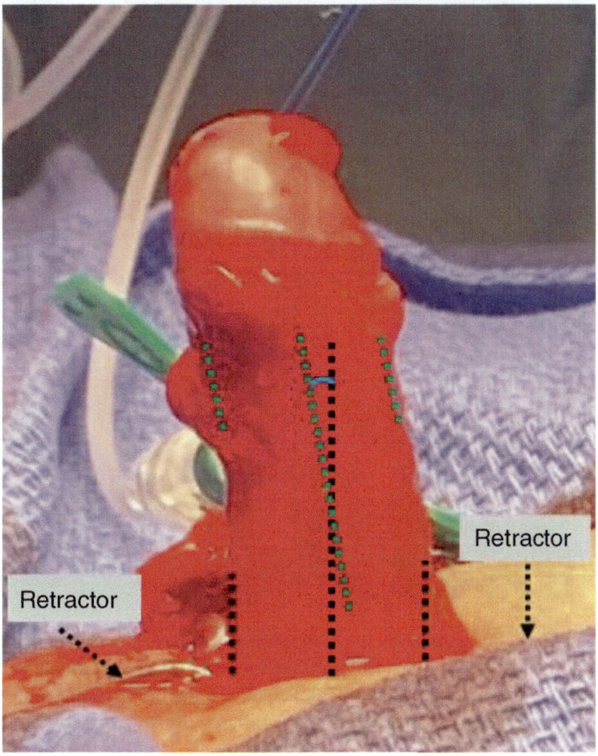

Fig. 6.4 Lateral view of the penile shaft during an erection test. Following degloving, two retractors are placed at the base of the penile shaft to allow full inspection of the penile shaft so as not to miss any proximal penile curvature

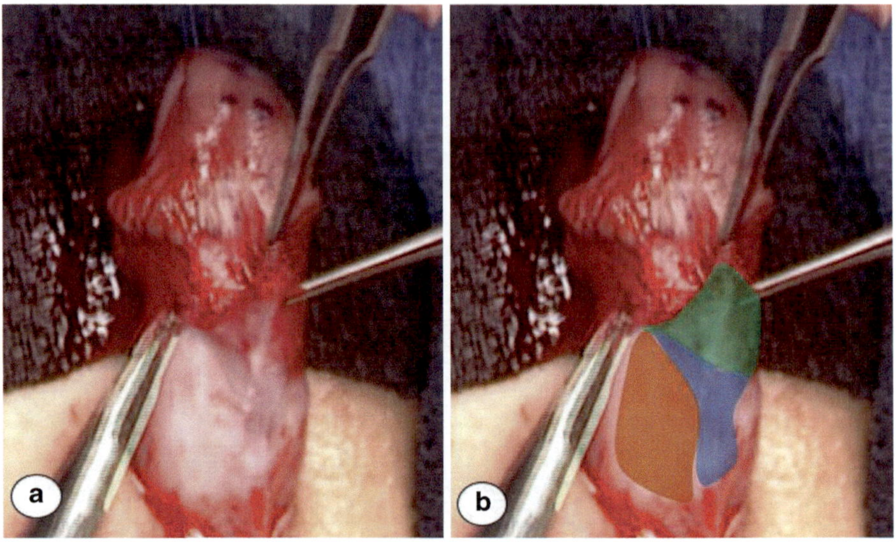

Fig. 6.5 A ventral picture of the penile shaft with the flap of the ventral dartos being prepared (**a**). The dissection goes all the way down to the Buck's fascia (shown in orange) (**b**) and just above the spongiosa of the urethra (shown in blue) to raise a robust well-vascularized dartos flap (green color)

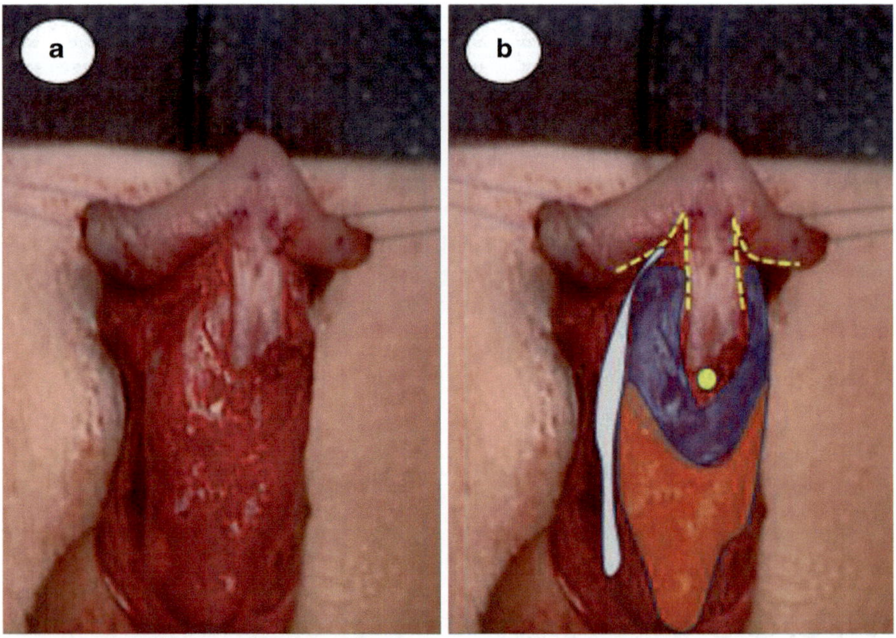

Fig. 6.6 Dissection of the U-shaped peri-urethral plate incision (**a**) is followed by appropriate glanular dissection, leading to the formation of wide glanular wings (yellow dotted lines) (**b**). The ventro-lateral dissection at the level superficial to the tunica albuginea (shown in light gray) results in the release of the lateral spongiosal flaps (illustrated in blue), which can aid in spongioplasty and allow tension-free glanuloplasty. Additionally, the Dartos flap is represented in orange

utilizing ventral transverse incisions of tunica albuginea (VTITA) is performed in cases of severe curvatures where phased repair is envisaged.

- The erection test is then repeated to determine that the curvature has been corrected.

6.4.5 Urethroplasty and Harvest of Inner Preputial Graft

- Similar to the TIP approach, a deep incision reaching the corpora cavernosa is done in the midline.
- A proportionate elliptical region of the stretched inner prepuce is defined and incised, thereby eliminating the dartos seen underneath. In cases of redo urethroplasty, an upper mucosal graft can help [29].
- The graft is then appropriately fitted to loosely cover the incised raw area. To assist this portion of the treatment, it is necessary to initially anchor the graft with four angular stitches.
- The graft does not need to be sutured to the mucosal borders of the incision, but rather, sub-epithelially (Fig. 6.7).
- An 8F Silastic stent is inserted into the bladder, and urethroplasty starting at the distal corners of the incised plate, 7-0 PDS running suture is utilized for the first layer of the urethroplasty.
- A second layer interrupted with 7-0 Vycril is then applied.
- The entire urethroplasty is then covered with a ventral dartos flap that has been previously prepared (Fig. 6.8).

6.4.6 Glanuloplasty

- The glanular wings are then mobilized laterally
- Glans wings are approached by subcuticular sutures of 6-0 or 7-0 polyglactin, resulting in a solid glans bridge beneath the neo-meatus [30]
- Catheter fixation is performed with 5-0 prolene using a technique that prevents para-meatal markings and migration

6.4.7 Skin Closure

- When possible, rotational preputial flaps are mobilized and approximated in the midline to create median raphe.
- The penis is coated with a Tegaderm and Coban® in a somewhat squeezed manner. The stent is permitted to drain freely in diapers for roughly 10 days before being removed.

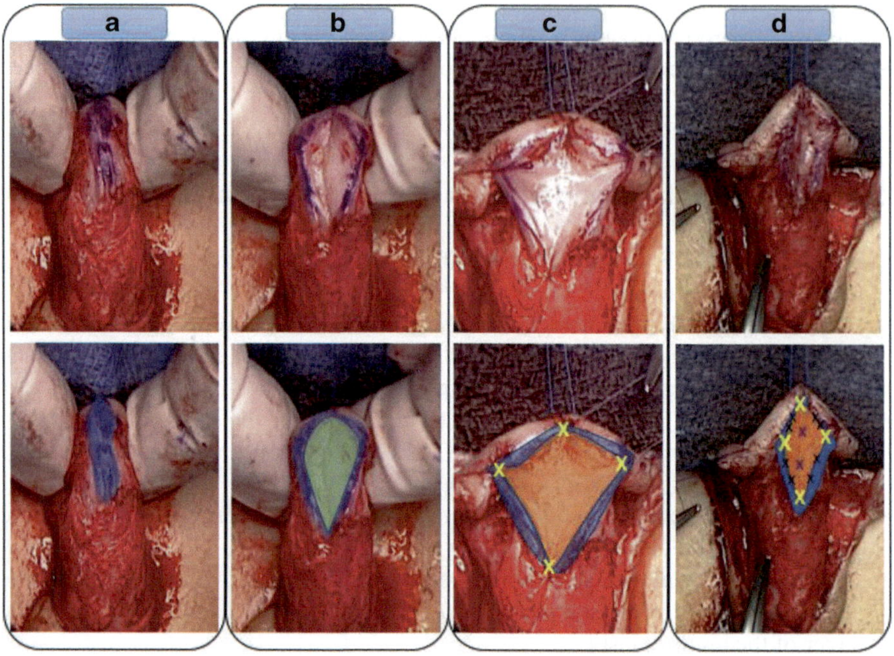

Fig. 6.7 Images depicting the steps of inner preputial graft fixation to the incised area of the urethral plate. (**a**) The urethral plate is colored blue, with the distal extent of the neo-meatus being determined to be distal to the original A point, which exits at the mucocutaneous junction. (**b**) The urethral plate (and glans) are deeply incised to the level of the corpora cavenosa. (**c**) Laying the inner mucosal preputial graft, beginning with four-point corner fixation (yellow crosses) (**d**) The graft is secured by two to three interrupted sutures at each of the four diamond-shaped limbs of the incised urethral plate (black crosses) and two to three midline quilting sutures (purple crosses)

6.5 Post-Operative Care

- To keep the Coban dressing for 24 hours
- The urethral catheter/stent to be removed after 5–7 days
- Antibiotic prophylaxis while the urethral catheter/stent in place

6.6 Tips and Tricks

- To put the stay suture dorsally in the glans well off the expected distal extent of the future neo-meatus [30].
- To enhance visibility of the urethral plate's margins, we color it with a marking pen.
- When incising the lateral borders of the urethral plate, Xylocaine with epinephrine (1:100.000) is injected in the spongiosum of the glans and sub-coronal area, underlying the marked incision line.

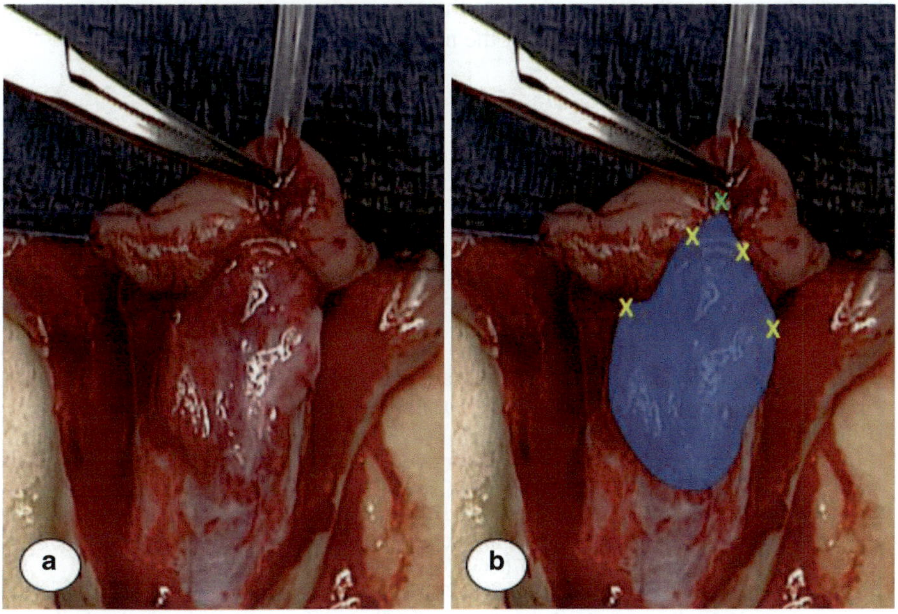

Fig. 6.8 (**a**) The ventral dartos flap is held in place by four sutures, the distal two of which are located in the grooves of the glanular wings (yellow crosses). (**b**) An extra "optional" fixation point can be done at the time of the distal glanular approximation suture

- Bevel the direction of the knife's tip laterally while incising the lateral borders of the urethral plate to reduce the risk of injury to a thin urethral plate.
- When anchoring the graft into the raw incised area, fix it to the underside of the incised urethral plate's medial borders.
- The use of a penile tourniquet during the graft suture prevents blood oozing, hence enhancing visibility during this delicate phase of the surgery [31].
- Throughout the skin closure, subepithelial threads are utilized to prevent the creation of suture tracks.

6.7 Results and Conclusion

There is no clear evidence to prove the superiority of DTIP over TIP [32]. A recent systematic review by Alshafei A, et al. showed a trend toward increased complications following TIP compared to DTIP, with development of urethrocutaneous in 9.4% (33/350) and 4.9% (13/267) after TIP and DTIP, respectively. Meatal stenosis occurred in 21.2% and 4.1% after TIP and DTIP, respectively [32, 33]. As observed in 17 patients in Gupta's [34] series, a large and bulky graft can lead to prolapse through the meatus, therefore adequate thinning and re-sizing of the graft is recommended to optimize the cosmesis of the neo-meatus.

References

1. Snodgrass W. Tubularized, incised plate urethroplasty for distal hypospadias. J Urol. 1994;151:464–5.
2. Mousavi SA, Aarabi M. Tubularized incised plate urethroplasty for hypospadias reoperation: a review and meta-analysis. Int Braz J Urol. n.d.;40:588–95.
3. Holland AJ, Smith GH, Cass DT. Clinical review of the "Snodgrass" hypospadias repair. Aust N Z J Surg. 2000;70:597–600.
4. Abbas TO, Braga LH, Spinoit AF, Salle JP. Urethral plate quality assessment and its impact on hypospadias repair outcomes: a systematic review and quality assessment. J Pediatr Urol. 2021; https://doi.org/10.1016/j.jpurol.2021.02.017.
5. Abbas TO, Charles A, Ali M, Salle JLP. Long-term fate of the incised urethral plate in Snodgrass procedure; A real concern does exist. Urol Case Reports. 2020:32. https://doi.org/10.1016/J.EUCR.2020.101216.
6. Abbas T, AlSalihi M, El-Hout Y, Ali M, AbdAlla E. General perioperative considerations. In: Abbas TO, editor. Hypospadiology. Singapore: Springer Nature Singapore; 2023. p. 53–65. https://doi.org/10.1007/978-981-19-7666-7_4.
7. Elbakry A, Hegazy M, Matar A, Zakaria A. Tubularised incised-plate versus tubularisation of an intact and laterally augmented plate for hypospadias repair: a prospective randomised study. Arab J Urol. 2016;14:163–70. https://doi.org/10.1016/j.aju.2016.03.004.
8. Hadidi AT. Functional urethral obstruction following tubularised incised plate repair of hypospadias. J Pediatr Surg. 2013;48:1778–83. https://doi.org/10.1016/j.jpedsurg.2012.10.071.
9. Abbas TO, Ali TA, Uddin S. Urine as a main effector in urological tissue engineering—a double-edged sword. Cells. 2020;9:538. https://doi.org/10.3390/cells9030538.
10. Kolon TF, Gonzales ET. The dorsal inlay graft for hypospadias repair. J Urol. 2000; https://doi.org/10.1016/S0022-5347(05)67603-3.
11. Mouravas V, Filippopoulos A, Sfoungaris D. Urethral plate grafting improves the results of tubularized incised plate urethroplasty in primary hypospadias. J Pediatr Urol. 2014;10:463–8. https://doi.org/10.1016/j.jpurol.2013.11.012.
12. Silay MS, Sirin H, Tepeler A, Karatag T, Armagan A, Horasanli K, et al. "Snodgraft" technique for the treatment of primary distal hypospadias: pushing the envelope. J Urol. 2012;188:938–42. https://doi.org/10.1016/j.juro.2012.04.126.
13. Gundeti M, Queteishat A, Desai D, Cuckow P. Use of an inner preputial free graft to extend the indications of Snodgrass hypospadias repair (Snodgraft). J Pediatr Urol. 2005;1:395–6. https://doi.org/10.1016/j.jpurol.2005.03.010.
14. Shimotakahara A, Nakazawa N, Wada A, Nagata S, Koga H, Takahashi T, et al. Tubularized incised plate urethroplasty with dorsal inlay graft prevents meatal/neourethral stenosis: a single surgeon's experience. J Pediatr Surg. 2011;46:2370–2. https://doi.org/10.1016/j.jpedsurg.2011.09.033.
15. Abbas T, McCarthy L. Foreskin and penile problems in childhood. Surg (United Kingdom). 2016:34. https://doi.org/10.1016/j.mpsur.2016.03.007.
16. Abbas TO. Evaluation of penile curvature in patients with hypospadias; gaps in the current practice and future perspectives. J Pediatr Urol. 2021; https://doi.org/10.1016/J.JPUROL.2021.12.015.
17. Abbas TO, Pippi Salle JL. When to graft the incised plate during TIP repair? A suggested algorithm that may help in the decision-making process. Front Pediatr. 2018;6:326. https://doi.org/10.3389/fped.2018.00326.

18. Abbas TO, Vallasciani S, Elawad A, Elifranji M, Leslie B, Elkadhi A, et al. Plate Objective Scoring Tool (POST); An objective methodology for the assessment of urethral plate in distal hypospadias. J Pediatr Urol. 2020;16:675–82. https://doi.org/10.1016/j.jpurol.2020.07.043.
19. Abbas TO. The Plate Objective Scoring Tool (POST): further reflections and extended applications. Res Reports Urol. 2021;13:783–91. https://doi.org/10.2147/RRU.S321188.
20. Abbas TO, Hatem M, Chandra P. Plate Objective Scoring Tool: a new preoperative indicator of penile curvature degree in children with distal hypospadias. Int J Urol. 2022; https://doi.org/10.1111/iju.14822.
21. Abbas TO, AbdelMoniem M, Khalil IA, Abrar Hossain MS, Chowdhury MEH. Deep learning based automated quantification of urethral plate characteristics using the plate objective scoring tool (POST). J Pediatr Urol. 2023; https://doi.org/10.1016/j.jpurol.2023.03.033.
22. Abbas T. Management of distal hypospadias: new insights and stepwise management algorithm. In: Abbas TO, editor. Hypospadiology. Singapore: Springer Nature Singapore; 2023. p. 67–80. https://doi.org/10.1007/978-981-19-7666-7_5.
23. Abbas T, Vallasciani S. Toward an ecosystem model of hypospadiology. In: Abbas TO, editor. Hypospadiology. Singapore: Springer Nature Singapore; 2023. p. 1–23. https://doi.org/10.1007/978-981-19-7666-7_1.
24. AbdulMoniem M, Abbas T, Khandakar A, Shuzan MNI, Chowdhury MH, Chowdhury MEH. Artificial intelligence in hypospadiology: role, applications, and benefits. In: Abbas TO, editor. Hypospadiology. Singapore: Springer Nature Singapore; 2023. p. 137–65. https://doi.org/10.1007/978-981-19-7666-7_10.
25. Abbas TO. An objective hypospadias classification system. J Pediatr Urol. 2022;18:481.e1–8. https://doi.org/10.1016/j.jpurol.2022.05.001.
26. Villanueva C, Abbas T. Penile curvature assessment in hypospadias. In: Abbas TO, editor. Hypospadiology. Singapore: Springer Nature Singapore; 2023. p. 93–102. https://doi.org/10.1007/978-981-19-7666-7_7.
27. Abbas TO, AbdelMoniem M, Chowdhury M. Automated quantification of penile curvature using artificial intelligence. Front Artif Intell 1AD;0:188. https://doi.org/10.3389/FRAI.2022.954497.
28. Baray SB, Abdelmoniem M, Mahmud S, Kabir S, Faisal MAA, Chowdhury MEH, et al. Automated measurement of penile curvature using deep learning-based novel quantification method. Front Pediatr. 2023;11:438. https://doi.org/10.3389/fped.2023.1149318.
29. Elifranji M, Abbas T, Vallasciani S, Leslie B, Elkadhi A, Pippi Salle JL. Upper lib graft (ULG) for Redo urethroplasties in children. A step by step video. J Pediatr Urol. 2020;0 https://doi.org/10.1016/j.jpurol.2020.06.029.
30. Abbas TO, Ali M. Urethral meatus and glanular closure line: normal biometrics and clinical significance. Urol J. 2018;15:277–9. https://doi.org/10.22037/uj.v0i0.4402.
31. Abbas TO, Pippi Salle JL. Dorsal Inlay TIP (DTIP). Hypospadias Surg. Cham: Springer International Publishing; 2022. p. 451–60. https://doi.org/10.1007/978-3-030-94248-9_27.
32. Alshafei A, Cascio S, Boland F, O'Shea N, Hickey A, Quinn F. Comparing the outcomes of tubularized incised plate urethroplasty and dorsal inlay graft urethroplasty in children with hypospadias: a systematic review and meta-analysis. J Pediatr Urol. 2020; https://doi.org/10.1016/j.jpurol.2020.01.009.
33. Spinoit A-F, Waterschoot M, Sinatti C, Abbas T, Callens N, Cools M, et al. Fertility and sexuality issues in congenital lifelong urology patients: male aspects. World J Urol. 2020; https://doi.org/10.1007/s00345-020-03121-2.
34. Gupta V, Yadav SK, Alanzi T, Amer I, Salah M, Ahmed M. Grafted tubularised incised-plate urethroplasty: an objective assessment of outcome with lessons learnt from surgical experience with 263 cases. Arab J Urol. 2016;14:299–304. https://doi.org/10.1016/j.aju.2016.09.002.

The Slit-Like Adjusted Mathieu (SLAM) Technique

7

Mohamed Fawzy and Ahmed T. Hadidi

Abstract

The Mathieu technique has withstood the test of time for almost 100 years with a study that reported a success rate of 100% in 204 consecutive patients. The major drawback of the original Mathieu technique is the final appearance of the glans (fist-mouth meatus that is not at the tip of the glans). The slit-like adjusted Mathieu technique (SLAM) avoids this drawback and results in a slit-like meatus at the tip of the glans. It is a reliable technique for correction of all distal and mid-penile hypospadias with persistent good results. The key modifications are: the design of a converging incision at the tip of the glans, V-excision from the tip of the meatal-based flap, and the technique of suturing. Multiple layer closure and careful attention to technical details contributed to 3% complication rate in primary distal hypospadias.

Keywords

Distal Hypospadias · Meatus · Urethral Plate · Urethroplasty · Flap · Chordee

Supplementary Information The online version contains supplementary material available at https://doi.org/10.1007/978-981-99-0795-3_7. The videos can be accessed individually by clicking the DOI link in the accompanying figure caption or by scanning this link with the SN More Media App.

M. Fawzy · A. T. Hadidi (✉)
Hypospadias Center, Sana Klinikum Offenbach, Offenbach am Main, Germany
e-mail: mohamed.fawzy@sana.de

T. O. Abbas (ed.), *Video Atlas of Hypospadias Surgery*,
https://doi.org/10.1007/978-981-99-0795-3_7

7.1 Introduction

Distal hypospadias is the commonest form of hypospadias (about 70%). Distal hypospadias may present in various forms as coronal, sub-coronal, mid penile, MIP, hypospadias with hypoplastic urethra. The majority of distal hypospadias have no chordee or superficial chordee that can be usually corrected by ventral degloving. However, the surgeon must be aware that some patients who may present with the meatus at the distal shaft may in fact have severe chordee that must be corrected before reconstructing new urethra and the penis should be classified as proximal hypospadias. Several techniques were described in the literature to repair distal hypospadias. It is advisable to learn at least the principles of the several techniques and apply the technique suitable for each patient. The SLAM technique described by Hadidi [1] is the main technique adopted for distal hypospadias in our center in Germany with the best outcome and suitable for most variants of distal hypospadias as well as complicated distal hypospadias especially after failed Tubularized Incised Plate (TIP). In this chapter, we will try to demonstrate the technique and the tips and tricks needed to get the best outcome using this technique.

7.1.1 Evolution of the Mathieu/Flip Flap/SLAM Technique

The classic Mathieu repair for distal hypospadias was first published in 1932 [2]. This renders Mathieu repair one of the oldest repairs described for distal hypospadias repair. Since then, several modifications have been described to improve the technique. The main drawbacks that made surgeons abandon Mathieu repair are fish-mouth meatus that is not at the tip, difficult glans closure around the neourethra, and high incidence of fistula. Most modifications done in this technique aimed at improving these three points. To obtain a slit-like meatus Barcat 1969 added a midline incision in the glans to bury the neourethra in the glans [3]. Others added hinging of the urethral plate to the technique [4, 5]. To achieve a meatus that is at the tip of the glans Hadidi described the Y-V glanuloplasty in 1996 [6], yet this modification failed to obtain a slit-like meatus. A slit-like meatus was first achieved in 2000 when Boddy and Samuel [7] first described the MAVIS technique (Mathieu and V incision sutured). During the past 25 years, there was gradual shift from the classic Mathieu technique to TIP technique promoted by Snodgrass since 1994 [8] because of the better cosmetic outcome of the meatus after TIP technique. The final modification done in Mathieu repair was described by Hadidi in 2012 as the SLAM technique [1], where three modifications were made to the original Mathieu repair and led to a dramatic improvement in the final cosmetic appearance, reduced complications and overcame the drawbacks of original Mathieu repair.

7.2 Indications

(A) All cases of distal hypospadias where the meatus lies distal to mid-shaft and mild to moderate degree of chordee <30 degrees that can be corrected without division of the urethral plate.
(B) Most complicated distal hypospadias where there is still enough skin to perform urethroplasty and close penile skin.
(C) MIP (Mega meatus with intact prepuce).

7.3 Steps of the Procedure

1. A U-shaped incision is outlined which differs from the classic Mathieu incision in that the distal ends of the U incision are converging and the widest point of the flap is at the meatal location Fig. 7.1.
2. The flap is elevated with the underlying fascia. This is important as this is the main blood supply to the flap.

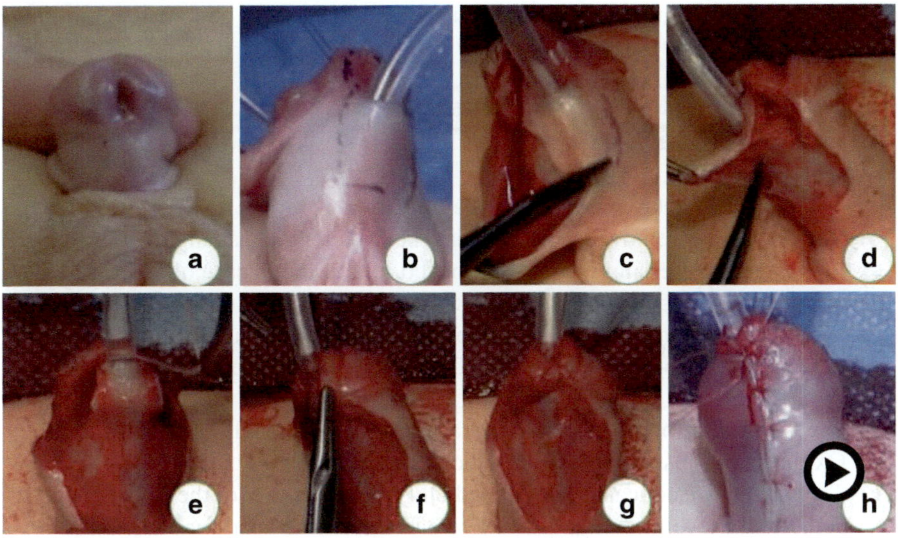

Fig. 7.1 Images illustrating the main intraoperative steps of the SLAM procedure for a coronal hypospadias (**a**). A U-shaped incision is indicated (**b**) where the distal limbs of the U incision are converging and the meatal location is where the flap is at its widest (**c**). The flap is raised along with the fascia beneath it (**d**). (**e**) Whenever feasible, the new urethra is reconstructed around a catheter of size F12 using three layers of sutures. A "V" is excised from the apex of the new urethra to create a meatus-like slit. (**f**) Both granular wings are sutured to a neo-urethra using interrupted mattress sutures (**g**). (**h**) Final look. SLAM procedure. (https://doi.org/10.1007/000-cn2)

3. The new urethra is reconstructed around a catheter size F12 whenever possible using three layers of sutures. Please notice that the urethra is not reconstructed to the very tip of the glans (leaving 3 mm from the incision).
4. A “V” is excised from the tip of the new urethra to achieve a slit-like meatus.
5. If the flap is thin or the fascia is underdeveloped, fashion a protective intermediate layer, using preputial fascia.
6. Both granular wings are sutured together around a neo-urethra using interrupted mattress sutures.
7. The technique can be successfully used when the meatus lies in the middle of the penis (so-called mid-penile hypospadias) by adopting the so-called “long lateral SLAM”, thus avoiding hair-bearing scrotal skin.

7.4 Postoperative Care

The catheter is left 1–2 days in most cases. In cases of mid-penile and recurrent hypospadias as well as cases of severe swelling postoperatively, it is preferred to leave the catheter for 7 days.

The wound surface is then covered with gentamicin ointment. An adhesive tape is used to compress the gauze, penis, and catheter against the abdomen to minimize the edema.

7.5 Postoperative Care

(a) The patient is freely mobile after the operation.
(b) The dressing is removed together with the catheter and usually there is no need to change the dressing unless it is soaked with urine in case of bladder spasms or suspected secondary hemorrhage.
(c) We advise the parents to use two diapers on top of each other for extra protection.
(d) A 2nd generation cephalosporin (Cefaclor) is continued postoperatively for 7–10 days.
(e) For pain-relief Ibuprofen and/or paracetamol are routinely used.
(f) Oxybutynin is used in cases of bladder spasms.
(g) The parents are educated that immediately upon removal of the dressing and the catheter the swelling might be severe and there is no need for panicking.
(h) The follow-up schedule is after 3 months, 1 year, 3 years, and 5 years to be continued till the child is 15 years old.
(i) During the follow-up visits the patients are examined for meatal shape and position, fistulas, and recurrent chordee. Patients and parents are questioned for micturition problems, if double streams are noticed, overall satisfaction, continence in older children, and sexual performance in sexually active older patients. Uroflowmetry is done in selected cases and postvoiding residual in cases with manifestations of obstruction.

7.6 Tips and Tricks

(A) SLAM technique is not feasible in patients with chordee >30 degrees where urethral bed needs to be divided in order to correct the curvature.
(B) The original meatus should be distal to mid-shaft to avoid including hair-baring skin of the scrotum in the flap, however in some cases of proximal hypospadias SLAM technique is still feasible. This can be achieved by extending the flap laterally (in an oblique manner) at the base of the penis (Long lateral SLAM). In this case care should be given to avoid rotation of the penis during closure.
(C) The presence of a hypoplastic urethra can be dealt with in two ways. Either incision of the hypoplastic urethral till normal urethra is reached, or designing a flap that can be flipped over the hypoplastic urethral without incising it. The latter is the preferred choice in our center as it saves time and reduces the urinary diversion time.
(D) If the hypospadias meatus is stenotic, it should be incised before designing the flap till it accommodates the 12 fr. Catheter to avoid future strictures proximal to the neourethra.
(E) The major advantage of SLAM technique is that the width of the urethral bed does not play a major role and can be as narrow as 3 mm. The narrow bed can be compensated for by preparing a wide skin flap.
(F) Proper mobilization of glandular wings to achieve larger wings is a key factor in the success of the SLAM technique, especially in cases with flat glans.
(G) The urethroplasty is performed over a 12 fr. Catheter. This ensures a wide neourethra and minimizes the risk of stenosis and stricture with healing.
(H) In some cases, with severe hypoplastic urethra and/or bifurcation of corpus spongiosum the flap is very thin. In this case an extra layer is used from preputial dartos fascia or proximal penile dartos fascia as an extra protective layer to enhance the blood supply of the flap.
(I) The starting point of urethroplasty is 3 mm proximal to the original meatus, so that the knot remains away from the neourethra, which minimizes the risk of infection and subsequent fistula formation.
(J) The urethroplasty is performed using a cutting needle as it makes it easier to go through the dermis of the flap as in skin incisions.

7.7 Results and Conclusion

Between 2005 and 2019 SLAM technique was performed on 2679 patients in our center. 2026 of them showed regularly in the follow-up. Satisfactory results were obtained in 1898 patients (95%). Recorded complications included 79 patients with fistula, 30 patients with meatal stenosis, and 19 patients with glandular dehiscence [9]. SLAM technique was also used in 161 patients with MIP where a second layer was obtained from ventral preputial fascia with good cosmetic results and surgical outcome compared to Pyramid technique [10]. SLAM technique can be also very useful in recurrent hypospadias and after failed TIP repair as it does not include a re-incision in the fibrotic urethral plate and the neourethra will be built using healthy penile skin.

References

1. Hadidi AT. The slit-like adjusted Mathieu technique for distal hypospadias. J Pediatr Surg. 2012;47(3):617–23. https://doi.org/10.1016/j.jpedsurg.2011.12.030. PMID: 22424366.
2. Mathieu P. Traitement en un temps de l'hypospade balanique et juxta-balanique. J Chir. 1932;39:481.
3. Barcat J. Symposium sur l'hypospadias. 16th meeting of the French Society of Children's Surgery. Ann Chir Infant. 1969;10:287.
4. Rich MA, Keating MA, Snyder HM, Duckett JW. Hinging the urethral plate in hypospadias meatoplasty. J Urol. 1989;142(6):1551–3. https://doi.org/10.1016/s0022-5347(17)39161-9. PMID: 2685370.
5. Aminsharifi A, Taddayun A, Assadolahpoor A, Khezri A. Combined use of Mathieu procedure with plate incision for hypospadias repair: a randomized clinical trial. Urology. 2008;72(2):305–8. https://doi.org/10.1016/j.urology.2008.02.034. Epub 2008 May 27. PMID: 18502484.
6. Hadidi AT. Y-V Glanuloplasty: a new modification in the surgery of hypospadias. Kasr El Aini Med J. 1996;2:223–33.
7. Boddy S, Samuel M. A natural glanular meatus after 'Mathieu and a V incision sutured': MAVIS. BJU Int. 2000;86(3):394–7. https://doi.org/10.1046/j.1464-410x.2000.00758.x. PMID: 10930947.
8. Snodgrass W. Tubularized, incised plate urethroplasty for distal hypospadias. J Urol. 1994;151(2):464–5. https://doi.org/10.1016/s0022-5347(17)34991-1. PMID: 8283561.
9. Hadidi AT. The Slit-Like Adjusted Mathieu (SLAM) Technique. In: Hadidi AT, editor. Hypospadias surgery. Cham: Springer; 2022. https://doi.org/10.1007/978-3-030-94248-9_22.
10. Duckett JW, Keating MA. Technical challenge of the megameatus intact prepuce hypospadias variant: the pyramid procedure. J Urol. 1989;141(6):1407–9. https://doi.org/10.1016/s0022-5347(17)41325-5. PMID: 2657110.

The Glanular-Frenular Collar (GFC) Technique

8

Hüseyin Özbey

Abstract

A clear understanding of the normal anatomy of the penis is essential for anatomical reconstruction of hypospadias. It is necessary to know that the male urethra is NOT a uniform tubular structure and the glanular urethra differs from the penile urethra in that it forms a fossa (navicularis) with a specific shape, with different boundaries, attachments, and elasticity. The fibrous ligamentous framework of the penis is the main component of this difference. Details of penile anatomy that have been completely overlooked in the history of hypospadias surgery include the "septum glandis", the tunica albuginea, the distal ligament, the navicular fossa, and the flow-dynamics of urine in the male urethra (Özbey and Kumbasar, Turk J Urol. 43:525–9, 2017; Henle, Anatomischer Hand-Atlas zum Gebrauch im Secirsaal (Band 6), 1877; Özbey, J Anat. 234:728–9, 2019; Özbey H, Arlı, Med Hypotheses. 140:109642, 2020). I believe that the surgical process for hypospadias should guide two distinct concepts of surgical repair reserved for the glanular and penile urethra. The Glanular-Frenular Collar (GFC) technique simulates the embryological development of

This chapter specifically addresses a new concept for reconstruction of the glanular urethra. Issues related to the etiology and elimination of the ventral curve are not discussed.

Supplementary Information The online version contains supplementary material available at https://doi.org/10.1007/978-981-99-0795-3_8. The videos can be accessed individually by clicking the DOI link in the accompanying figure caption or by scanning this link with the SN More Media App.

H. Özbey (✉)
Department of Pediatric Surgery, Division of Pediatric Urology and Andrology, I.M. Sechenov First Moscow State Medical University, Moscow, Russia

Yücetarla Cad, Tunaboylu Sok, Bakırköy, İstanbul, Turkey

T. O. Abbas (ed.), *Video Atlas of Hypospadias Surgery*,
https://doi.org/10.1007/978-981-99-0795-3_8

the urethra and aims to provide the structural and functional anatomical features of the glanular and penile urethra in hypospadias (Özbey and Etker, J Pediatr Urol. 13:34e1–6, 2017; Özbey H, J Pediatr Urol 20:539–40, 2024).

Keywords

Penis · Anatomy · Hypospadias · Septum glandis · Tunica albuginea · Fossa navicularis · Distal ligament · Urine flow dynamics

8.1 Introduction

The "septum glandis" is a fine fibrous tissue surrounding and holding the glanular urethra (fossa navicularis) in the midline with its upper and lower median septum. Although this information was first published in 1877 by Dr Jacob Henle, we had to uncover the same information after 140 years, using magnetic resonance imaging (MRI) [1–6]. According to our findings in both clinical and MRI studies: (1) the corpus spongiosum gradually ends where it meets the fossa navicularis, and after this level extensions of its tunica albuginea (septum glandis) cover the fossa navicularis, (2) the glans penis is NOT the expanded end of the corpus spongiosum, (3) the ventral surface of the glans is also NOT the extension of the "urethral plate" as in the penile urethra, which is surrounded by the corpus spongiosum, (4) the glans doesn't circumferentially cover the glanular urethra and the wings of the glans are separated by this fine fibrous-connective tissue (septum glandis), (5) the septum glandis together with its epithelial extension, the frenulum, forms the ventral wall of the glanular and subcoronal urethra, and (6) the extensions of the tunica albuginea of the corpora cavernosa form the distal (corpora-glans) ligament [1, 2, 7]. The distal ligament provides a strong connection to the corpora cavernosa, which contributes to the flexibility and rigidity of the glans penis and to bear the buckling pressure created during sexual intercourse [8]. The lower median septum is also the ventral connection of the glans to the corpus spongiosum (ventral shaft of the penis) and contributes to the glans stability.

By analyzing the dynamics of urine flow in the male urethra, we showed that the wider caliber of the navicular fossa than the penile urethra should provide an increase in pressure and a decrease in the velocity of the urine flow. The wave-like shape of the urine is the result of the navicular form of the glanular urethra with its vertical, elliptical opening covered by the fibroelastic septum glandis. We considered the FN and SG as "flow control chamber" to control the flow of the urine exiting the urethra [4]. This information, which forms the basis of the GFC technique, was also first introduced to hypospadias surgery by the author of this chapter.

8.2 Indications

The GFC technique can be used in all forms of hypospadias, either to create a glanular urethra alone or to create the penile and glanular urethra together. It can also be used in failed hypospadias repairs when there is a limited amount of foreskin available as the GFC technique involves two distinct approaches to urethral reconstruction. The GFC technique doesn't involve glans dissection and aims to keep glans tissue intact. The subepithelial glans approximation in the original GFC technique has been replaced with an internal approximation suture. As in normal anatomy, the formation of a loose connective tissue (septum and frenulum) between the wings of the glans provides space for the re-formation of the fossa navicularis and the elasticity required for its functional anatomy [5].

8.3 Steps of the Procedure (Fig. 8.1)

- The GFC technique starts with the separation of the outer and inner prepuce and degloving of the penis as previously described [9] (Fig. 8.1). The separation of the outer and inner prepuce enables the penis to be anatomically degloved according to its fibrous layers (dartos, Buck's fascia, and the tunica albuginea).
- The inner prepuce is modeled retaining its surfaces around the ventral glans for use in forming the septum and frenulum. In this way, the boundaries of the future glanular urethra, which will form the navicular fossa, are determined.
- A holding suture is placed to the inner preputial collar approximately 10–15 mm from the glans. This suture is pulled over the glans to expose the inner surface of the collar. The edges of the collar and its subepidermal layers are sutured midline (7/0 polydioxanone) to form a dense mesenchymal tissue (septum glandis) and frenulum (Glanular-Frenular Collar; GFC) (Fig. 8.2). The collar is pulled down and sutured to the penile foreskin, either with or without preserving the remainder of the foreskin

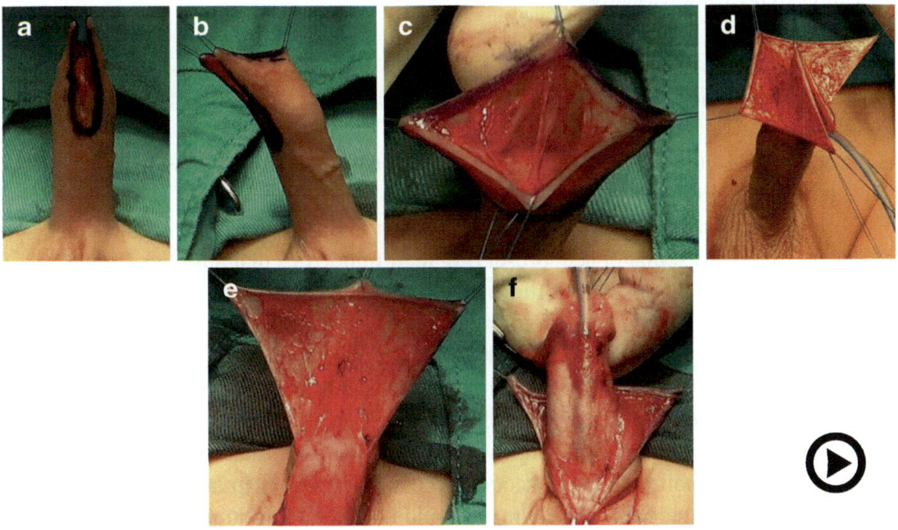

Fig. 8.1 Separation of the outer and inner foreskin and degloving of the penis for the GFC technique. GFC procedure. (https://doi.org/10.1007/000-cn3)

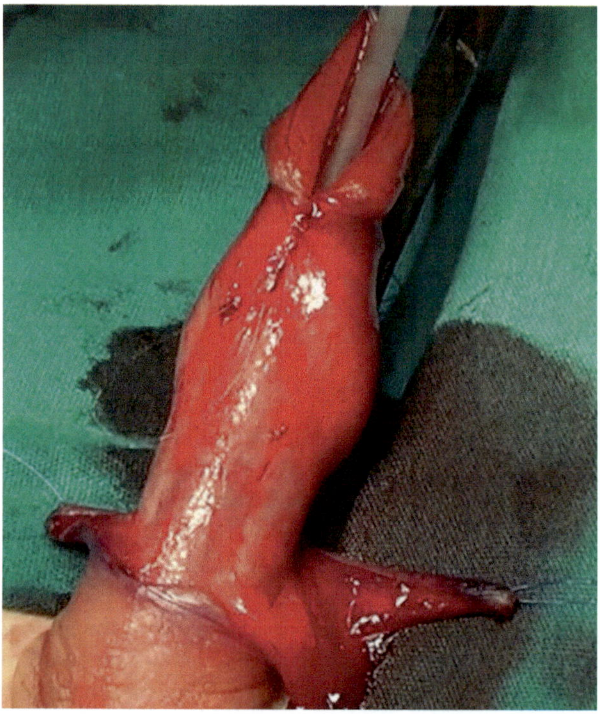

Fig. 8.2 The main maneuver of the GFC technique is to pull the collar (inner foreskin) over the glans to expose its inner surface and work from its inner side

- The glans wings are approximated with a (5/0 polyglactin) suture from the inside of the collar (internal approximation), without glans incision. The collar is pulled down and sutured to the penile foreskin, either with or without preserving the remainder of the foreskin

8.4 Tips and Tricks

- Proper placement of the holding sutures is critical to proper dissection for foreskin modeling (Fig. 8.1a, b).
- Following the natural border between the outer and inner foreskin allows entry into the relatively avascular space, preserving their major vascular supplies (Fig. 8.1c–f).
- If the relaxation incision to the urethral plate is necessary, it should NOT be extended to the anterior glans surface [11].
- The most important maneuver of the GFC technique is to pull the collar over the glans to expose its inner surface and to reconstruct the ventral wall (septum and frenulum) of the glanular urethra (Fig. 8.2).
- Internal approximation of the glans wings is another important maneuver of the GFC technique, eliminating glans dissection. The internal approximation suture should be placed exactly where the glans wings should have their maximum apposition.

Video – Hypospadias Repair with the Glanular-Frenular Collar (GFC) Technique

8.5 Results and Conclusion

The male urethra is NOT a uniform tubular structure. The ventral wall of the glanular urethra is formed by the median primordial fascial tissues that form a septum (glandis), and the frenulum. Glanular urethra is not covered by the corpus spongiosum and the glans is NOT an anterior expansion of the corpus spongiosum. A midline incision of the glans should be avoided as this type of incision can cause iatrogenic damage to the distal ligament and may be the cause of erectile dysfunction [10, 11]. It is clear that formation of a normal glanular urethra, with its fossa navicularis, "septum glandis" and frenulum are important indicators of an anatomically functional and aesthetically normal looking hypospadias reconstruction [12–14] (Fig. 8.3).

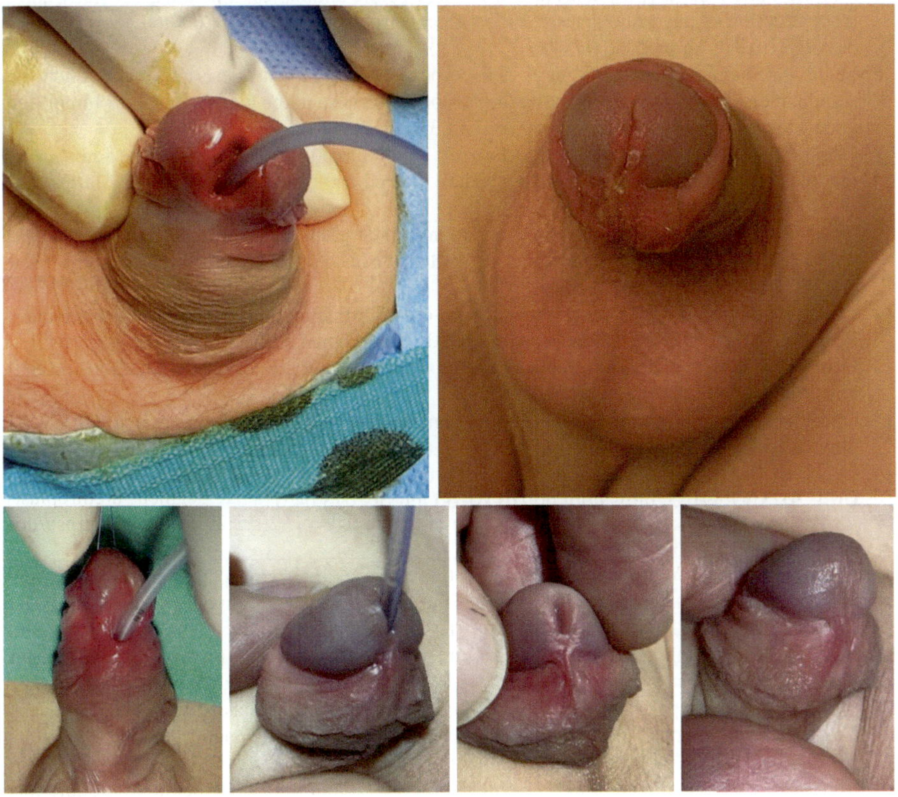

Fig. 8.3 Pre- and postoperative views of two patients operated with the GFC technique

References

1. Özbey H, Kumbasar A. Glans wings are separated ventrally by the septum glandis and frenulum penis: MRI documentation and surgical implications. Turk J Urol. 2017;43:525–9. https://doi.org/10.5152/tud.2017.00334.
2. Henle J. Anatomischer Hand-Atlas zum Gebrauch im Secirsaal (Band 6). Eingeweide. Braunschweig: Available via University Library Heidelberg; 1877. Available from: http://digi.ub.uni-heidelberg.de/diglit/henle1877bd6/0093
3. Özbey H. The mystery of Jacob Henle's 'septum glandis'. J Anat. 2019;234:728–9. https://doi.org/10.1111/joa.12965.
4. Özbey H, Arlı OT. "Fossa navicularis" and "septum glandis": a flow control valve for the male urethra? Med Hypotheses. 2020;140:109642. https://doi.org/10.1016/j.mehy.2020.109642.
5. Özbey H, Etker S. Hypospadias repair with the glanular-frenular collar (GFC) technique. J Pediatr Urol. 2017;13:34e1–6. https://doi.org/10.1016/j.jpurol.2016.09.016.
6. Özbey H, Devecioğlu D, Staroverov O. A closer look at iatrogenic hypospadias. Andrologia. 2021;53:e13803. https://doi.org/10.1111/and.13803.
7. Van der Putte SCJ. Hypospadias and associated penile anomalies: a histological study and a reconstruction of the pathogenesis. J Plast Reconstruct Aesthet Surg. 2007;60:48–60. https://doi.org/10.1016/j.bjps.2006.05.020.
8. Shafik A, Shafik AA, Asaad S, et al. The corporo-glans ligament: description and functional significance of a ligament connecting the corpora cavernosa to the glans penis. Int J Impot Res. 2004;16:220–3. https://doi.org/10.1038/sj.ijir.3901057.
9. Özbey H, Ayryan E, Staroverov O, Morozov DA. Anatomical modeling of the foreskin for the reconstruction of glanular hypospadias. J Pediatr Urol. 2021;17:335–7. https://doi.org/10.1016/j.jpurol.2021.03.023.
10. Husmann DA. Erectile dysfunction in patients undergoing multiple attempts at hypospadias repair:Etiologies and concerns. J Pediatr Urol. 2021;17:166e1–166.e7. https://doi.org/10.1016/j.jpurol.2020.12.002.
11. Özbey H, Morozov D. Hypospadias surgery, erectile dysfunction and the distal ligament. J Pediatr Urol. 2021;17:592–3. https://doi.org/10.1016/j.jpurol.2021.06.003.
12. Özbey H. The facts and misconceptions in hypospadias surgery. J Pediatr Urol. 2020;16:408–9. https://doi.org/10.1016/j.jpurol.2020.02.022.
13. Özbey H. The facts and misconceptions in glans penis anatomy. Differentiation. 2020;113:27. https://doi.org/10.1016/j.diff.2020.03.005.
14. Özbey H. Further misconceptions in glans penis anatomy and hypospadias surgery. J Pediatr Urol. 2023;19:391–3. https://doi.org/10.1016/j.jpurol.2023.04.035.

Glandular Urethral Disassembly (GUD) Technique

9

Antonio Macedo Júnior and Emanuelle Lima Macedo

Abstract

Glandular Urethral Disassembly (GUD) technique has been previously described and consists of a combination of two well-established maneuvers: minimal urethral mobilization and glandular disassembly from the corpora cavernosa as performed in the treatment of epispadias (Macedo et al. J Pediatr Urol. 16(3):401–3, 2020; Macedo et al. Int Braz J Urol. 46(6):1072–4, 2020; Macedo et al. J Pediatr Urol. 17(5):690.e1–6, 2020). It has the advantage of being versatile enough to treat primary and redo distal hypospadias. We acknowledge that this technique should be limited for coronal and subcoronal subtypes, with the urethral meatus no longer than 1 cm from the coronal area.

Keywords

Hypospadias · Distal hypospadias · Glanular urethral disassembly · GUD

Supplementary Information The online version contains supplementary material available at https://doi.org/10.1007/978-981-99-0795-3_9. The videos can be accessed individually by clicking the DOI link in the accompanying figure caption or by scanning this link with the SN More Media App.

A. M. Júnior
NUPEP/CACAU Pediatric Urology Department, Federal University of São Paulo, São Paulo, SP, Brazil

E. L. Macedo (✉)
Albert Einstein Medical School, São Paulo, Brazil

T. O. Abbas (ed.), *Video Atlas of Hypospadias Surgery*,
https://doi.org/10.1007/978-981-99-0795-3_9

9.1 Introduction

Distal hypospadias represent the most frequent presentation of hypospadias. The TIP repair is regarded as the preferred procedure by most pediatric urologists but the efficacy of this technique has been increasingly questioned. We propose the **GUD technique (glandular urethral disassembly)**, an aggressive partial glandar disassembly in association with minor urethral mobilization to treat distal hypospadias forms [1]. The combination of these two steps avoids the need for urethroplasty and suture lines, minimizing the risk for fistulas. The aggressive glans mobilization and disconnection from the corpora offer great mobility and capability of refurbishing it [2]. We also noticed that reconfiguration of glans enabled at the end a much more conical aspect. The merit of the procedure is the combination of minor mobilization of the urethra with down adjustment and rotation of the glans medially.

9.2 Indications

Primary and redo distal hypospadias forms: coronal and subcoronal.

9.3 Steps of the Procedure

- The technique consists of subcoronal circumcision to expose distal dysplastic urethra. In order to avoid damage to distal urethra that frequently is thin and membranous, the U-shaped incision is conducted below to the hypospadiac meatus where the skin is robust enough.
- After the penile shaft is degloved we can observe a bridge of skin bound to the thin distal urethra, similar to a flip-flap or a Mathieu flap. This minor skin flap is used only to traction the urethra during the distal mobilization from the corpora and is discarded at the end of the procedure (Fig. 9.1a–c). This procedure, differently from the classic Koff technique, requires minor urethral mobilization that we believe will avoid urethral retraction and compromise of blood supply.
- Laterally to distal spongious tissue at the Y urethra, we incise the Buck's fascia and superficial tunica albuginea on both sides releasing the urethra from the corpora and giving mobility to two flaps of spongiosum tissue that can be joined in midline to reinforce the urethra. We follow the lateral plane of dissection to the urethra cranially on both sides and converge above the meatus to outline an inverted Y-shaped incision.
- The glans is then entirely opened in the midline (Fig. 9.1d). The glans disassembled from the corpora and opened in the midline shows in this moment two glandular wings that will embrace the mobilized urethra subsequently and can be rotated downwards (Fig. 9.1e, f).
- The urethra normally can be easily lifted cranially and repositioned distally to the tip of the glans (Fig. 9.1g) with three posterior anchor stay sutures with PDS 5.0 at 11, 12, and 1 o'clock. We remove at this moment the skin bridge at ventral

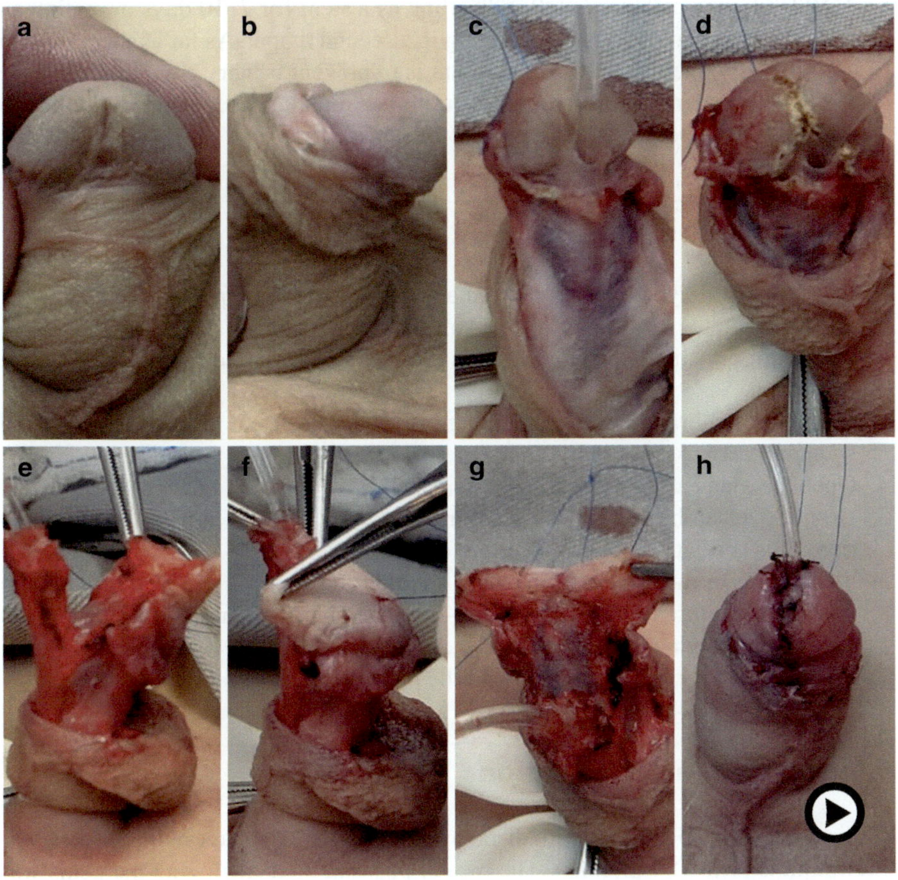

Fig. 9.1 The GUD technique in detail, (**a**) Coronal hypospadia, (**b**) Mild ventral curvature, (**c**) Penile skin degloved, exposing Y-shape spongious defect, notice that a mini "Mathieu-like" flap was designed to manipulate the urethra, (**d**) Inverted Y-shape glans incision to open it widely in the midline, (**e**) Urethra was disassembled from the glans and mobilized not more than 2 cm, (**f**) Urethra is lifted upwards and glans rotated downwards, (**g**) Notice the aggressive disassembly of the glans from the corpora and division of it in the midline, (**h**) End aspect, nice conical shape glans format. GUD procedure. (https://doi.org/10.1007/000-cn4)

distal urethra used solely to handle the urethra and avoid touching the urethra with forceps.

- The neomeatus is completed with interrupted PDS 6.0, and the glans is reconstructed embracing the urethra with three subcutaneous PDS 5.0 sutures (Fig. 9.1h).
- The redundant ventral foreskin is discarded, there is no need to create a barrier layer of dartos flap interposing the mobilized urethra to the glans. We use a tourniquet for glanular dissection and hemostasis control. After glans reconstruction, its new conical conformation is clear and the urethra is centrally displaced.

- A 10 F silicone catheter is left indwelling as a stent for 7–10 days providing an incontinent urinary diversion dropping in a second diaper. As far as there is not a urethroplasty, the reason to keep a stent is to prevent urinary complaints in case of glandular edema compressing the urethra. A bioclusive dressing is applied to the shaft of the penis concluding the procedure.

9.4 Tips and Tricks

1. Only for distal hypospadias, coronal and subcoronal, both primary or redos.
2. Do not touch the urethra, provide a "mini Mathieu flap" of skin below the native meatus just to hold the urethra, this skin flap is discarded at the end of the procedure.
3. Incise the urethra lateral to the spongiosum Y-type defect to rotate and make a spongioplasty.
4. Open the glans as a book (inverted Y-incision).
5. Do not over-mobilize the urethra to avoid retraction, only two cm of mobilization. This is related to case selection (distal forms).
6. The sutures of the urethra to the glans should run from 0–4 and from 8–12 h. Do not fix the urethra to the glans from 5–7 h to avoid down migration of meatus in case of partial glans dehiscence.
7. Leave a stent for 7–10 days to avoid the patient's discomfort.

9.5 Results and Conclusion

We have treated 205 patients with distal hypospadias. Median age at the surgery was 22.4 months (1 to 184 months). The meatal position after degloving the penis was coronal at 149 cases, subcoronal at 54 and 2 patients presented with megameatus and intact foreskin. The penile curvature evaluated by penoscrotal digital compression showed that 153 patients had no curvature, 35 had it but less than 30°, 4 had curvature between 30–45°, and 3 had more than 45°. Curvature resolved completely in all cases by degloving the penis and detaching paraurethral chordee [3].

Three patients had mild penoscrotal transposition in addition to hypospadias. Twenty-eight patients were treated as a secondary repair, mainly to fix coronal fístulas. These patients were treated according to the same principle for primary cases.

We found complications in seven patients (3.4%) consisting of six fistulas (3%) and three glans dehiscence (1.8%). Two patients had both complications. Follow-up was 27 months (1 to 58 months) and the median follow-up time was 26 months.

Mitchell & Blagi and Perovic et al. reported on complete penile disassembly for epispadia repair as a way to complete release of the rotation of the penis and treat dorsal chordee bringing the urethra to a more functional location [4]. We were inspired by this procedure when we started proposing extensive partial glandar disassembly in association with urethral mobilization. The rationale for this procedure is to avoid sutures and a formal urethroplasty, except sutures at the urethra meatus to reposition the urethra distally without tension. The partial glandar disassembly procedure can also be regarded as a way to create a more conical and cosmetical glans. We agree that the procedure is much more aggressive in the glans but once the incision follows the lateral Buck's fascia incision, no major bleeding occurs, having a tourniquet applied.

We acknowledge that this procedure is intended only to distal hypospadias (coronal and subcoronal). We stress that the GUD procedure can be performed irrespectively of any urethral plate "quality" as it does not require a minimum glans width as the TIP repair. Moreover, there is no room for preoperative testosterone treatment. The absence of suture and urethroplasty avoids practically the risk of the feared coronal fistula after surgery.

References

1. Macedo A Jr, Ottoni SL, Leal da Cruz M. The GUD technique: glandular urethral disassembly for distal hypospadias repair. J Pediatr Urol. 2020;16(3):401–3.
2. Macedo A Jr, Ottoni SL, Garrone G, Liguori R, Mattos RM, da Cruz ML. The GUD technique: glandar urethral disassembly. An alternative for distal hypospadias repair. Int Braz J Urol. 2020;46(6):1072–4.
3. Macedo A Jr, Ottoni SL, Di Migueli RDD, de Mattos RM, Garrone G, Leal da Cruz M. A different approach to distal hypospadias repair: the GUD (glandular urethral disassembly) technique. J Pediatr Urol. 2021;17(5):690.e1–6.
4. Mitchell ME, Bägli DJ. Complete penile disassembly for epispadias repair: the Mitchell technique. J Urol. 1996;155(1):300–4. PMID: 7490875.

Urethral Mobilization Procedure

10

William Fox and Patrick H. McKenna

Abstract

Urethral mobilization has been reported previously in the literature, however the modifications suggested by McKenna are distinct. This technique removes the risk of common postoperative complications such as urethral fistula since there is no suture line. The development of wide glanular flaps with a flair provides an excellent meatal cosmetic result while decreasing the risk of meatal stenosis. During the procedure the urethra is mobilized from the bottom up rather than the top down. This preserves the blood supply by leaving the spongiosal tissue intact. This procedure, although technically more difficult than a standard hypospadias repair, provides an option for repair of distal hypospadias, redo hypospadias, and can be utilized in all cases including proximal hypospadias to decrease the length of vascularized flaps. This procedure is particularly helpful in patients with stenotic TIP procedures who lack excess preputial skin. In redo procedures it usually results in only one operation as opposed to multiple.

Supplementary Information The online version contains supplementary material available at https://doi.org/10.1007/978-981-99-0795-3_10. The videos can be accessed individually by clicking the DOI link in the accompanying figure caption or by scanning this link with the SN More Media App.

W. Fox (✉)
University of Illinois College of Medicine Rockford, Rockford, IL, USA
e-mail: wfox3@uic.edu

P. H. McKenna (✉)
GU Reconstructive Center Mercyhealth, Rockford, IL, USA

Surgery, University of Illinois College of Medicine Rockford, Rockford, IL, USA

T. O. Abbas (ed.), *Video Atlas of Hypospadias Surgery*,
https://doi.org/10.1007/978-981-99-0795-3_10

Keywords

Hypospadias repair · Urethral mobilization · Chordee · Glans flaps · Cosmesis

10.1 Introduction

A successful hypospadias repair must address all associated abnormalities while also correcting the primary defect. The elasticity and proximal blood supply of the urethra allows for safe mobilization of the tissue. Distal urethral mobilization was first introduced by Beck, and this has been duplicated by Koff, Atala, Macedo [1–4]. McKenna et. al was the first to extend the use of this technique to patients with severe chordee, redo hypospadias, and more proximal hypospadias cases [5]. These advancements in urethral mobilization results in excellent cosmesis and low complication rate when compared to previous techniques. Urethral mobilization allows for curvature correction by releasing the attachment between the corporal bodies and spongiosum while also moving the meatus distally. The changes suggested by McKenna in mobilization for the first time allow this procedure to be utilized in more severe forms of hypospadias and is different from any of the other reported distal mobilization techniques. It should not be included in the discussion of other urethral mobilization techniques for it is a new procedure.

Urethral mobilization was first reported by C. Beck in 1898, however it is unclear if it was a true urethral mobilization [1]. Beck only performed the procedure on two patients, and one patient was not entirely successful due to the proximal location of the meatus. Koff et. al presented their findings in hypospadias repair, however this was for only distal repairs [2]. In addition, the urethra was mobilized from the top-down, and there was a 10% meatal stenosis rate. Koff later presented a modified Barcat technique, however this technique utilized flaps and there was a suture line after the operation [6]. Atala et. al reported their technique as well, however they used dorsal plication in cases and there were instances of meatal retraction [3]. Macedo et. al recently presented the GUD technique, and this is a modification of a distal hypospadias repair technique [4]. The commonality of each of these approaches is that they apply to distal, rather than more proximal defects or redo procedures. All approaches work from the top down and are only successful in distal cases. All are quite different from the technique presented here in this chapter.

Our operation is especially well-suited for patients with prior operations and little excess preputial skin avoiding the need for preputial skin or mucosal graft. Native urethra is the ideal tissue for hypospadias repair since it represents the normal urethral tissue. Since there are no suture lines, urethral mobilization removes the risk of urethral fistula. When utilizing the technique described in the chapter video, meatal stenosis is zero. Most mid-to-distal hypospadias cases are amenable to this procedure. This technique is particularly useful redoing failed distal repairs, with the most common being stenotic TIP procedures. The entire previous repair and scar can be excised and replaced by native urethra. In addition, urethral mobilization in penoscrotal and perineal repairs significantly shortens the length of the required vascularized preputial skin flaps needed for the repair. Urethral mobilization is technically more difficult than other techniques.

10.2 Indications

This procedure has broad indications:

1. It is clearly indicated in patients with distal hypospadias
2. Patients with distal hypospadias with moderate to severe chordee
3. Patients with atretic urethras and significant chordee up to the midshaft
4. Redo hypospadias procedures
5. Patients with deficient preputial skin with/without chordee
6. Particularly helpful in patients with stenotic TIP procedure
7. In all forms of hypospadias that are more severe, urethral mobilization can be used to move the meatus from the perineum or penoscrotal area to the midshaft. This allows the surgeon to utilize a much smaller graft or flap than if the urethra had not been mobilized

10.3 Steps of the Procedure

1. 8Fr pediatric feeding tube is passed into the urethra to evaluate tissue quality. Tractional sutures are placed bilaterally at the lateral corners of the dorsal hood. Preplanned "Firlit" flaps are marked for later frenulum repair at closure.
2. Circumferential incision is made to create preputial skin flaps. Dissection is carried down to the avascular plain dorsal and continued ventral until the penis is fully degloved.
3. Curvature correction is begun by excising any dysplastic scar tissue from the ventral side of the penis. Chordee is then assessed via visual inspection, palpation, and artificial erection. If there is persistent chordee or the meatus must be moved distally, proceed with the urethral mobilization.
4. The plane between the spongiosum and corporeal bodies is carefully developed in the midshaft, where the spongiosum is normal, to mobilize the urethra. A vessel loop is used for gentle traction on the spongiosum (Fig. 10.1). It is key to start in the middle of the urethra and not distally as others have done in the past. The plane is developed proximally and carried distally as needed to gain the required urethral length. If chordee is still present, the corporal bodies can be separated in the midline and rolled out. If persistent chordee persists after the ventral dissection and corpora incision, fairy cuts can be made on the corporal bodies. Fairy cuts are rarely required. Once the chordee is proven to be corrected by artificial erection, the urethral mobilization can be completed to give adequate length to reach the distal glans. Plication techniques are rarely if ever used.
5. Wide glans flaps are developed with a small flare dorsally to allow greater mobility at closure. The urethra is advanced to the tip and fixed with 5-0 vicryl. A single 4-0 polydioxanone suture is placed to advance and anchor the urethra to the corporal bodies in the distal shaft to advance and fix the urethra and minimize tension at the meatus. The meatus is anchored with 5-0 vicryl suture. Excise the glanular tissue and incise the corporal bodies at the tip to make a space for the urethra to fit into the glans (Fig. 10.2). This decreases the risk of urethral

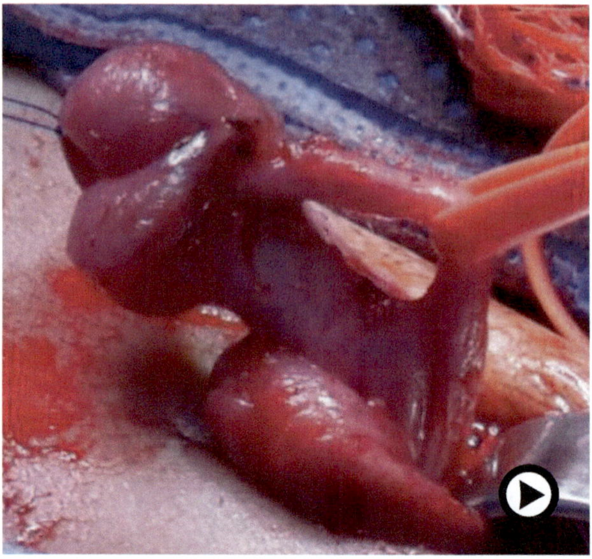

Fig. 10.1 The urethra has been mobilized from the bottom up, and a vessel loop has been placed around the urethra. Urethral mobilization procedure. (https://doi.org/10.1007/000-cn5)

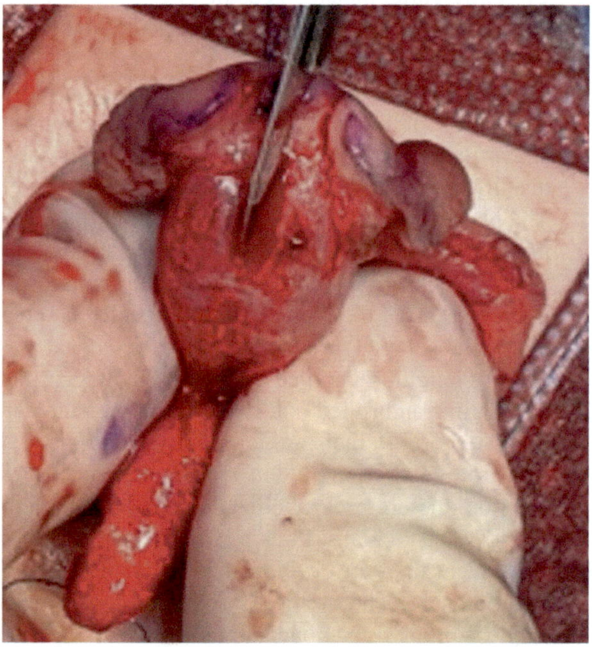

Fig. 10.2 The incision of the corporal bodies to make a space for the urethra

stenosis. The glans is closed over the urethra tension-free with a combination of a subcuticular 4-0 polydioxanone and 6-0 vicryl suture. The meatus is matured circumferentially with the 6-0 vicryl suture.

6. If the meatus cannot be moved to a normal anatomic location by urethral mobilization alone, you can employ a combination of glans flaps laid into the urethra dorsally.
7. The preplanned preputial skin flaps are rotated ventrally. The skin is then closed with a combination of 6-0 vicryl and 4-0 chromic suture.

10.4 Postoperative Care

The patient receives ancef on the day of surgery. Then switched to keflex for 7 days as an outpatient. We use an 8 Fr silastic tube, which stays in for 6 days. But if it comes out early, no tube is replaced. We use a mepilex silver-impregnated dressing to dress the operative site which stays on for 24 hours. Bacitracin is used on the tip of the penis until the dressing comes off. We encourage the family to avoid significant physical activity such as toys patients will straddle. We use a double diaper technique while the stent is in place. Once the stent is out on post op day 6, we utilize sitz baths 3×/day for 5 days with 1 oz betadine solution. We follow up at 2 weeks, 3 months after the 2 weeks, then 6 months after that visit, and check a post-void residual with a bladder scan. Patients are discharged at that point. They are told to contact us if they have dysuria, difficulty voiding, or UTI. We have had no known late complications with follow-up in some patients as long as 20 years.

10.5 Tips and Tricks

- Avoid the use of a tourniquet
- Avoid the use of grafts
- Ensure the surgical team is educated about what is needed for a good outcome
- Correct chordee without dorsal plication
- Generous frenula collar
- Mobilization of the urethra from the bottom up
- Wide glans flaps with relaxing lateral flair
- Advance and fix the urethra so there is no tension on the meatus
- Remove tissue and separate corporal bodies to make hole for glanular urethra which is combined with wide midline glans flap
- Modification to meatal reconstruction

10.6 Results and Conclusion

When done correctly, this procedure allows for excellent results and low complications. The results of this technique were previously presented in McKenna et. al, and it showed a singular case of fistula formation (1.2%), however this patient presented with a bleeding disorder and hematoma [3]. There were zero cases of post-operative meatal stenosis and all patients emptied their bladder effectively [3]. This technique is distinct from previous publications discussed in this book chapter. Our technique extends the use of urethral mobilization to much more severe forms of hypospadias including redo procedures, proximal hypospadias, and cases with severe chordee. It is important to ensure that when mobilizing the urethra, start from the bottom up. If the surgeon starts from the top they end up dissecting into the wrong surgical plane, and the vascular supply of the urethra is compromised. Additionally, the urethra must be advanced and fixed to the corporal bodies to avoid meatal tension upon closure.

References

1. Beck C. A new operation for balanic hypospadias. New York Med J. 1898;67:147.
2. Koff SA. Mobilization of the Urethra in the Surgical Treatment of Hypospadias. J Urol. 1981;125(3):394–7. https://doi.org/10.1016/S0022-5347(17)55048-X.
3. Atala A. Urethral mobilization and advancement for midshaft to distal hypospadias. J Urol. 2002;168(4 Pt 2):1738–41; discussion 1741. https://doi.org/10.1097/01.ju.0000023971.96439.b8. PMID: 12352348.
4. Macedo A Jr, Ottoni SL, Garrone G, Liguori R, Mattos RM, da Cruz ML. The GUD technique: glandar urethral disassembly. An alternative for distal hypospadias repair. Int Braz J Urol. 2020;46(6):1072–4. https://doi.org/10.1590/S1677-5538.IBJU.2018.0835. PMID: 32167733; PMCID: PMC7527101.
5. Koenig JF, Kottwitz M, McKenna PH. Urethral mobilization for distal and mid shaft hypospadias with chordee. J Urol. 2013;190(4 Suppl):1545–8. https://doi.org/10.1016/j.juro.2013.02.038. Epub 2013 Feb 20. PMID: 23454409.
6. Koff SA, Brinkman J, Ulrich J, Deighton D. Extensive mobilization of the urethral plate and urethra for repair of hypospadias: the modified Barcat technique. J Urol. 1994;151:466–9.

Part III

Procedures for the Repair of Proximal Hypospadias

Staged Preputial Graft (SPG) Repair

11

Tariq O. Abbas and J. L. Pippi Salle

Abstract

Proximal hypospadias remains difficult to treat. This chapter's purpose is to illustrate staged preputial graft (SPG) repair. In cases of proximal hypospadias in which the spongiosa bifurcation is below the pubic bone or the penile curvature is greater than 45 degrees, an SPG may be utilized.

Keywords

Proximal hypospadias · Corporotomy · Curvature · Preputial graft · Staged repair

11.1 Introduction

Proximal hypospadias accounts for around 20% of all primary cases, and its management remains difficult [1–3]. The urethral plate is frequently hypoplastic, narrow, fibrotic, and short, which contributes to the severity of the penile curvature [4]. Yet, there has been no agreement on the best management plan for proximal hypospadias [5, 6], in part due to disagreement in characterizing its severity [7, 8]. The debate over single-stage correction versus phased surgery for proximal hypospadias has raged on for the past two decades, with credit shifting back and forth.

Supplementary Information The online version contains supplementary material available at https://doi.org/10.1007/978-981-99-0795-3_11. The videos can be accessed individually by clicking the DOI link in the accompanying figure caption or by scanning this link with the SN More Media App.

T. O. Abbas (✉) · J. L. P. Salle
Pediatric Urology Section, Sidra Medicine, Doha, Qatar
e-mail: tabbas@sidra.org

T. O. Abbas (ed.), *Video Atlas of Hypospadias Surgery*,
https://doi.org/10.1007/978-981-99-0795-3_11

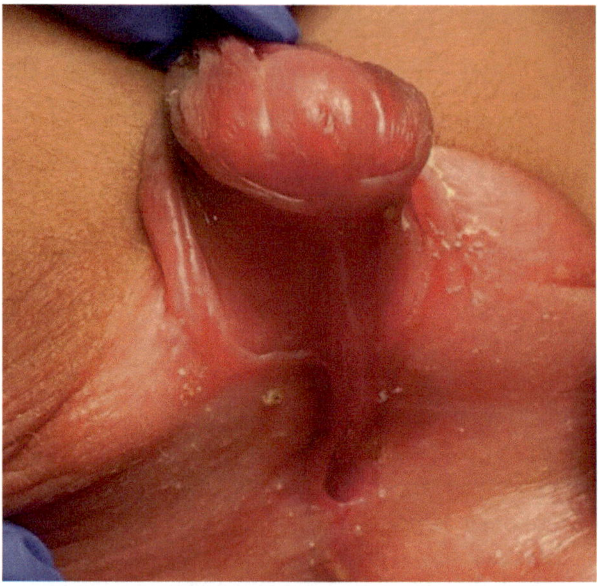

Fig. 11.1 Proximal hypospadias where the meatus is scrotal and spongiosa bifurcation is below the pubic bone

11.2 Indications

1. Staged preputial graft can be employed in proximal hypospadias cases where the spongiosa bifurcation is proximal to penoscrotal junction based on meatal position classification (hypospadias severity Grade 3 in Abbas 2022 classification) [7] Fig. 11.1 *or*
2. The penile curvature is >45 degrees.

11.3 Video Demonstration

Factors	Findings
Age at surgery (months)	13
Gestational age (weeks)	36
Birth weight (g)	1850
Gestational risks (e.g., maternal co-morbidities, IVF, Twin)	Invitro fertilization (IVF)
Family history	None
Testosterone (if yes, reason, and protocol used)	Glans 11 mm, 2 mg/kg/dose 12, 8, and 4 weeks prior to surgery
Any features of DSD (e.g., undescended testes)	None

11.4 Steps of the Procedure

11.4.1 First Stage

1. Following the degloving of the penile shaft skin, the residual fibrous chordee tissue is excised, and an artificial erection test is performed to assess for any remaining penile curvature [9–11].
2. If there is still penile curvature, the urethral plate is detached and moved, removing all the fibrous/dysplastic tissue on the underside (Fig. 11.2).

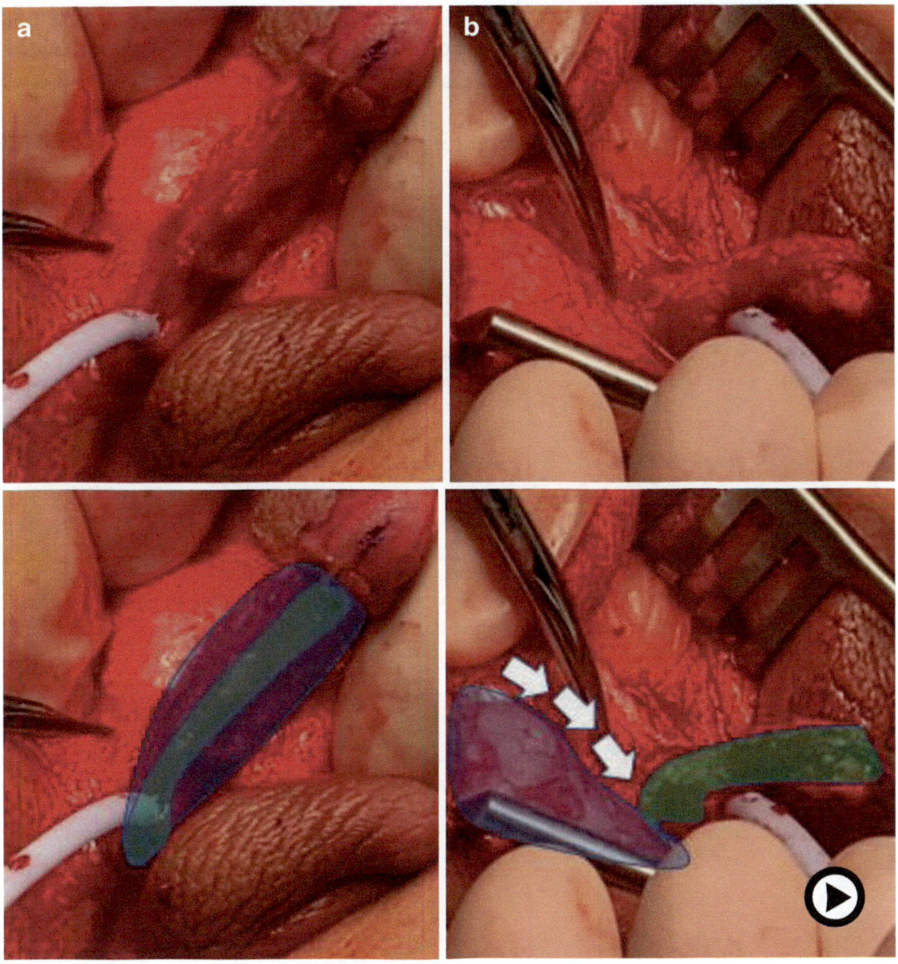

Fig. 11.2 (**a**) Dissection of the urethral plate when severe curvature (>45 degrees) persists after skin degloving. Blue color highlights the corpora and the green reflects the urethral plate (**b**). SPG repair (https://doi.org/10.1007/000-cn6)

3. Erection test is repeated and, if penile curvature >45 degrees, three ventral transverse incisions of the tunica albuginea are performed at the site of greatest penile curvature without the use of a tourniquet. Avoiding entry into the corporal erectile tissue is crucial. The albuginea should be incised while keeping the thin outer layer of the erectile tissue intact. Subsequently, an erection test is conducted again (Fig. 11.3).
4. To ensure proper grooving and the formation of the future orthotopic meatus, the glans is spatulated deeply.
5. The graft or the mobilized proximal urethral plate covers the glans cleft and the ventral raw region, which includes the VTITA. Three longitudinal lines of absorbable suture should be stitched to the corpora to avoid hematoma formation from occurring during the graft process. Near the graft's boundaries, the skin is smoothed out. The graft is immobilized and pressure is applied by tying the long sections of stitches to a Vaseline gauze dressing, which acts as a tie-over (Fig. 11.4).
6. If penoscrotal transposition is present it is corrected at this point.

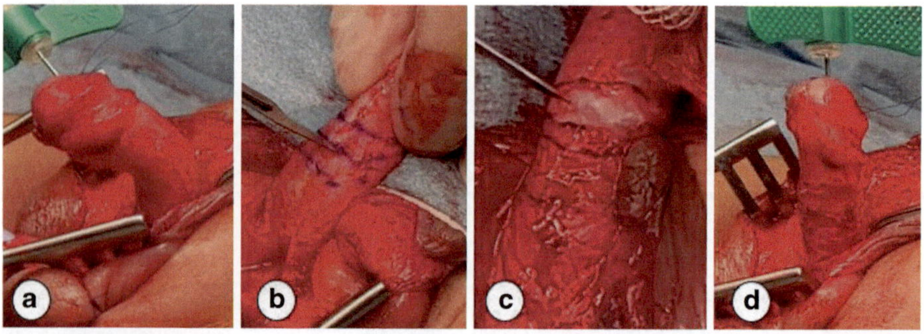

Fig. 11.3 Correction of ventral penile curvature >45 degrees. (**a**) Erection test after division of the urethral plate (70 degrees in this case); (**b**, **c**) Ventral transverse incisions of tunica albuginea (VTITA); (**d**) Erection test after penile curvature correction with VTITA

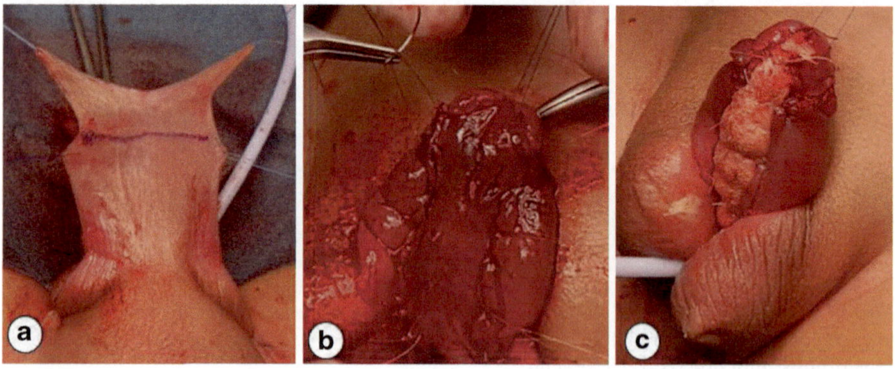

Fig. 11.4 A preputial (**a**) graft harvest, (**b**) fixation, and (**c**) tie-over dressing with Vaseline gauze

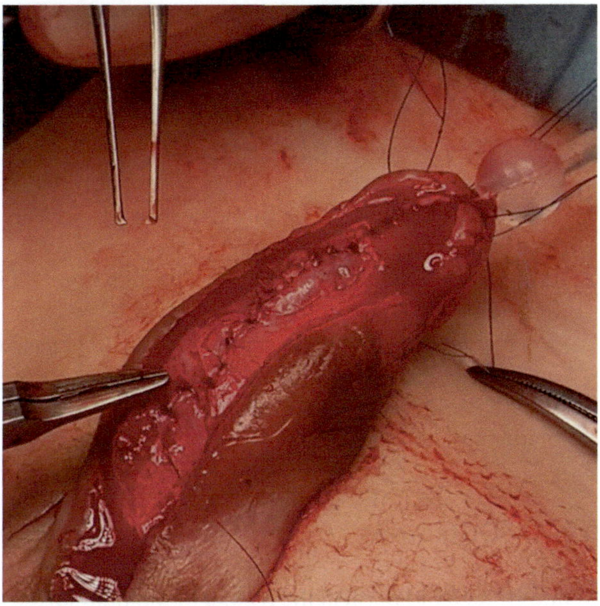

Fig. 11.5 Urethroplasty during second stage repair using interrupted 5-0 or 6-0 Polydioxanone suture over an 8 F silastic catheter

11.4.2 Second Stage

After six to twelve months have passed since the first step, or whenever the graft is soft and ready for tubularization, the second stage is often executed. Here are the steps:

1. To begin, the presence of residual curvature is evaluated by conducting an erection test. Recurrence of curvature necessitates thorough penile degloving and a new erection test. Do ventral lengthening again if the angle is greater than 45 degrees. To fix a dorsal plication if the angle is 20–45 degrees. In most cases, moderate curvature can be self-corrected with tubularization alone, without the requirement for dorsal plication.
2. The second step in urethroplasty is to place a single layer of interrupted 5-0 or 6-0 Polydioxanone suture over a flexible indwelling catheter (Fig. 11.5).
3. To prevent fistula formation, it is common practice to execute a tunica vaginalis flap as a second layer of coverage.
4. At last, the skin is closed.

11.5 Post-Operative Care After the First Stage

1. Dressing and indwelling catheter are left in place for five days and then removed in the outpatient clinic without sedation.
2. Vacuum physiotherapy begins around the third week after surgery. It involves performing 10 pumps while holding a vacuum for 3 seconds, twice a day, for a period of 4–6 months

3. After the second stage, a silastic catheter is left in place for 14 days.
4. Uroprophylaxis is administered while the catheter/stent is in situ.

11.6 Tips and Tricks

1. If the incision is too deep in the corpora, the application of a tourniquet during VTITA might prevent bleeding.
2. If mild residual penile curvature is present after VTITA it is corrected by a midline dorsal plication stitch.
3. It is important to regularly evaluate the penile curvature following penile degloving, as this procedure typically results in an improvement in curvature.
4. In order to prevent the creation of skin sinuses, the skin is closed using subcuticular stitches.

11.7 Outcomes

While Bracka did publish the results of the first 600 cases in 1995 utilizing his two-stage repair method, the benefits of sequencing the repairs were not recognized for over ten years [12]. In research conducted by Snodgrass et al., complications involving urethro-cutaneous fistulae and glans dehiscence were the most common, accounting for 23% of the cases, in 43 boys with penile curvature angles greater than 30 degrees after staged hypospadias treatment [13, 14]. Thirteen and fourteen in a study conducted by Pippi Salle et al., 140 boys with proximal hypospadias were studied over a 10-year period. Out of them, 60 boys received SGR, and 75 percent underwent ventral lengthening with VTITA. Despite being the most severe instances, these boys nonetheless achieved a success rate of 72 percent [15].

References

1. Spinoit A-F, Waterschoot M, Sinatti C, Abbas T, Callens N, Cools M, et al. Fertility and sexuality issues in congenital lifelong urology patients: male aspects. World J Urol [Internet]. 2020.
2. Abbas T, McCarthy L. Foreskin and penile problems in childhood. Surg (United Kingdom) 2016;34(5).
3. Gopal M, Abbas T, Salle JLP. Management of proximal hypospadias: current challenges and future directions. In: Abbas TO, editor. Hypospadiology [Internet]; 2023. p. 81–91.
4. Wani SA, Baba AA, Mufti GN, Rashid KA, Bhat NA, Buch M, et al. Bracka verses Byar's two-stage repair in proximal hypospadias associated with severe chordee: a randomized comparative study. Pediatr Surg Int [Internet]. 2020;36(8):965–70.
5. Subramaniam R, Spinoit AF, Hoebeke P. Hypospadias repair: an overview of the actual techniques. Semin Plast Surg [Internet]. 2011;25(3):206–12.
6. Abbas TO Hypospadiology: current challenges and future perspectives. 2023. 190 p.
7. Abbas TO. An objective hypospadias classification system. J Pediatr Urol [Internet]. 2022;18(4):481.e1–8.

8. Villanueva C, Abbas T. Penile curvature assessment in hypospadias. In: Abbas TO, editor. Hypospadiology [Internet]; 2023. p. 93–102.
9. Abbas TO. Evaluation of penile curvature in patients with hypospadias; gaps in the current practice and future perspectives. J Pediatr Urol [Internet]. 2021.
10. Abbas TO. The rising need for preoperative objective quantification of curvature in patients with hypospadias. J Pediatr Urol [Internet]. 2021;17(4):599–600.
11. Abbas TO, AbdelMoniem M, Chowdhury M. Automated quantification of penile curvature using artificial intelligence. Front Artif Intell [Internet]. 1AD;0:188.
12. Manzoni G, Bracka A, Palminteri E, Marrocco G. Hypospadias surgery: when, what and by whom? BJU Int [Internet]. 2004;94(8):1188–95.
13. Snodgrass W, Bush N. Staged tubularized autograft repair for primary proximal hypospadias with 30-degree or greater ventral curvature. J Urol [Internet]. 2017;198(3):680–6.
14. Bethell GS, Chhabra S, Shalaby MS, Corbett H, Kenny SE, BAPS NOAH Contributors. Parental decisional satisfaction after hypospadias repair in the United Kingdom. J Pediatr Urol [Internet]. 2020;16(2):164.e1–7.
15. Pippi Salle JL, Sayed S, Salle A, Bagli D, Farhat W, Koyle M, et al. Proximal hypospadias: a persistent challenge. Single institution outcome analysis of three surgical techniques over a 10-year period. J Pediatr Urol [Internet]. 2016;12(1):28.e1–7.

Byars Flaps for Staged Urethroplasty

12

Christopher J. Long, Aseem R. Shukla, and Mark R. Zaontz

Abstract

Management of proximal hypospadias is a challenge for all surgeons. It presents unique challenges to distal variants and the surgical approach is modified accordingly. There are many different variations on the theme for managing these patients, although there has been a shift away from single-stage repair to multi-stage repair due to concerns for worse outcomes and a higher complication rate. For the 2-stage repair, the principles are the same – correction of the penile curvature at the first stage in addition to creating a supple skin bed on the ventral penile shaft suitable for urethroplasty at the second stage. We proceed with a single ventral corporotomy for ventral curvature and cover this with dorsal-based

Supplementary Information The online version contains supplementary material available at https://doi.org/10.1007/978-981-99-0795-3_12. The videos can be accessed individually by clicking the DOI link in the accompanying figure caption or by scanning this link with the SN More Media App.

C. J. Long (✉)
Pediatric Urologic Surgical Reconstruction, Philadelphia, PA, USA

Division of Urology, Department of Surgery, The Children's Hospital of Philadelphia, Philadelphia, PA, USA

Perelman School of Medicine at the University of Pennsylvania, Philadelphia, PA, USA
e-mail: Longc3@chop.edu

A. R. Shukla · M. R. Zaontz
Division of Urology, Department of Surgery, The Children's Hospital of Philadelphia, Philadelphia, PA, USA

Perelman School of Medicine at the University of Pennsylvania, Philadelphia, PA, USA
e-mail: Shuklaa@chop.edu; zaontz@chop.edu

T. O. Abbas (ed.), *Video Atlas of Hypospadias Surgery*,
https://doi.org/10.1007/978-981-99-0795-3_12

Byars flaps in order to achieve proper ventral penile shaft skin coverage. We prefer flaps over grafts due to the ample blood supply, which aids the healing process.

Keywords

Hypospadias · Proximal hypospadias · 2-stage repair · Byars flaps

12.1 Introduction

A discussion of surgical technique should begin with an anatomic assessment and particular indications. Our institution has a long-standing history of preferring a single-stage approach to proximal hypospadias via an island onlay or Duckett interposition tube [1]. Honest assessment of our results indicated that we weren't meeting the patient outcomes we intended [2]. The 2-stage repair is now our treatment of choice for proximal or severe hypospadias. [3, 4] Proximal hypospadias extends beyond the overly simplistic categorization of the meatus. Inclusion of the width of the glans, quality of the glans groove, the degree of penile curvature, and the ventral penile skin development are necessary components of the initial evaluation. A shallow glans groove and, in particular, severe ventral penile curvature is approached in an algorithmic process that results in a staged approach with increased severity. Management of curvature drives the staged surgical procedure decision for us. If the penis is straightened by degloving alone or has mild curvature after degloving, which we define <30 degrees, we typically perform a dorsal plication and single stage repair. In some patients with poor quality ventral shaft skin, however, we will perform a staged repair. The focus of this video chapter is on the patient with more than 30 degrees of ventral curvature after penile degloving. Testosterone is administered to patients with unfavorable anatomy, specifically a small glans width (14 mm or less), a narrow groove, or a smaller penis [5]. The urethral plate is divided and if still curved (>30 degrees) a ventral lengthening procedure is performed.

12.2 Indications

Patients with severe hypospadias. Indications vary by patient but we specifically focus on patients with severe curvature, hypoplastic ventral skin, and/or poor quality of the glans and urethral plate (Fig. 12.1a, b). Patients with severe penile curvature are those that have sequentially gone through penile degloving, division of the urethral plate, and still have significant curvature, which we define as 30 degrees or more. Patients with poor-quality ventral shaft tissue are more of a subjective assessment. If there is a hypoplastic urethra that is located at the midshaft of the penis or more proximal, we proceed with a 2-stage repair. If the glans groove is poor and not amenable to primary closure with a Thiersch Duplay approach or dorsal inlay graft repair, this is another indication for a 2-stage repair.

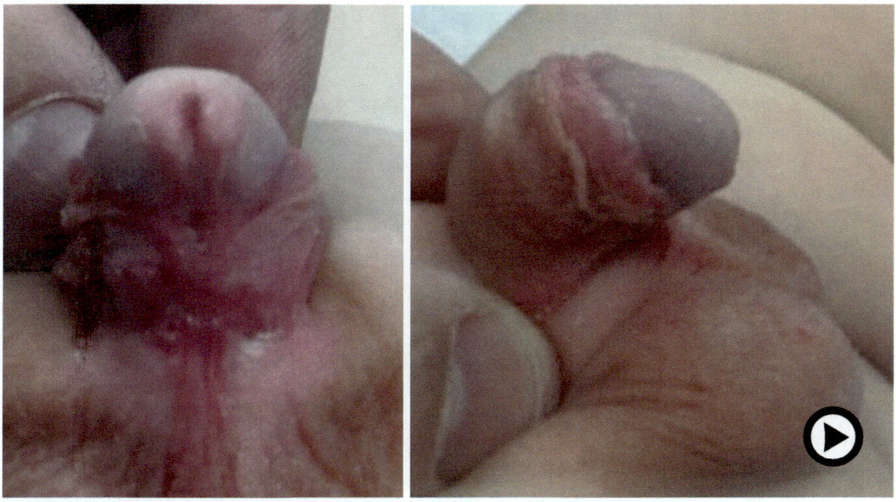

Fig. 12.1 Patient with proximal hypospadias, with a ventral (left panel) and lateral view (right panel) provided. Dermal graft corporoplasty. (https://doi.org/10.1007/000-cn8)

12.3 Video Demonstration

First-stage video is of a 10-month-old male with a history of proximal hypospadias. Both testes were descended and no genetic workup was performed. Second-stage video was the same patient, 45 mm urethroplasty with left tunica vaginalis barrier layer coverage.

12.4 Steps of the Procedure

12.4.1 Anatomy Assessment, Penile Degloving

- 4-0 Prolene holding suture is placed in the glans.
- Urethra is calibrated with a Bougie a Boulie, quality of urethral plate tissue assessed.
- Ventral and dorsal incisions are marked. Ventral incision is extended to just distal to the hypoplastic urethra. Dorsally a chevron incision is made, angled down to generate Firlit flaps to rotate ventrally, creating a circumferential mucosal collar.
- Penis is degloved using a combination of cautery and scissors. Catheter is placed in the urethra for identification purposes. Dissection is carried superficial to Buck's fascia, trying to stay in an avascular plane (Fig. 12.2).

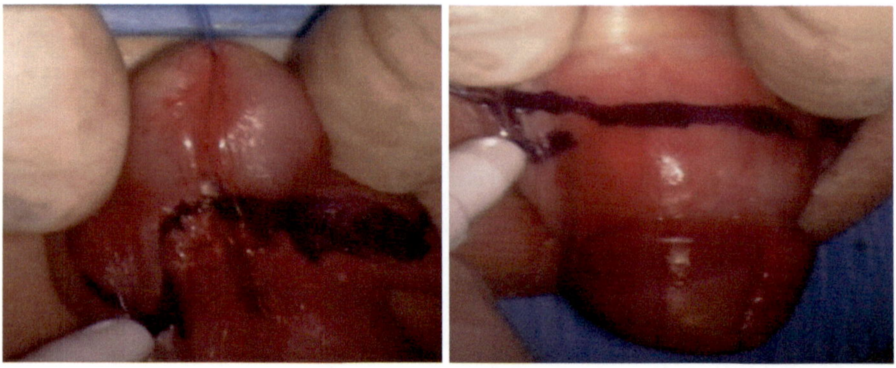

Fig. 12.2 Left panel with a view of the ventral incision, meatus is proximal to the marked line. Right panel shows the dorsal marking, extending down on the lateral border in an angled fashion

Fig. 12.3 Artificial erection with the penis degloved

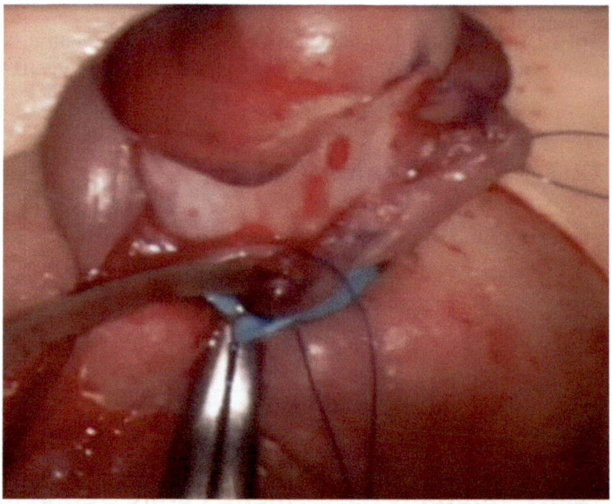

12.4.2 Artificial Erection

- Erection test is performed with tourniquet in place, 25G butterfly needle, and injectable saline. In this video the urethra has been divided and mobilized proximally, a tourniquet is in place, and there is 45 degrees of ventral penile curvature (Fig. 12.3)

12.4.3 Ventral Corporotomy

- Single, transverse ventral corporotomy incision is marked and made
- This is done with tourniquet in place to maintain a bloodless field

- Corporotomy is made and developed, extending from 9 to 3 o'clock positions to free the ventral tethering
- Graft is harvested (dermal or tunica vaginalis) with a slightly larger volume to allow for proper fit
- Graft sutured in water water-tight fashion
- Artificial erection is repeated to ensure curvature has resolved (Figs. 12.4, 12.5 and 12.6)

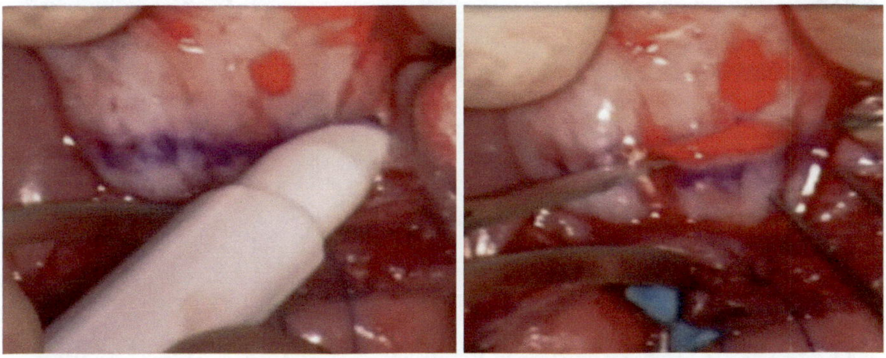

Fig. 12.4 We prefer to make a single ventral corporotomy opposite the point of maximal curvature. Care is taken to perform an artificial erection to identify the proper location. We also perform the artificial erection without the tourniquet to ensure that proximal penile curvature is not missed. The ventral corporotomy is made through the tunica but care is taken to avoid injury to the erectile tissue. A midline septum is incised, if it isn't it can contract and lead to persistent curvature

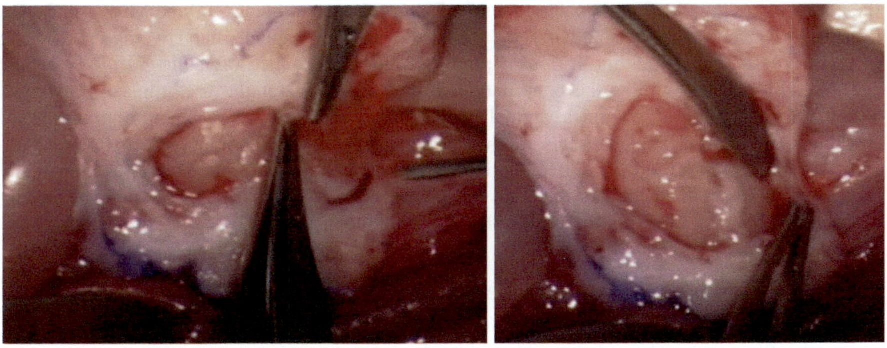

Fig. 12.5 A midline septum is incised, if it isn't it can contract and lead to persistent curvature (left panel). The margins of the corporotomy are freed such that the graft can be sutured to the tunica but the erectile tissue is spared (right panel)

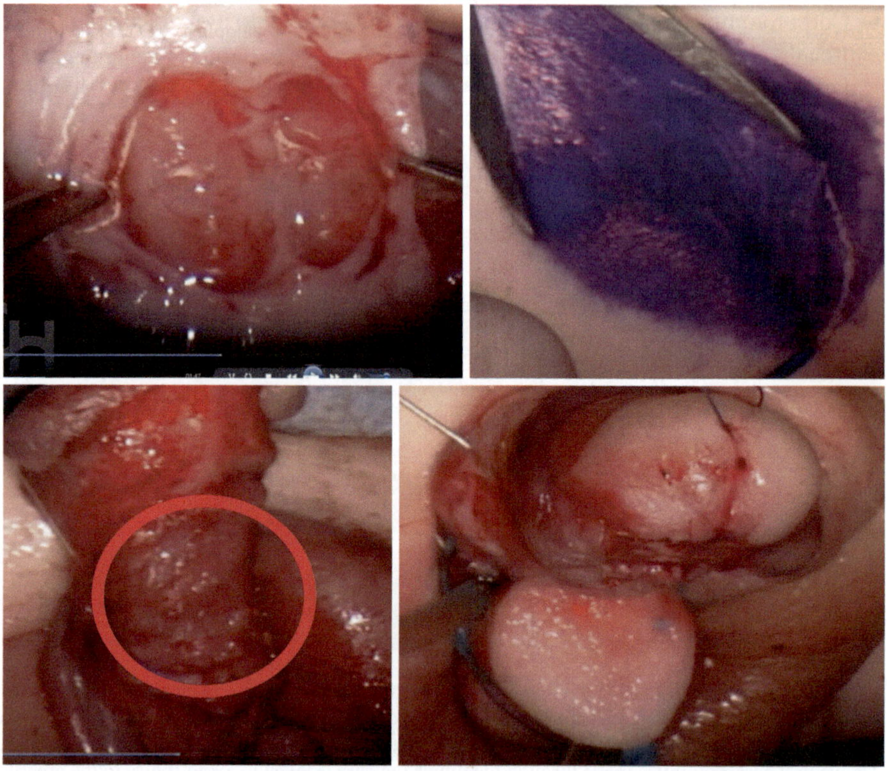

Fig. 12.6 Ventral defect after full mobilization and division of the midline septum. The size of the graft is then measured and harvested. We prefer a dermal patch graft harvested from the groin, in the point of the crease to minimize post-surgical scarring. The graft is harvested 20% larger than the corporotomy to allow for some contraction. Two of the co-authors (CJL and MRZ) prefer the dermal graft due to its thicker consistency and to allow tunica vaginalis flap coverage at the time of urethroplasty. One co-author of this chapter, ARS, prefers a tunica vaginalis graft to cover the corporotomy and will utilize the contralateral tunica vaginalis for the urethroplasty coverage. Whether for dermal graft or tunica vaginalis, four quadrant sutures are placed to align the graft, trimming it as needed. The quadrants are then closed separately in a running, water-tight fashion. Red line in the bottom left panel depicts the borders of the sutured graft. Once closed artificial erection is repeated to ensure that the penis is straight (bottom right panel). Some patients require a concomitant dorsal plication suture to fully straighten the penis

12.4.4 Byars Flap Skin Closure

- Byars flap is developed from the dorsal, redundant prepuce which is incised in the midline
- Dartos is aligned across the corporotomy
- Glans is incised in the midline and flap is extended into this defect to create a proper urethral groove

- Dartos is removed from the flap, essentially creating a graft, within the glans defect
- Skin flaps are then sutured in the midline to cover the ventral penile shaft defect (Figs. 12.7, 12.8 and 12.9)

The bandage is kept simple. A Foley catheter is placed into the urethra for 3–5 days. A compression dressing with Tegaderm for 3–5 days is placed on the penile shaft. Some surgeons prefer a Coban dressing around the Tegaderm for 24–48 hours to prevent hematoma formation, while others prefer a Duckett pressure dressing where gauze and telfa are placed over the entire repair with tegaderm for three days. Finally, the Falkowski-Firlit X-shaped Elastic dressing can be used. The skin flaps are carefully maintained to ensure proper healing and to prevent contracture. Beginning 3–4 weeks after surgery penile massage is performed with Vaseline, massaging the flap to ensure that the penis is straight and that the skin heals evenly. We do find that this can prevent flap contracture and is continued for 3–4 months after surgery with each diaper change.

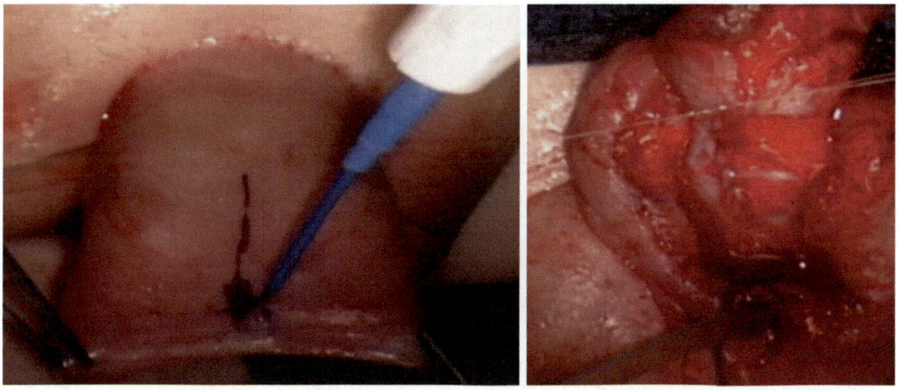

Fig. 12.7 Once the penis is straight, we direct our attention to the ventral penile skin coverage. We typically approach this in one of two ways. Our most common, traditional approach has been the Byars flap. The redundant dorsal foreskin is incised in the midline, to the point of a proper circumcision skin fit and approximated dorsally. If penile concealment is present then we place stitches to anchor the penis at the 12, 5, and 7 o'clock position, from the deep dermal layer to Buck's fascia. Alternatively, an island flap can be harvested from the inner preputial skin and rotated ventrally, avoiding a ventral midline suture line that can lead to scarring. The dartos is approximated across the corporal graft to aid in closure and to help the overlying ventral shaft skin. The dorsal-based skin flaps that have been transposed are then secured to the ventral surface of the penis. The flap is secured longitudinally from the urethral meatus and extends distally into the mobilized glans. We try to lay preputial skin around the meatus to prevent incorporation of scrotal skin at the second stage. Quilting of the flap can be performed to prevent postoperative hematoma formation, particularly within the glans. The quilting also stabilizes the proposed neourethral skin to prevent angulation or buckling of the future neourethra after the flap is tubularized for the future neourethra

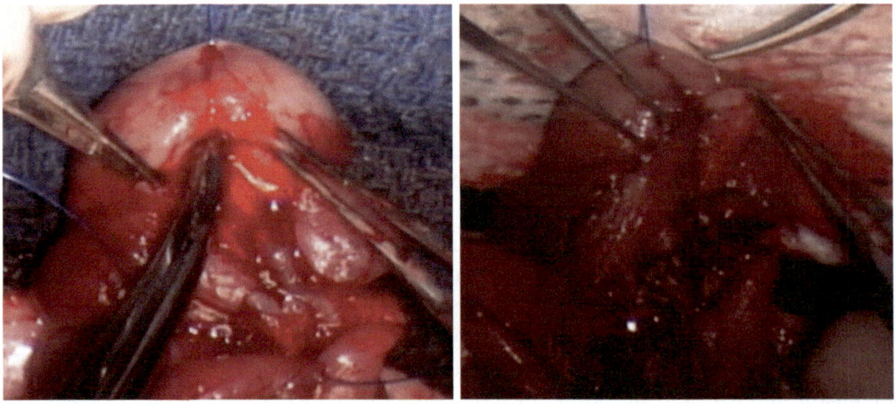

Fig. 12.8 The glans is incised in the midline to create a deep groove. We try to remove the dartos on the skin within the glans to prevent a bulky urethral plate that challenges closure. If an island flap is utilized, we flatten and secure the pedicle flap across the corporotomy to prevent bulking of the ventral flap. This maintains perfusion while creating an even flap for urethral closure

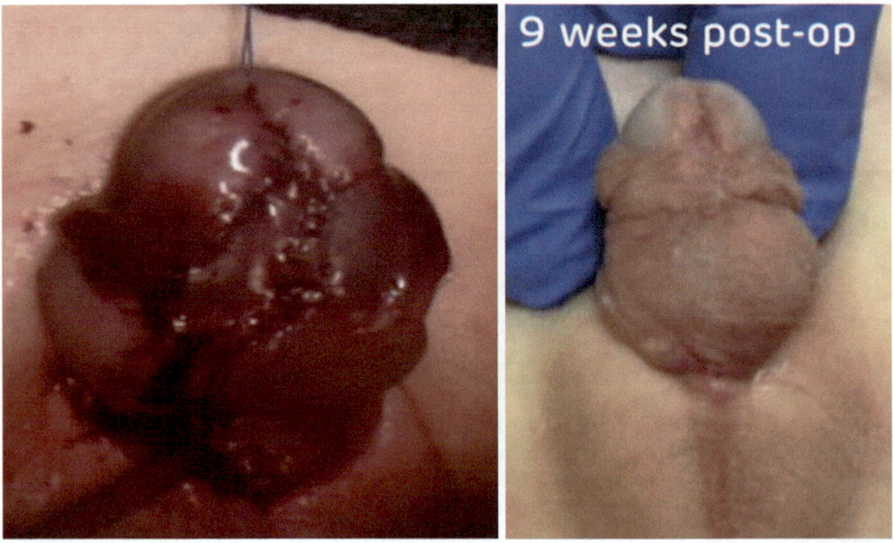

Fig. 12.9 Picture of the penis at the end of the procedure (left panel) and at the 9 week postop visit (right panel)

12.4.5 Second-Stage Repair

- Urethra is calibrated to ensure no contracture
- Penis is examined to rule out scar tissue
- Artificial erection is performed to rule out recurrent curvature
- Ventral U-shaped incision is marked and incised (Fig. 12.10)

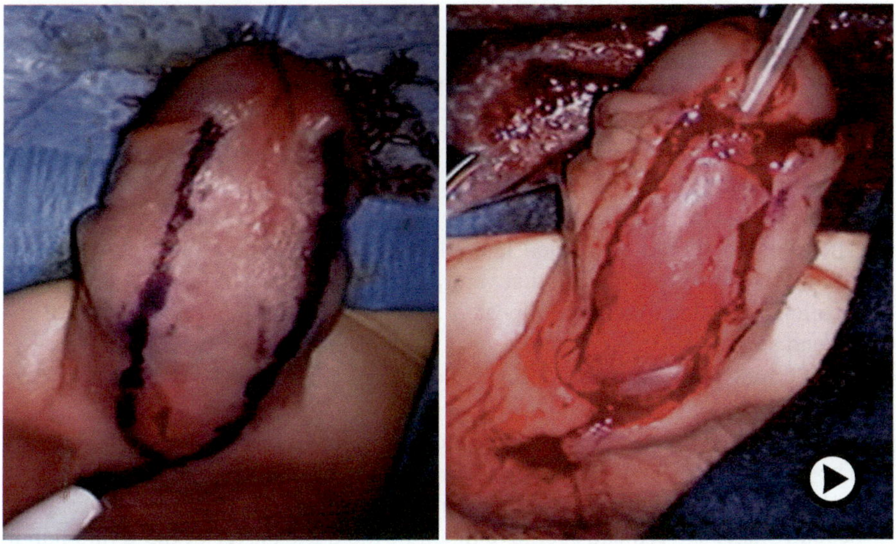

Fig. 12.10 A U-shaped incision is marked along the ventrum of the penis and incised (left panel). The flaps are gently mobilized to ensure a tension-free closure. The final urethral catheter is placed and then first layer closure is performed in a running, subcuticular fashion. Care is taken to advance the urethra to a point that is an optimal balance of a distal, functional location but also one which will not narrow within the glans. Some patients end with a coronal meatus while others can be advanced into the glans, often as a function of the glans width. A second running urethroplasty closure, done in a Lembert fashion, is performed to fully close the urethra. If there is sufficient dartos present this can be brought across the repair as a barrier layer. Often, we will harvest a tunica vaginalis flap from the scrotum to drape across the urethroplasty due to its excellent blood supply (right panel). When performed we place a pexy suture to maintain the testicle location within the dependent scrotum and make sure to mobilize the flap to the level of the external ring to prevent tension on the penis, which can result in penile torsion. Second stage urethroplasty. (https://doi.org/10.1007/000-cn7)

12.5 Postoperative Care

A period of 6–12 months is given prior to second-stage urethroplasty, as determined by the flap healing process. Most of the repair is performed at the time of the first stage. The catheter is sutured in place and typically left for 7–10 days. We again maintain a simple dressing with a Tegaderm on the penile shaft for 3–5 days. We typically only administer antibiotics at the time of surgery, although we have administered at the time of catheter removal if left in for longer periods of time. Pain control is maintained with a combination of Tylenol, Ibuprofen, and oxybutynin.

Follow-up is continued through puberty. We ask parents to monitor for erections and the urinary stream for any concerns. Uroflowmetry is done as patient's age to ensure proper emptying and stream. Patients can have concerns of slowed urinary stream, post-void dribbling, or a need to milk the urethra, particularly if a longer urethroplasty is performed.

12.6 Tips and Tricks

- A key part of the procedure is to decide when to proceed with a 2-stage repair, based on the patient's specific anatomy.
- The single ventral corporotomy should be performed opposite the point of maximal curvature, the midline septum should be mobilized, and the edges of the tunica should be mobilized to facilitate a tension-free graft closure.
- The incision should be carried laterally to the point where the penis "hinges" slightly posteriorly to ensure that ventral tension has been released.
- Artificial erection should be repeated after graft closure and at the start of the second stage.
- If a dermal graft is used a 2-layer closure should be performed to minimize scarring.
- The epidermal layer should be removed off of the dermal graft.
- The glans should be incised to create a recipient bed for flap placement.
- Bulky graft tissue should be avoided in the glans which can limit closure at the second stage. We typically remove much of the dartos layer of the Byars flap to create a deep groove.
- A compression dressing is key to maintain hemostasis and to obtain proper wound healing.
- Flap massage can help prevent contracture and to get an even healing across the skin.
- A 2-layer running urethroplasty helps minimize fistula formation.
- Barrier layers should be utilized to maintain a healthy urethroplasty repair.
- Tunica vaginalis flap, if utilized, should be mobilized to the level of the external ring to prevent penile tethering.

12.7 Conclusions

A single ventral corporotomy has a high success rate for correcting severe penile curvature. The average increase in ventral penile length is 1.6 mm. The overlying skin coverage should be done with a well-perfused flap to prevent skin contracture. Multiple layer urethroplasty should be performed in order to maintain water-tight closure.

We want to recognize Emma Walsh for her significant contributions to video editing for this chapter, her expertise is invaluable.

References

1. Shukla AR, Patel RP, Canning DA. The 2-stage hypospadias repair. Is it a misnomer? J Urol. 2004;172:1714–6; discussion 6
2. Long CJ, Chu DI, Tenney RW, Morris AR, Weiss DA, Shukla AR, et al. Intermediate-term followup of proximal hypospadias repair reveals high complication rate. J Urol. 2017;197:852–8.

3. Lucas J, Hightower T, Weiss DA, Van Batavia J, Coelho S, Srinivasan AK, et al. Time to complication detection after primary pediatric hypospadias repair: a large, single center, retrospective cohort analysis. J Urol. 2020;204:338–44.
4. Long CJ, Canning DA. Hypospadias: are we as good as we think when we correct proximal hypospadias? J Pediatr Urol. 2016.
5. Mittal S, Eftekharzadeh S, Christianson SS, Hyacinthe N, Tan C, Weiss DA, et al. Quantifying glans width changes in response to preoperative androgen stimulation in patients undergoing hypospadias repair. J Urol. 2022;207:1314–21.

Onlay Island Flap for the Repair of Hypospadias

13

Gerhard Reinaldi Situmorang, Putu Angga Risky Raharja, Arry Rodjani, and Irfan Wahyudi

Abstract

The dorsal prepuce has been integral in urethral reconstruction for hypospadias, initially introduced by Asopa and popularized by Duckett. Asopa et al. utilized the preputial flap in severe hypospadias, while Elder et al. adapted it for distal and midpenile cases without chordee, proving its efficacy in proximal cases as well. This technique offers advantages by utilizing readily available, hairless, and adequately sized dorsal prepuce, often discarded otherwise. The onlay island flap repair technique thus presents a sustainable and clinically significant solution for hypospadias management.

Keywords

Hypospadias · Urethral reconstruction · Dorsal prepuce · Onlay island flap

---

Supplementary Information The online version contains supplementary material available at https://doi.org/10.1007/978-981-99-0795-3_13. The videos can be accessed individually by clicking the DOI link in the accompanying figure caption or by scanning this link with the SN More Media App.

G. R. Situmorang (✉) · P. A. R. Raharja · A. Rodjani · I. Wahyudi
Department of Urology, Faculty of Medicine, Universitas Indonesia, Cipto Mangunkusumo Hospital, Jakarta, Indonesia
e-mail: gerhard.reinaldi01@ui.ac.id

T. O. Abbas (ed.), *Video Atlas of Hypospadias Surgery*,
https://doi.org/10.1007/978-981-99-0795-3_13

Key Points

- Onlay island flap repair technique is a versatile and effective option for urethral reconstruction in hypospadias, using the dorsal prepuce as a resourceful solution.
- It is usually used for primary distal hypospadias, with good cosmetic outcome and low complication rates.
- Onlay island flap urethroplasty can also be used for mid- and proximal hypospadias, with good results.
- Complication rates of onlay island flap repair range from 10% to 33%, with comparable results to other urethroplasty techniques.

13.1 Introduction

Use of dorsal prepuce for urethral reconstruction in hypospadias was first described by Asopa and further popularized by Duckett [1–3]. Asopa et al. used the preputial flap as a tube in a single-stage repair of severe hypospadias where urethral plate needs to be transected [1]. Elder et al. modified the technique and used the prepuce as a vascularized onlay island flap for distal and midpenile hypospadias without chordee [2]. However, onlay island flap has been well proven to be used for proximal hypospadias, as well [4]. The use of the onlay island flap repair technique presents an advantage by making use of the dorsal prepuce [5]. This prepuce is typically available, hairless, and of adequate size to construct the deficient urethral plate. Additionally, this prepuce is often discarded, making it a resourceful solution to the reconstructive process [5].

13.2 Indications

Onlay island flap urethroplasty is usually used for primary distal hypospadias, along with tubularized incised plate (TIP), dorsal inlay graft, and Mathieu repair. Onlay island flap urethroplasty for primary distal hypospadias had good cosmetic outcome and a low associated complication [6]. Onlay island flap urethroplasty also had good outcome in distal hypospadias patients with narrow urethral plate ($\leq$6 mm) [5, 7]. Onlay island flap is also a viable option for one-stage repair of mid- and proximal hypospadias, and has shown to yield good results [4].

13.3 Steps of the Procedure

13.3.1 Patient Preparation

The surgery is performed under general anesthesia with/without caudal anesthesia. After retracting the foreskin and cleaning the coronal sulcus, a traction suture is placed at the dorsum of the glans penis distally with 5/0 polypropylene suture for handling. A thorough examination is performed to assess the site and size of the meatus, presence of chordee, glans configuration, urethral plate depth and width, and dorsal hood availability.

13.3.2 Marking Drawing

A small metal sound is introduced into the meatus, and the thickness of the corpus spongiosum is assessed. The points where the corpus spongiosum is thickest are marked. If necessary, thin skin in the ventral aspect of the urethra may be excised. A U-shaped marking along the lateral margins of the urethral plate and a circumferential subcoronal design are also marked (Fig. 13.1a, b).

13.3.3 Penile Degloving and Orthoplasty

The penile skin is degloved from the corporeal bodies in both the ventral and dorsal aspects by carefully dissecting the avascular plane between Buck's fascia and the dartos fascia (Fig. 13.1c). Any inelastic dartos is excised to correct the chordee. To evaluate the curvature of the penis, a penile erection test is performed. If necessary, dorsal plication of the penis may be performed to correct the curvature. However, if the curvature is very pronounced, it may be necessary to dissect the urethral plate off the corpora cavernosa, and then perform staged urethroplasty using either a flap or graft.

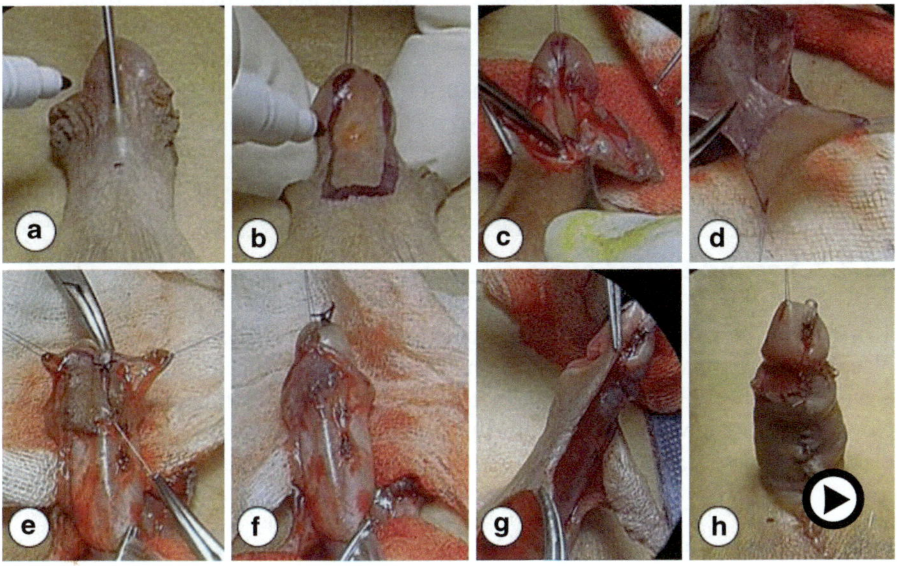

Fig. 13.1 Marking of the ventral penile incision design (**a**, **b**) followed by penile skin degloving (**c**). The onlay preputial flap is then marked and prepared maintaining the vascular pedicle attached then laterally rotated to be fixed on the native urethral plate (**e**, **f**). Skin closure is performed using Byars flaps (**g**, **h**). Onlay island flap reconstruction (https://doi.org/10.1007/000-cn9)

13.3.4 Harvesting Dorsal Preputial Island Flap

After correcting the penile curvature, the distance between the urethral meatus and the tip of the glans is measured, as well as the width of the urethral plate. The width of the urethral plate plus the onlay flap should be adjusted based on the age of the patient to ensure sufficient caliber of the urethra. However, a total width of 12–14 mm is typically chosen [4]. The dorsal foreskin is marked, and a superficial incision is made through the skin of the flap only, leaving the pedicle intact (Fig. 13.1d). The pedicle is then freed down to the base of the penile shaft to allow the flap to be transposed ventrally and rotated 90 degrees (Fig. 13.1e).

13.3.5 Preparation of the Glans

To prepare the glans for glansplasty, parallel incisions are made to outline the urethral plate, and the glans is mobilized laterally to allow for closure over the reconstructed urethra. A tourniquet may be applied to the base of the penis to reduce bleeding during dissection.

13.3.6 Suturing of the Flap

The onlay flap is rotated ventrally and approximated parallel to the urethral plate. The edges are sutured together using a running 6/0 polydioxanone or poliglecaprone suture on the right side from the meatus to the tip of the glans. A silastic stent or an 8 Fr silicone catheter is inserted into the urethral meatus for stenting. The remaining flap and urethral plate are then sutured with inverted interrupted sutures until reaching the tip of the glans in a symmetrical fashion. The distal portion of the flap used for the urethroplasty is trimmed as necessary. If a silastic stent was used, percutaneous cystostomy may be necessary for urinary diversion.

13.3.7 Second-Layer Coverage

To cover the new urethra, a second layer of onlay island flap is used and sutured in place with interrupted 6/0 polydioxanone or poliglecaprone suture. It is important to ensure that the onlay island flap is tension-free to avoid torsion of the penis. However, if the new urethra can be fully covered with glans tissue during glansplasty, the second-layer coverage from the flap may be unnecessary.

13.3.8 Glansplasty

The glans wings' flaps are then wrapped around the neourethra and approximated with 5/0 poliglecaprone or 6/0 polyglactin suture in interrupted subcuticular fashion to create a slit-like appearance of the glanular meatus. The skin of the glans is then closed with interrupted 6/0 sutures.

13.3.9 Wound Closure

Modified Byars' flap is used for skin closure with interrupted 5/0 polydioxanone or poliglecaprone suture (Fig. 13.1g, h). Any excessive redundant skin is discarded. A compressive dressing is applied and left in place for 5–7 days.

13.4 Tips and Tricks

13.4.1 Patient Selection

Optimal patient selection is important to achieve the best results with onlay island flap urethroplasty. This technique can be used for both distal and proximal hypospadias, and is effective even in cases with a shallow urethral plate. Studies have shown that urethral plate width is not a problem for this technique [5, 7]. However, patients with a small glans diameter may require hormonal therapy before the surgery. In cases of a small glans penis, the surgeon may opt to not perform glansplasty and instead perform urethroplasty until subcoronal.

13.4.2 Flap Design

The flap design should be rectangular in shape, with the length of the flap equal to the distance between the urethral meatus and the tip of the glans. The width of the flap should be adjusted based on the patient's age or penile size, as well as the width of the urethral plate. A total width of 12–14 mm (which includes both the urethral plate width and the onlay island flap width) is typically chosen. Choosing a larger width may result in a urethral diverticulum. A narrower width, on the other hand, may lead to a smaller caliber of the neourethra, which could result in stenosis. The design should also be marked on the tip of the inner prepuce, as it may be folded under the dorsal penile skin.

13.4.3 Mobilization of the Onlay Island Flap

During the mobilization of the onlay island flap, we may place traction sutures on the edges of the flap. The tension created by the traction enables us to identify the junction between the dartos fascia and the dorsal penile skin. The dartos fascia is dissected from the skin to preserve its vascular supply to the flap. It is important to avoid excessive use of diathermy, as it may compromise the vascularization of the flap. The dartos tissue should be kept as bulky as possible to ensure good vascularization of the flap. The dissection of the dartos tissue should continue until the flap can be transposed ventrally and rotated 90 degrees without causing torsion. Some authors may also perform midline splitting of the pedicle to allow for dorsal penile buttonholing of the island flap, which can help reduce penile torsion [5].

13.4.4 Suturing Technique

The suturing technique is crucial. We usually perform a continuous suture on the right side of the flap (if the flap is transposed from the right side). The bite of the suture should not be too small, and the distance between each bite should not be too far apart. The use of magnification is mandatory to achieve better results. The remaining flap and urethral plate are sutured with interrupted inverted fashion until a symmetrical tip of the glans is achieved on the left side. In our center, we usually perform the suture with 6/0 polydioxanone or poliglecaprone suture. Second-layer coverage with the dartos tissue of the flap may be necessary to reduce complications.

13.4.5 Postoperative Care

Postoperative care is as important as the intraoperative technique. We typically apply a compressive dressing after surgery. At our center, we often use stenting with a silastic stent and urinary diversion with cystostomy. However, it is also possible not to use a stent or to use urinary diversion with a catheter instead. The dressing is usually removed on postoperative day three or longer, depending on each case. An antibiotic ointment is regularly applied to the wound after removal of the dressing. The silastic stent is removed during postoperative day seven, and the cystostomy is usually removed two weeks later after confirming that the patient can urinate from the tip of the glans.

13.4.6 Surgeon Experience

The surgeon's experience is an essential factor that can affect the outcome of onlay island flap repair. Several studies have shown that the success rates of hypospadias repair are higher in the hands of experienced surgeons. It's important to note that the learning curve for onlay island flap repair can be steep, and it may take a surgeon some time to develop the skills and experience necessary to perform the procedure successfully.

13.5 Results

The overall complication rates of onlay island flap repair ranged from 10% to 33% [8–10]. In the studies which included only proximal defects, the overall complications increased to 31–33% [9, 10]. A study found comparable complication rates of onlay island flap and TIP urethroplasty [11]. In proximal hypospadias repair, onlay island flap might be better than TIP procedure [11]. A prospective study comparing the outcome of modified onlay island flap with that of the Mathieu urethroplasty for distal hypospadias repair showed significantly lower complication rate, and a better cosmetic outcome, urinary stream, and relatives' satisfaction for modified onlay island flap group [5]. Another prospective study comparing outcomes of onlay island flap with dorsal inlay graft showed comparable complications [12].

13.6 Conclusions

Onlay island flap repair technique using the dorsal prepuce is a viable option for urethral reconstruction in hypospadias, with good cosmetic outcomes and low complication rates, particularly for primary distal hypospadias. It can also be used for mid- and proximal hypospadias, with good results. The surgeon's experience is a critical factor that can affect the outcome of the procedure. Optimal patient selection, flap design, mobilization of the onlay island flap, and suturing technique are crucial for achieving good results. Further studies are necessary to compare the outcomes of onlay island flap repair with other urethroplasty techniques, particularly in proximal hypospadias repair.

Acknowledgments We would like to express our sincere gratitude to Jonathan Pratama Swannjo, MD, Pradipta, MD, Eka Setiawan Ananta Putra, MD, Dwidian Khresna Risanto, MD, and Rananda Anggakara Hendarmo, MD for their contributions on video editing.

References

1. Asopa HS, Elhence IP, Atri SP, Bansal NK. One stage correction of penile hypospadias using a foreskin tube. A preliminary report. Int Surg. 1971;55(6):435–40.
2. Elder JS, Duckett JW, Snyder HM. Onlay island flap in the repair of mid and distal penile hypospadias without chordee. J Urol. 1987;138(2):376–9. https://doi.org/10.1016/s0022-5347(17)43152-1.
3. Duckett JW. The island flap technique for hypospadias repair. Urol Clin North Am. 1981;8(3):503–11.
4. González R, Lingnau A, Ludwikowski BM. Results of onlay preputial flap urethroplasty for the single-stage repair of mid- and proximal hypospadias. Front Pediatr. 2018;6:19. https://doi.org/10.3389/fped.2018.00019.
5. ElGanainy EO. A modified onlay island flap vs. Mathieu urethroplasty for distal hypospadias repair: a prospective randomised study. Arab J Urol. 2015;13(3):169–75. https://doi.org/10.1016/j.aju.2015.06.005.
6. El-Helaly HAA, Youssof HA, Ibrahim HM, Aldaqadossi HAH, Abdalla OM, Dogha MM. Distal hypospadias repair: comparative study between snodgrass and transverse preputial onlay flap. J Pediatr Urol. 2022;18(5):610.e1–6. https://doi.org/10.1016/j.jpurol.2022.08.016.
7. Mohajerzadeh L, Mirshemirani A, Rouzrokh M, et al. Evaluation of onlay island flap technique in shallow urethral plate hypospadiasis. Iran J Pediatr. 2016;26(1):0–3. https://doi.org/10.5812/ijp.660.
8. Hollowell JG, Keating MA, Snyder HM 3rd, Duckett JW. Preservation of the urethral plate in hypospadias repair: extended applications and further experience with the onlay island flap urethroplasty. J Urol. 1990;143(1):91–8. https://doi.org/10.1016/s0022-5347(17)39878-6.
9. Wiener JS, Sutherland RW, Roth DR, Gonzales ETJ. Comparison of onlay and tubularized island flaps of inner preputial skin for the repair of proximal hypospadias. J Urol. 1997;158(3 Pt 2):1172–4. https://doi.org/10.1097/00005392-199709000-00123.

10. Demirbilek S, Kanmaz T, Aydin G, Yücesan S. Outcomes of one-stage techniques for proximal hypospadias repair. Urology. 2001;58(2):267–70. https://doi.org/10.1016/s0090-4295(01)01183-9.
11. Sujijantararat P, Chaiyaprasithi B. Comparative outcome between transverse island flap onlay and tubularized incised plate for primary hypospadias repair. Asian J Surg. 2009;32(4):229–33. https://doi.org/10.1016/S1015-9584(09)60399-7.
12. Aritonang J, Rodjani A, Wahyudi I, Situmorang GR. Comparison of outcome and success rate of onlay island flap and dorsal inlay graft in hypospadias reconstruction: a prospective study. Res Rep Urol. 2020;12:487–94. https://doi.org/10.2147/RRU.S266886.

The Lateral-Based Onlay (LABO) Flap Technique for Proximal Hypospadias Without Severe Chordee

14

Hanno Wirmer and Ahmed T. Hadidi

Abstract

The lateral-based onlay (LABO) principle is to suture the lateral foreskin to the urethral plate as an onlay flap or as a lateral meatal-based flap. It is suitable for patients with proximal hypospadias in the absence of deep chordee that necessitates division of the urethral plate. It has particular value in patients with small or flat glans. Multiple layer closure and careful attention to technical details was associated with 5% complication rate in primary proximal hypospadias.

Keywords

Hypospadias · Proximal · Penoscrotal · Small glans · Onlay · Flap · Urethroplasty

14.1 Introduction

Correction of proximal hypospadias remains a major challenge. However, distinction must be made between penoscrotal hypospadias without or with slight (<30°) chordee (grade III hypospadias), and proximal or perineal hypospadias with severe (>30°) chordee (grade IV hypospadias) that requires division of the urethral plate and suitable for the CEDU technique [1], the Koyanagi technique [2], or the Duckett

Supplementary Information The online version contains supplementary material available at https://doi.org/10.1007/978-981-99-0795-3_14. The videos can be accessed individually by clicking the DOI link in the accompanying figure caption or by scanning this link with the SN More Media App.

H. Wirmer · A. T. Hadidi (✉)
Hypospadias Center, Sana Klinikum Offenbach, Offenbach am Main, Germany
e-mail: hanno.wirmer@sana.de

T. O. Abbas (ed.), *Video Atlas of Hypospadias Surgery*,
https://doi.org/10.1007/978-981-99-0795-3_14

Island flap [3]; The urethral plate can be preserved in Grade III proximal hypospadias without severe chordee and the following techniques are commonly used; the onlay flap [4], the Thiersch technique [5], and the tubularized incised plate technique [6]. Higher rates of complications are reported in patients with small, flat glans [7, 8].

LABO technique is described in detail. It offers a good solution for patients with proximal hypospadias without severe chordee (grade III), and small flat glans, even when the urethral plate is narrow [9, 10].

14.2 Indications

LABO is recommended for proximal hypospadias without or with mild superficial chordee (<30°). It is of particular value in patients with small glans.

14.3 Video Demonstration

Factors	Findings
Age at surgery (month)	13
Gestational age (weeks)	40
Birth weight (g)	2900
Gestational risks	None
Family history	None
Testosterone (if yes, reason, and protocol used)	None
Any features of DSD	None

14.4 Surgical Technique

- A U-shaped incision is outlined. The 2 lateral incisions go very deep into the glans and converge distally. The left lateral incision stops at the coronal sulcus and continues distally in the prepuce at the muco-cutaneous junction and constitutes the medial border of the LABO flap. The flap is designed to have a wide base.
- The right incision is deepened starting near the coronal sulcus and the tip of the medial border is sutured to the urethral plate 2 mm proximal to the edge (A).
- The medial border of the LABO flap is sutured to the left edge of the urethral plate.
- The LABO flap is turned over catheter size F12 and the second apical suture is fixed 2 mm from the tip.
- Urethroplasty is completed using continuous subcuticular 6/0 Vicryl® suture on a cutting needle.
- A second and preferably third protective layer is employed from the penile fascia or dartos fascia from the scrotum.
- The glanular wings are approximated over catheter size F12 and the penile skin is closed (Fig. 14.1).

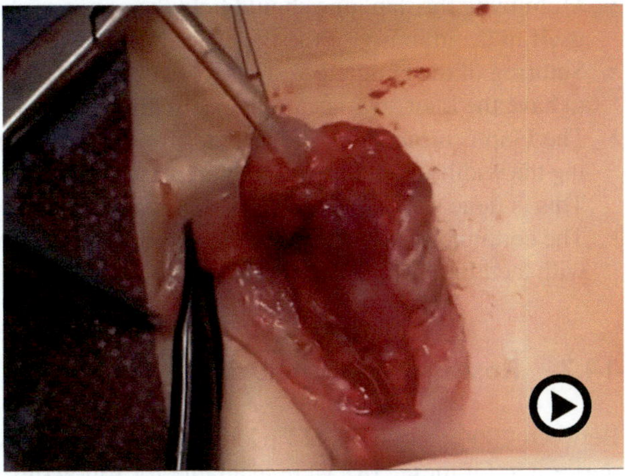

Fig. 14.1 LABO technique (https://doi.org/10.1007/000-cna)

14.5 Postoperative Care

(i) The catheter stays inserted for 7–10 days. Changes of the dressing are only performed if it becomes wet with blood or urine.
(ii) Antibiotic therapy with Cefaclor orally is continued until catheter removal.
(iii) Analgesia with Ibuprofen and Paracetamol.
(iv) Oxybutynin is given in case of bladder spasms.
(v) The follow-up schedule is after 3 months, 1 year, 3 years, and then every 2–3 years till the end of puberty.

14.6 Tips and Tricks

- The knots must not be tied too tight to avoid ischemia of the tissue.
- Instead of using a tourniquet, blood Hemostasis is better achieved by stretching the penis fixed at the tip over the left index finger and exerting dorsal pressure. This allows targeted hemostasis.
- Deep glanular incision and mobilization of the glanswings is essential for tension-free closure of the glans.
- The distal slanting of the paraurethral incision to the midline allows further mobilization of the glanswings.
- Bringing the flap 2 mm below the tip of the glans keeps the meatal edges free of sutures and further increases the diameter of the meatus.
- The V Incision from the ventral apex of the flap ensures a slit-like meatus.
- A narrow hypospadic meatus should be incised ventrally to accommodate a 12-French catheter.
- Urethroplasty over a 12-French catheter minimizes the risk of later occurring functional urethral obstruction.
- Care must be taken to elevate Buck's fascia with the flap as this constitutes the main blood supply.

- Mobilizing the flap, one should hold the opposite skin edge and not the flap skin itself to avoid injury of the flap.
- Suturing of the neourethra starts a few millimeters below the hypospadic meatus to have the knot away from the neourethra and avoid fistula.
- The Flap is turned over the catheter from left to right with two forceps, measuring the width actually required. Only then, the lateral border of the flap is incised. This is done step by step at 5–7 mm intervals.
- The continuous suturing of the neourethra is performed in a subcuticular manner with a cutting needle, which makes it easier to go through the dermis.

14.7 Results and Conclusion

Between 2004 and 2019, 214 patients were operated with the LABO technique in our center. Of these, 182 were available for follow-up. Patient age ranged between 8 months and 2 years (mean 11 months). All the patients had proximal hypospadias with flat or incomplete cleft glans and no deep chordee. Satisfactory results were achieved in 173 patients (95%). Two patients developed fistulae, four had glans dehiscence, two developed proximal diverticulum and one developed prolapsing skin outside the meatus 2 years after the urethroplasty. All complications were managed in one operation [9].

References

1. Hadidi AT. Perineal hypospadias: back to the future chordee excision & distal urethroplasty. J Pediatr Urol. 2018;14(5):424.e1–9. https://doi.org/10.1016/j.jpurol.2018.08.014. Epub 2018 Aug 23. PMID: 30297228
2. Koyanagi T, Matsuno T, Nonomura K, et al. Complete repair of severe penoscrotal hypospadias in 1 stage: experience with urethral mobilization, wing-flap-flipping urethropasty and "glanulomeato-plasty". J Urol. 1983;130:1150–4.
3. Duckett JW, Baskin LS. Hypospadias. In: Gillenwater JY, Grayback JT, Howards SS, Duckett JW, editors. Adult and pediatric urology. 3rd ed. St. Louis: Mosby-Year Book; 1996. p. 2549–89.
4. Elder JS, Duckett JW, Snyder HM. Onlay island flap in the repair of mid and distal penile hypospadias without chordee. J Urol. 1987;138:376–9.
5. Amukele SA, Weiser AC, Stock JA, et al. Results of 265 consecutive proximal hypospadias repairs using the Thiersch-Duplay principle. J Urol. 2004;172:2382–3.
6. Snodgrass W. Bush: tubularised incised plate for proximal hypospa-dias repair: continued evolution and extended application. J Ped Urol. 2011;7:2–9.
7. Snodgrass W, Cost N, Nakonezny P, et al. Analysis of risk factors for glans dehiscence after tubularised incised plate hypospadias repair. J Urol. 2011;185:1845–51.
8. Snodgrass W, Macedo A, Hoebeke P, et al. Hypospadias dilemmas: a round table. J Pediatr Surg. 2011;7:145–57.
9. Hadidi AT. Proximal hypospadias with small flat glans: the lateral-based onlay (LABO) flap technique. In: Hadidi AT, editor. Hypospadias surgery: an illustrated textbook. Cham: Springer; 2022. p. 237–48.
10. Hadidi AT. Proximal hypospadias with small flat glans: the lateral based onlay (LABO) flap technique: J Pediatr Surg. 2012;47:2151–7.

Combined Buccal Mucosa Graft (Watch Shape) with Onlay Skin Flap for Severe Hypospadias: One-Stage Repair

15

Marko Bencic, Borko Stojanovic, Abhishek Bhalerao, Marta Bizic, and Miroslav L. Djordjevic

Abstract

Severe hypospadias repair includes one-stage or two-stage reconstruction, depending on several hypospadiac parameters as well as surgeon's preference. Penile and glans size, degree of curvature, urethral plate development, and availability of penile skin dictate the surgical approach. One-stage procedures have the advantage of correcting all deformities and complete reconstruction in one surgery, where possible. We previously published technique using buccal mucosa graft combined with longitudinal island skin flap for one-stage severe hypospadias repair. However, in most severe cases transection of urethral plate does not lead to complete penile straightening. In those cases, additional correction of curvature is required. Mobilization of neurovascular bundle would compromise glans vascularization, and dorsal plication would additionally shorten the penis. That is why ventral grafting presents more suitable option, as a lengthening procedure. There are several options for grafting material, and we presumed that buccal mucosa graft could be specially fashioned to be used for grafting, and

---

Supplementary Information The online version contains supplementary material available at https://doi.org/10.1007/978-981-99-0795-3_15. The videos can be accessed individually by clicking the DOI link in the accompanying figure caption or by scanning this link with the SN More Media App.

M. Bencic · B. Stojanovic · M. Bizic · M. L. Djordjevic (✉)
School of Medicine, Department of Urology, University of Belgrade, Belgrade, Serbia

Belgrade Center for Urogenital Reconstructive Surgery, Belgrade, Serbia
e-mail: bencic@uromiros.com; stojanovic@uromiros.com; martabizic@uromiros.com; djordjevic@uromiros.com

A. Bhalerao
Belgrade Center for Urogenital Reconstructive Surgery, Belgrade, Serbia

T. O. Abbas (ed.), *Video Atlas of Hypospadias Surgery*,
https://doi.org/10.1007/978-981-99-0795-3_15

simultaneously for urethral plate creation as well, in selected cases. Urethroplasty is finalized with previously described dorsal longitudinal island skin flap, buttonholed on the ventral side.

Keywords

Hypospadias · Curvature · Buccal mucosa graft · Urethroplasty · Longitudinal island skin flap

15.1 Introduction

Hypospadias presents one of the most frequent congenital anomalies of male external genitalia and still presents a great challenge in research for the most suitable technique. Distal hypospadias repair currently presents a straightforward reconstruction with low rate of complications. In contrast to the distal forms, the optimal treatment of severe hypospadias is still controversial, and it is still debated whether to use single or staged repair [1–5]. The surgical goals remain – straight penis with appropriate length, good cosmetic outcome, voiding on the top with acceptable rate of complications. Two-stage repair is based on the initial correction of ventral curvature with creation of new urethral plate using preputial/penile skin flap or buccal mucosa graft, followed by urethroplasty in the second stage [6–8]. On the other side, one-stage surgery is challenging due to the lack of available tissue for reconstruction, especially in most severe cases. We present a one-stage technique for scrotal hypospadias repair, which is based on using a specially shaped buccal mucosa graft for simultaneous ventral tunica grafting and new urethral plate creation, in combination with longitudinal dorsal island skin flap [9].

15.2 Indications

(a) Proximal hypospadias (penoscrotal, scrotal).
(b) Severe ventral curvature (more than 70°), and significant curvature (more than 30°) after urethral plate transection.
(c) Short and fibrotic urethral plate.
(d) Small, clitoriform penis (Fig. 15.1).

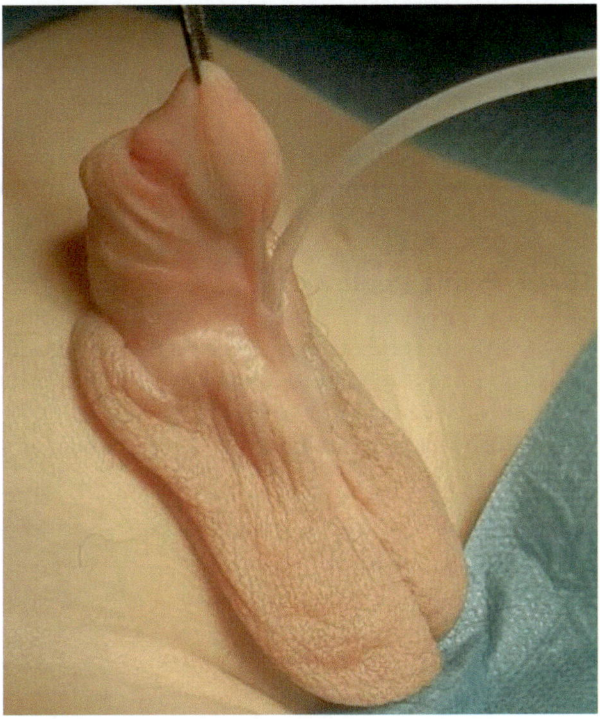

Fig. 15.1 Severe hypospadias with penoscrotal transposition. Short urethral plate with severe chordee is evident

15.3 Video Demonstration

Factors	Findings
Age at surgery (months)	32
Gestational age (weeks)	39
Birth weight (g)	3300
Gestational risk	None
Family history	None
Testosterone	Topical dihydrotestosterone, two times per day, starting six weeks before surgery, for the period of four weeks.
Any features of DSD	None

15.4 Steps of the Procedure

15.4.1 Suprapubic Catheter

- A 6Fr Nelaton catheter is introduced, and bladder is filled with saline. Suprapubic tube 9Fr is placed into the bladder and fixed to the skin with 3-0 Nylon suture.

15.4.2 Penile Degloving

- A 4-0 Vycril stay suture is placed on the dorsal side of the glans, in the midline.
- Incision lines are marked around hypospadiac meatus, along the urethral plate towards the coronal level (Fig. 15.2).
- Incision is made ventrally in a U-shaped fashion.

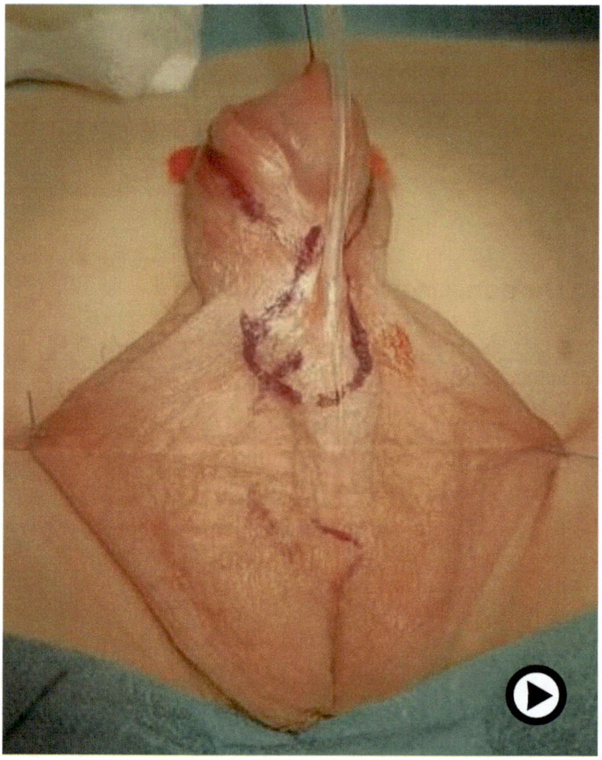

Fig. 15.2 Incised lines are marked. Catheter is placed in hypospadic meatus. Scrotum is spread for better exposure. Watch procedure (https://doi.org/10.1007/000-cnb)

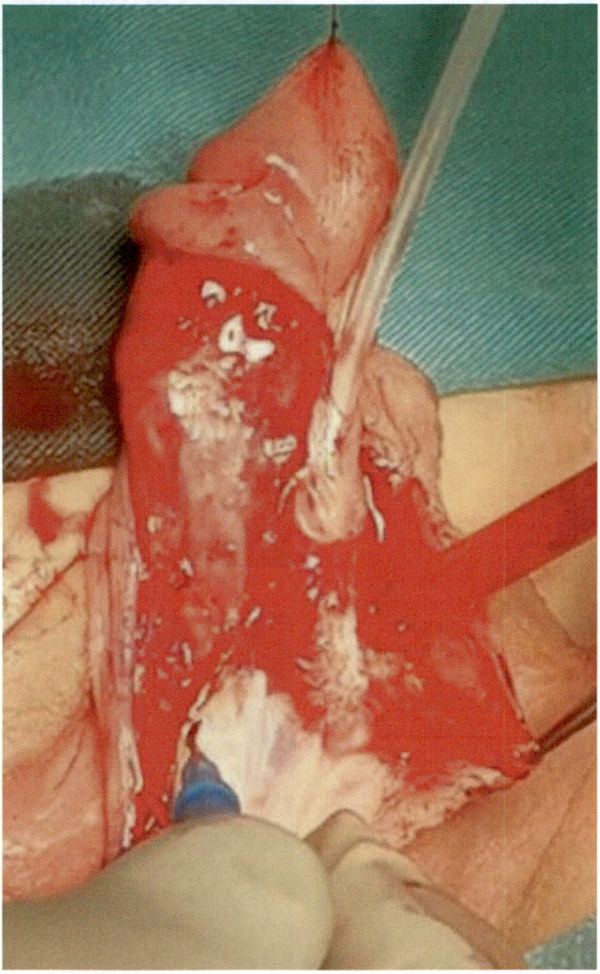

Fig. 15.3 Penile skin is completely dissected just above Buck's fascia layer. Proximal dissection is important to maximally release the penile shaft from fibrotic tissue

- Meticulous dissection around divergent spongiosal tissue is performed to avoid injury and excessive bleeding (Fig. 15.3).
- After complete degloving, artificial erection showed severe curvature with fibrotic and short urethral plate (Fig. 15.4). Insufficient ventral penile skin is obvious.

15.4.3 Urethral Plate Dissection

- Urethral plate is infiltrated with prepared solution of 0.25% bupivacaine in 1:100.000 epinephrine.

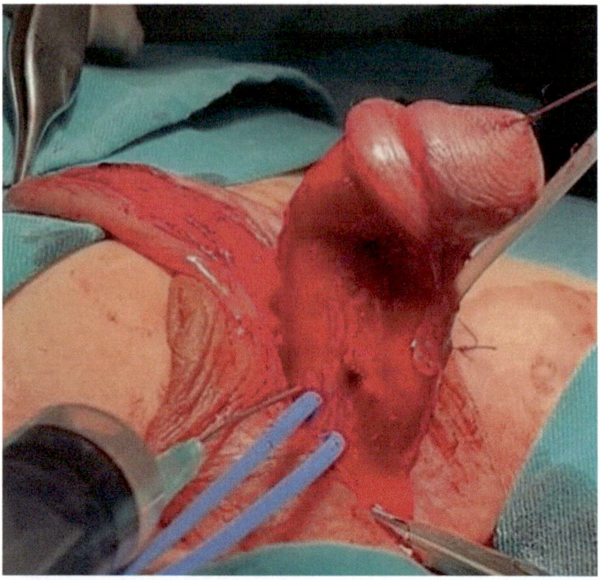

Fig. 15.4 Artificial erection confirmed severe penile curvature with fibrotic short urethral plate

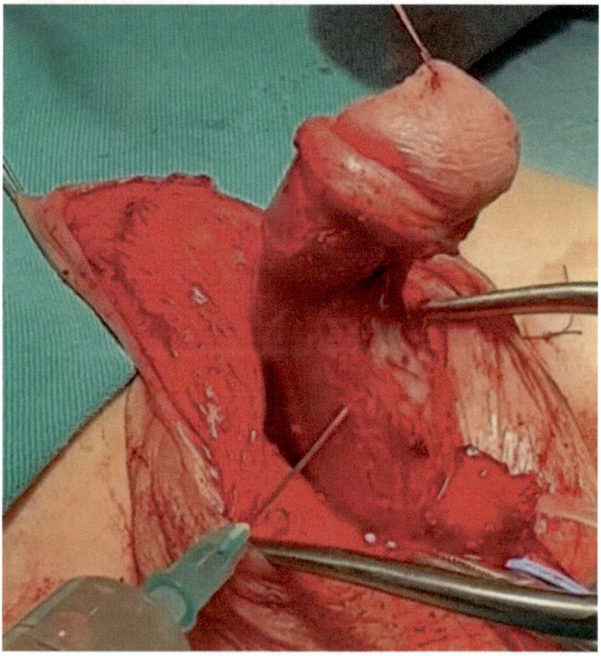

Fig. 15.5 Artificial erection after urethral plate division and urethral mobilization revealed remaining curvature of more than 30°

- The short urethral plate is divided, and unhealthy fibrotic tissue is radically excised distally, to the coronal level. Urethra is fully mobilized to the pre-bulbar level to achieve maximal penile length. In this way, penile shaft is completely released from fibrotic tissue and skin chordee (Fig. 15.5).

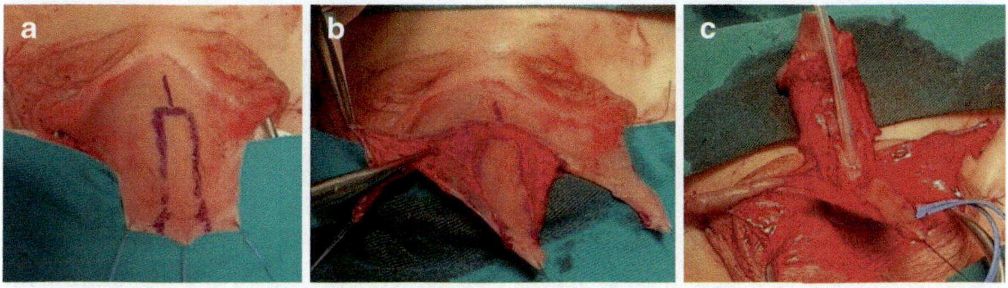

Fig. 15.6 (**a**) Longitudinal dorsal island skin flap is marked at the dorsal distal penile skin. (**b**) Mobilization of the flaps. (**c**) Longitudinal island skin flap is button-holed ventrally. Two lateral flaps will be used for penile shaft covering

15.4.4 Preparation of Longitudinal Dorsal Island Skin Flap

- Longitudinal island skin flap is designed on the dorsal penile skin.
- Meticulous sharp dissection is performed to avoid injury of the flap pedicle.
- Three well vascularized flaps are created from the dorsal penile skin: longitudinal island skin flap for urethroplasty, and two lateral flaps for penile skin reconstruction.
- Button-hole maneuver is used to transpose the longitudinal flap to the ventral side (Fig. 15.6).

15.4.5 Buccal Mucosa Harvesting

- The buccal mucosa graft is harvested from the left inner cheek, which is exposed using two stay sutures for the upper and lower lip.
- The external orifice of the parotid gland is marked, as well as incision lines.
- The length of the graft depends on the distance between the tip of the glans and the urethral meatus, while the width is 8–10 mm.
- The submucosa of the graft area is infiltrated with a solution of 0.25% bupivacaine in 1:200000 epinephrine for bleeding control.
- The graft is harvested using sharp dissection, with special care to preserve the integrity of the buccinator muscle and the underlying branches of the facial nerves.
- The donor site is carefully examined for bleeding and closed with a running suture 4-0 Vicryl. The mucosal graft is defatted and ready to use [10, 11].

15.5 Correction of Ventral Curvature with Simultaneous Urethral Plate Creation

- The point of maximal curvature on the ventral side is determined. Ventral grafting procedure is indicated to straighten the penis. In this way, mobilization of the neurovascular bundle and shortening of the penis are avoided.

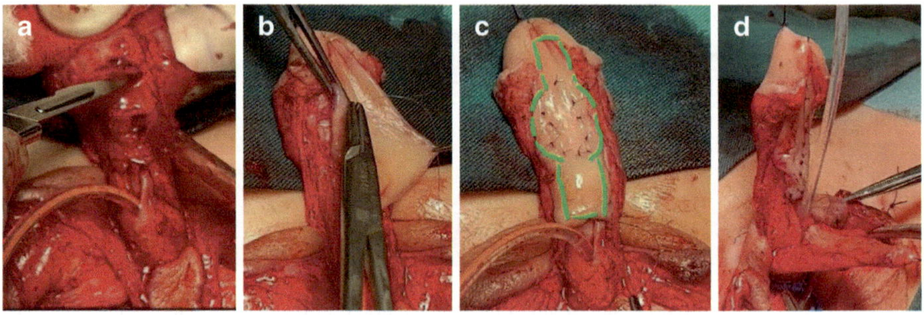

Fig. 15.7 (**a**) Tunica albuginea is opened, with edges additionally dissected from cavernosal sinusoids. (**b**) Graft is joined to tunica margin. (**c**) Defect of tunica albuginea is covered with spherical part of watch-shaped buccal mucosa graft. (**d**) Penis is completely straightened with newly formed urethral plate

- H-shaped incision of both tunica albuginea layers is performed. Additional careful mobilization of tunica edges from underlying erectile tissue is done to achieve proper suture site for buccal mucosa graft. Meticulous incision is done to avoid injury of corporal vascular structure.
- Previously harvested buccal mucosa graft is defatted and specially designed in a "watch shape" manner. The spherical part in the middle and two rectangular parts extending to opposite sides are created. The size of the graft and its parts depends on the position of tunical defect.
- The graft is joined proximally and distally to form the new urethral plate, and simultaneously straightening the penis by covering the defect of tunica albuginea.
- Spherical part of buccal mucosa graft is fixed to the edges of tunica albuginea using eight U-shaped interrupted sutures of Monocryl 6-0 (Fig. 15.7).

15.5.1 Urethroplasty

- A well-vascularized longitudinal island skin flap is button-holed ventrally and sutured to the edges of the buccal mucosa. Proximal edges are joined initially in order to form a funnel anastomosis, and continued distally by one-layer running suture, Monocryl 6-0, in a tension-free manner over a 6Fr silicone Foley catheter (Fig. 15.8).
- The catheter is left in place as a urethral stent and used for postoperative wetting of the buccal graft.
- Abundant pedicle of the flap is fixed laterally to Buck's fascia layer with interrupted Monocryl 6-0 sutures to cover all suture lines of the neourethra, preventing fistula formation.

15.5.2 Glansplasty

- The glans is opened in the midline to the tip of the future meatus, creating glans wings. The graft is gently stretched distally with its suture lines on the corpora.

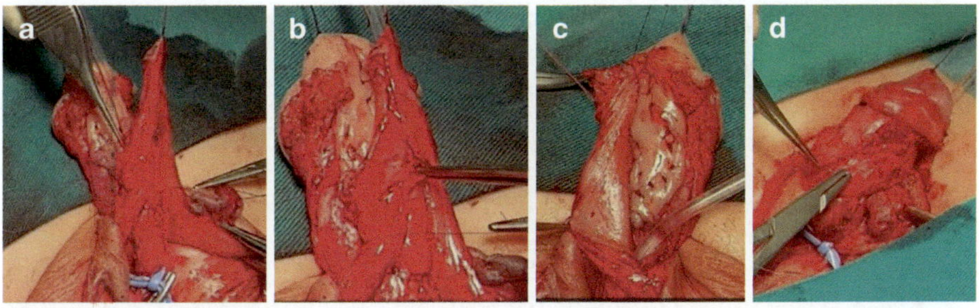

Fig. 15.8 (**a**) Well-vascularized longitudinal island skin flap is prepared for anastomosis. (**b**) Margin of the flap is joined with buccal mucosa graft with running suture. (**c**) Tension-free urethroplasty is done to create wide urethra. (**d**) Flap pedicle is spread and fixed laterally

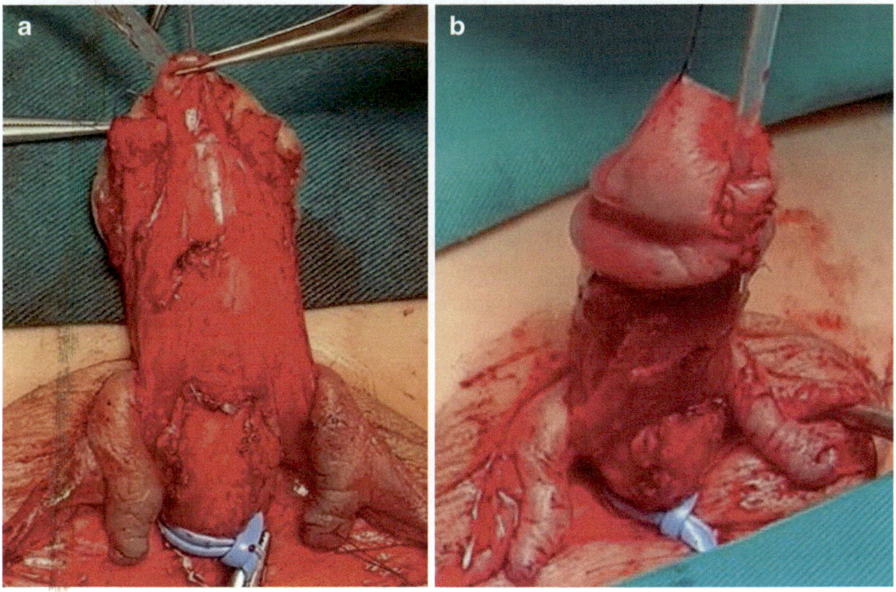

Fig. 15.9 (**a**) Abundant vascular pedicle covers neourethra and all suture lines. (**b**) Final appearance after glansplasty

- The distal portion of the graft is fixed to the tip of the glans, with Monocryl 6-0.
- Distal part of longitudinal skin flap is joined with distal part of the graft to form glandial neourethra and neomeatus, over a Foley catheter 6Fr.
- Glans wings are joined with one interrupted suture Monocryl 6-0, to form the corona. The most distal part of longitudinal island skin flap is fashioned as a double-faced flap and lateral edges are joined with glans wings with interrupted sutures for glans augmentation. In this way, conically shaped glans is created (Fig. 15.9).
- Glansplasty is performed with 6-0 Monocryl interrupted sutures.

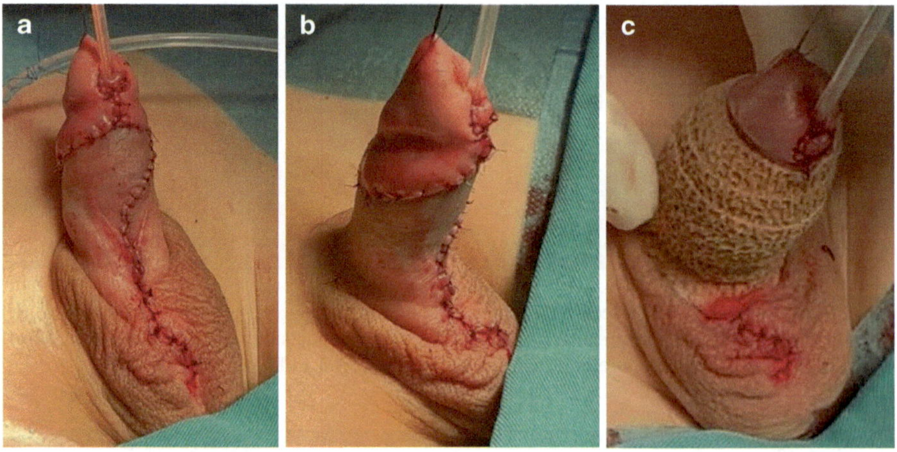

Fig. 15.10 (**a**) Result after surgery—ventral view. (**b**) Result after surgery—lateral view. (**c**) Coban dressing is placed

15.5.3 Penile Skin Reconstruction

- Penoscrotal angle is created. The penile shaft is reconstructed using two well-vascularized lateral skin flaps, with interrupted sutures Monocryl 6-0.
- The penis is coated with a thin gauze and Coban® elastic-adhesive bandage (Fig. 15.10).

15.6 Post-operative Care

- The Coban dressing is replaced on the third postoperative day and removed seven days after surgery.
- Urinary indwelling catheter is removed seven days after surgery.
- The suprapubic urinary catheter is removed two weeks after surgery.
- Antibiotic prophylaxis is prescribed while the suprapubic catheter is in place.

15.7 Tips and Tricks

- During degloving, use electrocautery to release penile shaft from fibrotic chordee, without injuring spongiosal body. Use sharp scissors to dissect penile skin from urethral meatus.
- After degloving, release the base of the penis ventrally from prescrotal adipose tissue.
- Use scalpel for precise opening of the tunica albuginea ventrally, and release edges for graft fixation.

- Preserve all blood supply when creating hole on the base of the longitudinal skin flap.
- Remove the most distal part of the skin (1 mm) when creating double-faced flap.
- Use skin flaps for penile skin reconstruction, with special care to avoid rotation of the penile shaft.

15.8 Results and Conclusion

In the period between July 2014 and December 2021, this technique is performed in 42 patients (aged from 10 to 24 months) with proximal hypospadias. Good outcome was achieved in 30 boys (83%). Urethral fistula occurred in 5 cases (12%) and was solved by minor repair. Meatal stenosis in 2 cases (4.5%) was successfully treated by temporary meatal dilatation. Straight penis was achieved in all cases based on vacuum device checking and parents' reports.

This one-stage repair of severe hypospadias has good outcome, with acceptable rate of complications [12, 13].

References

1. Gong EM, Cheng EY. Current challenges with proximal hypospadias: we have a long way to go. J Pediatr Urol. 2017;13:457–67.
2. Tijani KH, Idiodi-Thomas HO, Elebute OA, Alakaloko FM, Ojewola RW, Ademuyiwa AO. Two-stage flap repair of severe hypospadias: usefulness of the tubularized incised plate urethroplasty. J Pediatr Urol. 2017;13:483.e1–5.
3. Bracka A. Hypospadias repair: the two stage alternative. Br J Urol. 1995;76:31–41.
4. Hensle TW, Kearney MC, Bingham JB. Buccal mucosa grafts for hypospadias surgery: long-term results. J Urol. 2002;168:1734–6.
5. Wu Y, Guan Y, Wang X, Wang C, Ma X, Guan H. Repair of proximal hypospadias with single-stage (Duckett's method) or Bracka two-stage: a retrospective comparative cohort study. Transl Pediatr. 2023;12(3):387–95.
6. AbouZeid AA, Medhat Shahin AE, Elsadek M, Dahab MM, Amra HS, Shokry SS. Urethral plate substitution in two-stage hypospadias repair: grafts versus flaps. J Pediatr Surg. 2023;58(10):2027–33.
7. Castellan M, Gosalbez R, Devendra J, Bar-Yosef Y, Labbie A. Ventral corporal body grafting for correcting severe penile curvature associated with single or two-stage hypospadias repair. J Pediatr Urol. 2011;7:289–93.
8. Hayashi Y, Kojima Y, Mizuno K, Nakane A, Kato T, Kurokawa S, Kamisawa H, Maruyama T, Kohri K. Demonstration of postoperative effectiveness in ventral lengthening using a tunica vaginalis flap for severe penile curvature with hypospadias. Urology. 2010;76:101–6.
9. Djordjevic ML, Majstorovic M, Stanojevic D, Bizic M, Kojovic V, Vukadinovic V, Korac G, Krstic Z, Perovic SV. Combined buccal mucosa graft and dorsal penile skin flap for repair of severe hypospadias. Urology. 2008;71:821–5.
10. Markiewicz MR, Margarone JE III, Barbagli G, Scaannapieco FA. Oral mucosa harvest: an overview of anatomic and biologic considerations. EAU-EBU Update Ser. 2007;5:179–87.
11. Dubey D, Kumar A, Mandhani A, Srivastava A, Kapoor R, Bhandari M. Buccal mucosa urethroplasty: a versatile technique for all urethral segments. BJU Int. 2005;95:625–9.

12. Djordjevic ML, Stojanovic B, Agrawal K. Hypospadias. In: Agrawal K, Mahajan RK, editors. Textbook of plastic, reconstructive, and aesthetic surgery volume IV: reconstruction of trunk, genitalia, lower limb, and maxillofacial trauma. Noida: Thieme Medical and Scientific Publishers Pvt. Ltd; 2019. p. 167–92.
13. Djordjevic ML, Bizic M, Stojanovic B, Bencic M, Kojovic V, Korac G. Buccal mucosa graft for simultaneous correction of severe chordee and urethroplasty as a one-stage repair of scrotal hypospadias (watch technique). World J Urol. 2019;37(4):613–8.

Koyanagi Procedure

16

Valeska Bidault, Daniela Gorduza, Delphine Demede, and Pierre Mouriquand

Abstract

Perineal hypospadias represents the most severe form of proximal hypospadias, posing significant challenges in surgical repair due to its complex anatomical features. Various surgical approaches have been devised with the aim of restoring normal penile function and achieving satisfactory cosmesis. These techniques primarily focus on either preserving the urethral plate or transecting it. Despite numerous attempts, existing surgical methods have demonstrated a notable incidence of complications and the need for redo surgeries. Koyanagi's pioneering one-stage urethroplasty with parameatal foreskin flap, initially introduced in 1983, showed promising initial outcomes but encountered higher-than-expected complication rates upon further evaluation. Nonetheless, the Koyanagi technique remains a viable option for addressing severe hypospadias in experienced hands. This abstract outlines our center's approach to the Koyanagi technique, detailing procedural steps, invaluable insights, and our center's outcomes, contributing to the ongoing discourse on hypospadias repair strategies.

Supplementary Information The online version contains supplementary material available at https://doi.org/10.1007/978-981-99-0795-3_16. The videos can be accessed individually by clicking the DOI link in the accompanying figure caption or by scanning this link with the SN More Media App.

V. Bidault (✉) · D. Demede · P. Mouriquand
Paediatric Surgery and Urology Department, Centre for Rare Diseases of Genital Development From Fetus to Adulthood, Université Claude Bernard Lyon 1, Hospices Civils de Lyon, Hôpital Femme Mère Enfant, Lyon, France
e-mail: valeska.bidault@chu-lyon.fr; delphine.demede@chu-lyon.fr

D. Gorduza
Paediatric Surgery Department, Centre Hospitalo-universitaire de Saint-Etienne, Hôpital Nord, Saint-Etienne, France
e-mail: daniela.gorduza@chu-st-etienne.fr

T. O. Abbas (ed.), *Video Atlas of Hypospadias Surgery*,
https://doi.org/10.1007/978-981-99-0795-3_16

Keywords

Perineal hypospadias · Urethroplasty · Koyanagi technique · Surgical outcomes

Key Points

- Perineal hypospadias results from marked hypoplasia of ventral tissues of the penis, that compels the surgeon to transect the urethral plate in order to achieve complete straightening of the penile shaft before reconstruction of the urethra.
- The Koyanagi technique, in its original version or with Hayashi modification, provides the ventral aspect of the penis with well-vascularized parameatal foreskin flap in order to reconstruct the transected urethra in a single-step procedure.
- Precise drawing of incisions, careful dissection, and ventral transposition of the foreskin flap with its vascular pedicle and quilting of the neo-urethra to the corpus cavernosa ensure the surgeon of the best surgical outcomes.
- Complication rate remains high (75%) but similar to other techniques used for proximal hypospadias (Cloutier-Bracka 2-step procedure, Duckett Island Flap). Glans dehiscence, fistula, urethral stricture, and urethrocele represent the most frequent complications.
- Overall satisfactory result occurs in 2/3 of cases after Koyanagi and eventual re-do surgeries. Parents should be aware that most cases require at least 2 operations.

16.1 Introduction

The perineal hypospadias is the most severe form of proximal hypospadias and the most challenging to repair. It is defined as a development arrest of the genital tubercle with a proximal division of the corpus spongiosum and a marked hypoplasia of the tissues forming the ventral aspect of the penis, usually associated with an important ventral curvature [1] (Fig. 16.1). Many surgical techniques have been described for perineal hypospadias trying to achieve normal penile functions and good cosmesis. The principle of these techniques is related to the possibility of preserving the urethral plate (Onlay, long Tirsch-Duplay or TIP) or transecting the urethral plate (Koyanagi, Duckett Island flap or 2 stages repair with Bracka procedure). Unfortunately, all the surgical techniques showed a high rate of complications and redo surgeries [2–10].

The one-stage urethroplasty with parameatal foreskin flap was first described by Koyanagi in 1983 [11], with promising preliminary results. With time, this technique started to gain popularity among pediatric urologists. The authors tried to generalize the technique for all forms of hypospadias [12]. Few modifications were described [13–18]. The technique revealed a high rate of complications, higher than previously stated although few studies evaluated the outcome on a long-term basis.

Nevertheless, the use of Koyanagi technique is an option for the most severe forms of hypospadias with a reasonable success rate in experimented hands. We describe our technique with its steps, our tips and tricks, and outcomes in our center.

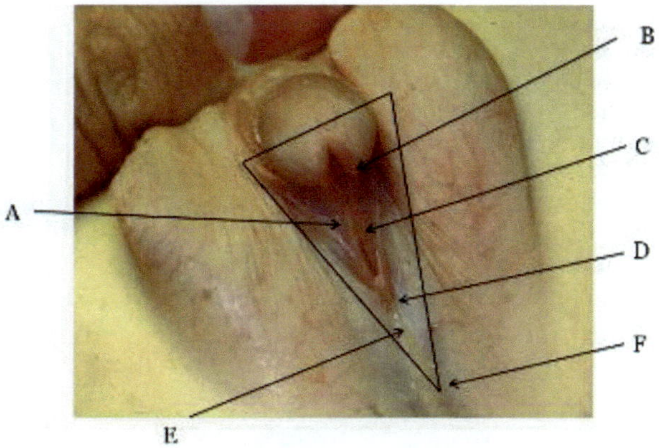

Fig. 16.1 Ventral triangular defect in severe proximal hypospadias: proximal hypospadias is caused by a developmental arrest of the tissues forming the ventral aspect of the genital tubercle, responsible for severe hypoplasia of ventral tissues (**a**) with open glans (**b**), small hypoplastic urethral plate (**c**) and various degrees of chordee. The ventral triangular defect characterizes hypospadias with: at the tip of the triangle the division of the corpus spongiosum (**f**), and on each side the pillars of the spongiosum that will join the basis of the open glans (**b**). The urethral meatus (**d**), located downstream the division of the corpus spongiosum (**f**) with a part of thin urethra not surrounded by corpus spongiosum (**e**) is indeed not a good criterion to define hypospadias severity

16.2 Indications

All proximal hypospadias that require transection of the urethral plate (no preservable urethral plate) are eligible to Koyanagi repair. The Koyanagi procedure is a one-stage procedure aiming at straightening the penis; reconstructing the defective urethra with well-vascularized tissues mobilized from the ventral, lateral, and dorsal aspects of the genital tubercle with their blood supply; refashioning the skin around the genital pedicle. Koyanagi urethroplasty provides enough well-vascularized tissues to build a large urethral tube without spoiling skin covering of the penis, even in case of severe hypoplasia of preputial skin. It appears thus a valuable alternative to two-stage procedures [19] (Cloutier-Bracka urethroplasty). It also avoids circular urethral anastomosis, which are known to be source of specific complications in long-term hypospadias follow-up (stenosis, urine dribbling, urethrocele).

To confirm whether the urethral plate could be preserved or not, a simple test can be done, consisting in laying the penis on the abdomen of the child. If it cannot lay flat on the abdomen, and keeps on twisting back and forth, what we call "jerk movement" of the genital tubercle, it indicates that the urethral plate is too short and has to be transected to straighten the shaft of the penis (Fig. 16.2). In these cases, Koyanagi technique is a valuable choice, and our preferred technique for penile reconstruction.

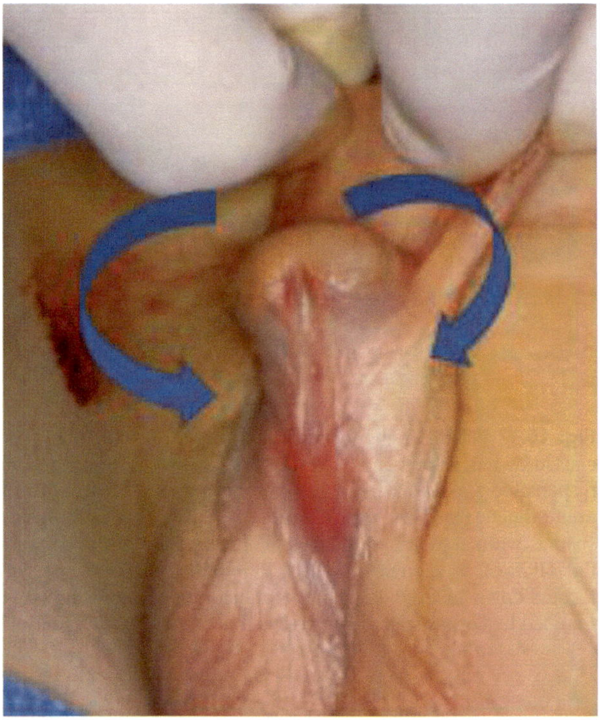

Fig. 16.2 Jerk movement of the genital tubercle: when the penis is lifted up, it cannot lay flat on the anterior abdominal wall, and twists on each side and the other

16.3 Steps of the Procedure

16.3.1 Incision Lines

Under general anesthesia and a caudal bloc, incision lines are drawn around the glans and at the junction between foreskin and dorsal penile skin (Fig. 16.3).

16.3.2 Mobilization of Tissues for Urethroplasty

Secondarily, the ventral, lateral, and dorsal tissues of the penis are mobilized with their blood supply (Fig. 16.4).

Then, a coronal circumferential incision is realized with transection of urethral plate just below the glans (Fig. 16.5). The urethral plate is lifted and detached from the ventral aspect of the penis. The hypoplastic fibrous tissue (dysplastic spongiosum) sitting on the ventral aspect of the corpora is removed which permits to achieve a straight penis in most cases and stops the "jerk" movement of the penis which then can lay still without rotation.

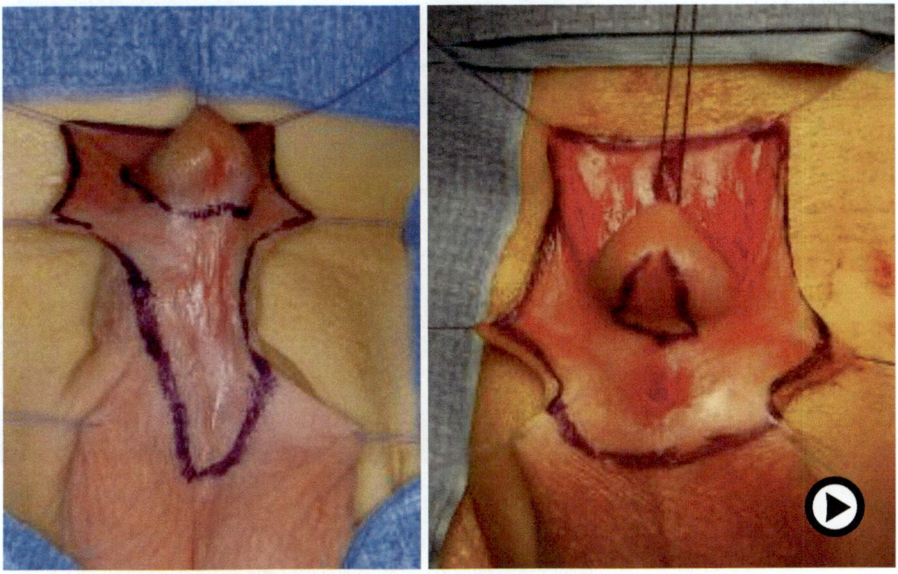

Fig. 16.3 Incision lines. At the base of the glans, a circumcision incision is drawn (left). Glans wings will be separated on the midline of its ventral aspect (right). Koyanagi procedure (https://doi.org/10.1007/000-cnc)

After a full mobilization down to the base of the genital tubercle of the ventral, lateral, and dorsal penile tissues with their blood supply, an artificial erection test is performed and, if the curvature persisted, a dorsal plication (Nesbitt or Tunica Albuginea Plication (TAP)) is performed (Fig. 16.6). All this dissection part is made without any tourniquet around the penis, as the dissection starts way back into the perineal area and does not allow the positioning of the tourniquet proximal enough to reduce the blood loss.

16.3.3 Transfer of the Tissues to the Ventral Aspect of the Genital Tubercle and Positioning of the Neo-urethra

After tissue mobilization, a vertical buttonhole is created through the dorsal pedicle to transfer all tissues ventrally (Fig. 16.7). The dorsal part of the graft can either be divided along the midline (Koyanagi) or left intact like a bridge joining the 2 lateral grafts (Hayashi). A theoretical advantage of this technical variation would be to allow a better blood supply of the distal segment of the graft. The neo-urethral plate is then refashioned suturing together the medial edge of each lateral skin flaps using interrupted 7/0 PDS stitches (Fig. 16.8).

The neo-urethral plate is also tacked down ("quilting") onto the ventral aspect of the corpora cavernosa to avoid prolapse of the reconstructed urethra.

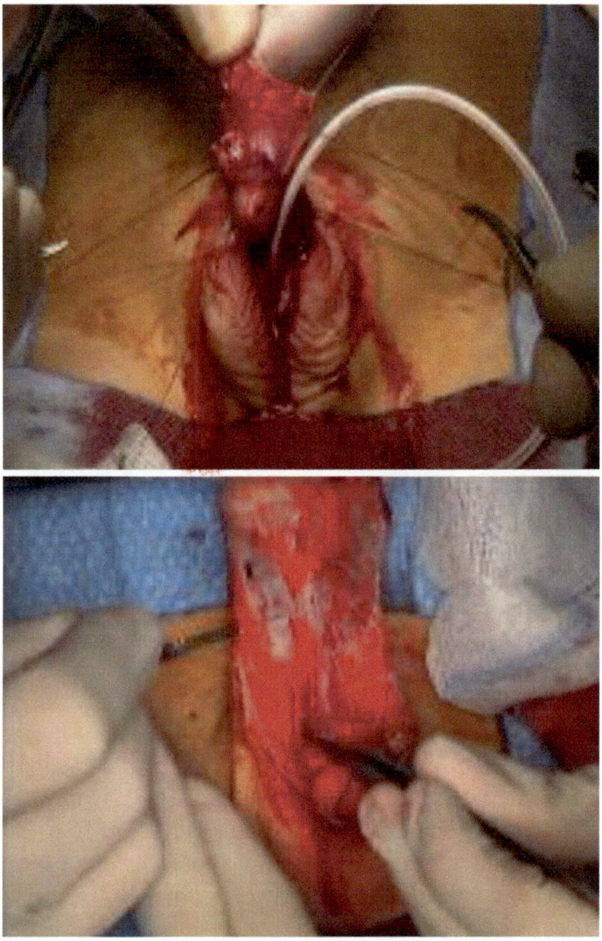

Fig. 16.4 Mobilization of ventral (upper), and dorsal (lower) tissues of the genital tubercle

16.3.4 Urethral Plate Tubularization and Penile Skin Covering

Once the urethral plate is reconstituted up the Glans sulcus (corona), it is tubularized in a Duplay fashion around a size 8 Fr silastic bladder catheter which will be left in place for at least 10 days. Proximal spongioplasty can be then performed when enough corpus spongiosum is available around the native urethra, covering the native meatus and the proximal part of the urethroplasty, while the rest of the neo-urethra is covered with vascular pedicles of the foreskin flaps and approximated on the ventral midline. Most surgeons prefer to leave the neomeatus at the base of the glans as the glans crossing can significantly increase the urethral voiding pressures and subsequently dilate the penile neourethra (urethrocele). If this option is used, the glans wings are left apart, and the penis covered with the remaining skin (Fig. 16.9).

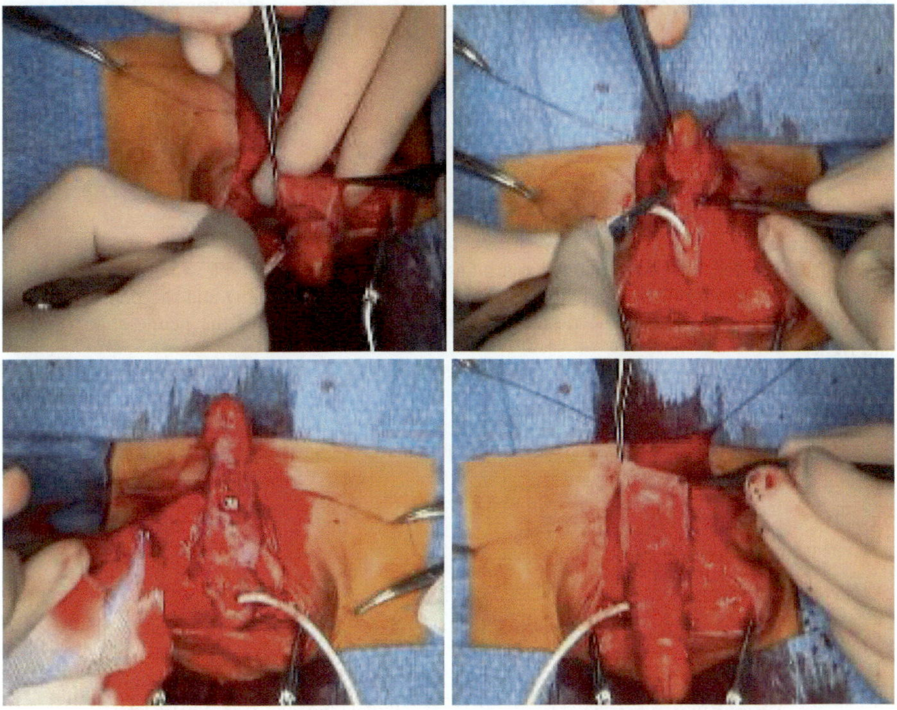

Fig. 16.5 Circumcision (up left) and urethral plate incision (up right) with total mobilization of the tissues at the base of the genital tubercle (down)

Fig. 16.6 Erection test

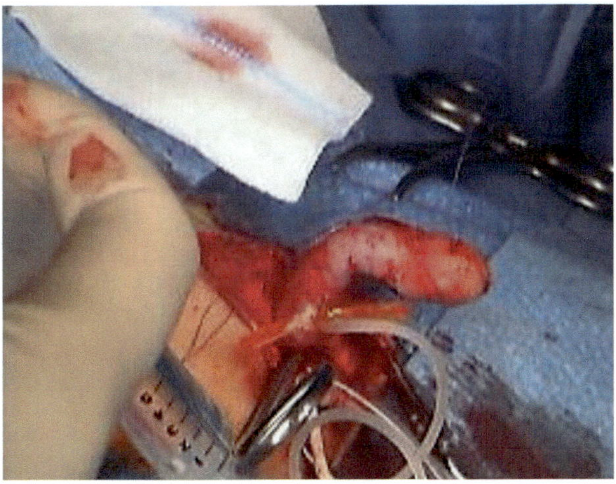

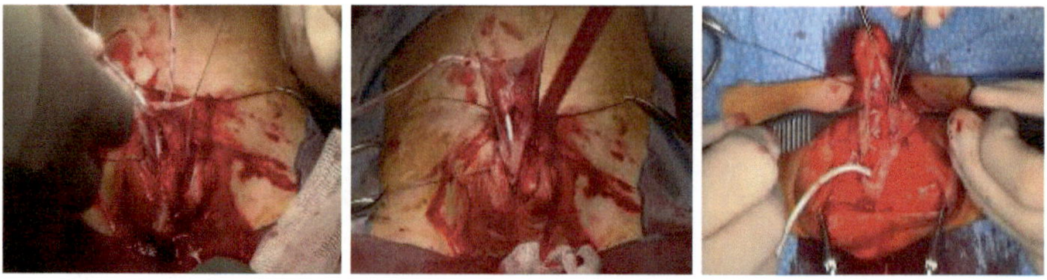

Fig. 16.7 Transfer of all tissues to the ventral aspect of the genital tubercle: a buttonhole incision is made in the middle of the pedicle of the dorsal preputial graft (left) and the penis is passed through this hole to transfer the tissue graft on the ventral aspect of the penile shaft (middle and right)

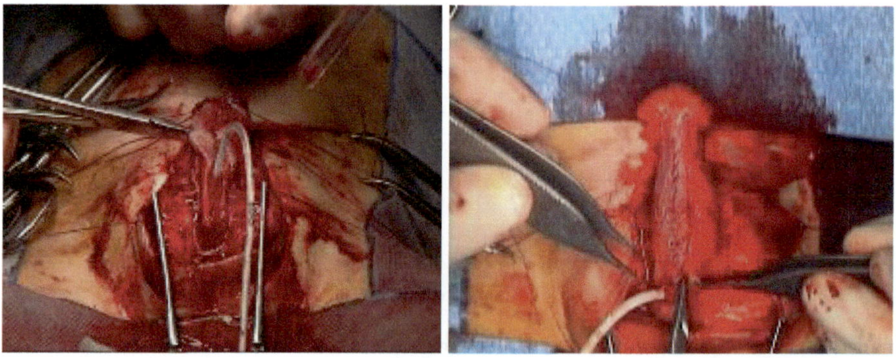

Fig. 16.8 Suturing the lateral flaps of the graft (left) together to reconstitute the urethral plate (right)

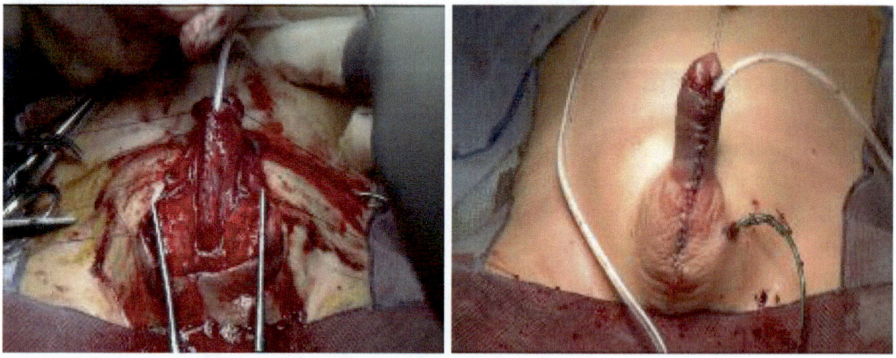

Fig. 16.9 Tubularizing urethroplasty (left) and final aspect after skin covering (right)

A daisy dressing is then applied around the penis, using hyaluronic acid and silver sulfadiazine cream, silicon tulle dressing, elastic bandage, and daisy-shaped divided elastic adhesive tape (Elastoplast ™). The urethral catheter is secured by a transglanular non-resorbable suture (Fig. 16.10).

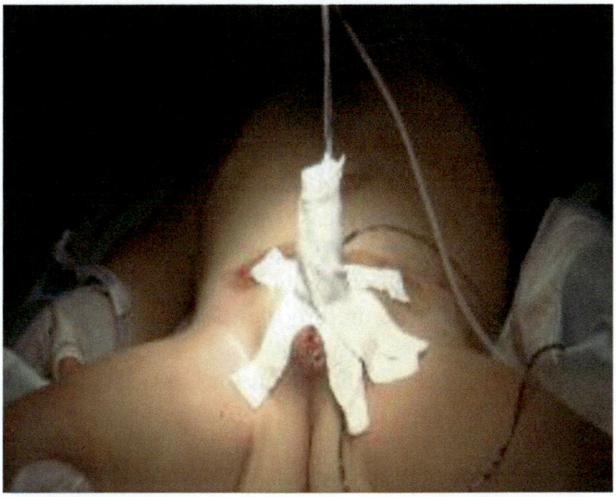

Fig. 16.10 Daisy dressing

Post-operative protocol: The patient is usually discharged 2 or 3 days after surgery. The urethral stent and the dressing are removed usually at day 10 to 14 post-operatively. A suprapubic catheter is often placed to secure the bladder drainage, particularly if the urethral meatus is initially located in the scrotal area. Oxybutinin and antibiotic prophylaxis (trimethoprim/sulfamethoxazole) are prescribed until removal of the urinary catheter.

Regarding follow-up, the patients are seen 2 to 4 months after surgery then, 1 year and at puberty. Most are seen more often due to potential complications.

16.4 Step-by-Step Video of the Procedure

16.4.1 Tips and Tricks

Koyanagi procedure can be easily standardized, and some steps are mandatory to obtain satisfactory postoperative results, as shown in the video above. To summarize, here are some advices we think may help pediatric urologists master this technique, regardless of initial severity of perineal hypospadias.

- Draw precisely incision lines to ensure that you cover all the available tissues for further urethral reconstruction.
- Develop large vascular pedicles for foreskin flaps while mobilizating ventral, lateral, and dorsal preputial tissues.
- Section the urethral plate to straighten the penis, perform artificial erection test, and add dorsal plication if needed.
- Create a vertical midline button hole in the vascular pedicle of the graft to transfer tissues toward the ventral aspect of the penis to prevent harming of the blood supply.
- Do not use any tourniquet during this surgery, as dissection will be conducted down to the perineum to mobilize all the tissues.

- Suture medial edges of the lateral skin flaps with interrupted stitches of 7/0 PDS and quilt the reconstituted urethral plate onto the corpus cavernosa to prevent further prolapse of neo-urethra, then tubularize it around a size 8 catheter using the same suture material.
- Cover the neo-urethra by spongioplasty on the proximal segment and by suturing vascular pedicle around it, and use the remaining skin to cover the penis.
- To avoid pressure increase into the neo-urethra through the glans crossing of the distal urethroplasty, leave the neo-meatus at the base of the glans and suture the distal end of the neo-urethral plate to the edges of each glans wing. This will decrease further urethrocele development and urethral ballooning during micturition.
- Leave a silastic urethral stent for a few days, and a daisy dressing to complete hemostasis.

16.5 Results and Conclusion

During 14 years, 91 patients with proximal hypospadias underwent Koyanagi urethroplasty in our center by expert senior surgeons.

The mean age at surgery was 21.4 months (9–132 months). Of 86 patients with a mean follow-up of 6 years (12–177 months) (5 loss of follow-up), 31 (36%) required a complementary dorsal plication.

Twenty-one patients (24%) had a satisfactory outcome with only one procedure, straight penis, apical or glanular meatus, no urinary problem and adequate cosmetic aspect. Sixty-six patients (76%) had complication after the initial reconstruction. The most common complication encountered was dehiscence of the urethroplasty (51 patients out of 86 (59.3%)). Ten patients encountered urethrocutaneous fistula (11.6%) and 11 patients urethral stenosis (12.7%), with 4 urethral diverticulum or urethrocele.

Of 63 patients who underwent a second procedure, 29 required further surgical attention due mostly to stenosis of the reconstructed urethra.

Twenty patients (23%) required 3 or more procedures. Average number of surgeries per patient in this series was 2.3.

Regarding overall satisfaction, 55 over 86 patients (63.95%) had satisfactory result after the last operation, but evaluation remains essentially subjective lying upon patients, parents, and surgeon views.

After the first description of Koyanagi technique and publishing of its first series [12], this technique started to gain acceptance among pediatric urologists. In the literature, the complication rate is variable, from 16% to 77% [9, 12, 17, 20, 21]. Koyanagi et al. published their rate of complication after using this technique in 70 patients of 47%, mostly fistulae [12]. Our series reveals more frequent urethral dehiscence, but similar rates of urethral fistula and urethral stricture to other published series, but with longer follow-up.

The following table shows a review of complication rates in the literature for Koyanagi technique (Table 16.1).

Table 16.1 Complications after Koyanagi technique according to the literature

Study	Population (N)	Follow up (months)	Rate of complication (%)	Urethro-cutaneous fistula (%)	Urethral stenosis (%)	Urethral diverticulum (%)	Dehiscence (%)
Koyanagi et al. [12]	70	–	47	21	9	–	–
Emir et al. [16]	20	34	20	20	–	–	–
Sugita et al. [17]	151	72	16	12.6	2	–	–
Catti et al. [9]	26	25	61.5	19.2	34.6	26.9	42.3
Catti et al. [9]	31	34	61.3	38.7	16.1	16	19.3
Acimi et al. [15]	43	28	77	39.5	–	9	–
Our series (Lyon 2023)	*86*	*72*	*76*	*11.6*	*12.7*	*4.6*	*59.3*

In hypospadiology, few techniques have been developed and have proven their reliability in reconstructing a functional urethra when urethral division is mandatory to straighten the penile shaft. Besides the Koyanagi technique, other techniques are reported to treat perineal hypospadias such as the Asopa-Duckett tube or the two-stage urethroplasties.

In the literature, the rate of complications after staged repair (Cloutier Bracka) is variable from 3% to 68% [5–7, 22–25], but most often exceeds 35% [2, 5, 7, 19, 22]. Most frequent complications are fistulae after tubularization of the neo-urethra.

For similar severe hypospadias using Duckett technique, the rate of overall complication ranges from 33% to 100% [4, 24–30], most of them being fistulae of the neo-urethra. Interestingly, a systematic review over 20 years reported by M Castagnetti et al. showed that the rate of complication between Koyanagi and Duckett is comparable (37.9% for Duckett and 31.9% for Koyanagi technique) [31].

To conclude, Koyanagi technique for proximal hypospadias reveals high rate of complications, higher than previously stated. However, a quarter of patients had only one surgery in our series. Cosmetic after reconstruction was acceptable despite high rate of re-operation.

Overall, Koyanagi technique remains a valuable approach for proximal hypospadias repair, and displays similar results with other techniques published in the late decades, mainly Duckett tubularized preputial island foreskin flap and staged urethroplasty.

Long-term study is essential to fully evaluate the real outcome of reconstructive surgical technique as many complications could appear many years after reconstruction, particularly after puberty.

References

1. Mouriquand P, Mure PY. Current concepts in hypospadiology. BJU Int. 2004;93(s3):26–34. https://doi.org/10.1111/j.1464-410X.2004.04706.x.
2. Salle JLP, Sayed S, Salle A, et al. Proximal hypospadias: a persistent challenge. Single institution outcome analysis of three surgical techniques over a 10-year period. J Pediatr Urol. 2016;12(1):28.e1–7. https://doi.org/10.1016/j.jpurol.2015.06.011.
3. Braga LHP, Pippi Salle JL, Lorenzo AJ, et al. Comparative analysis of tubularized incised plate versus onlay island flap urethroplasty for penoscrotal hypospadias. J Urol. 2007;178(4 Pt 1):1451–6; discussion 1456-1457. https://doi.org/10.1016/j.juro.2007.05.170.
4. Hueber PA, Diaz MS, Chaussy Y, Franc-Guimond J, Barrieras D, Houle AM. Long-term functional outcomes after penoscrotal hypospadias repair: a retrospective comparative study of proximal TIP, Onlay, and Duckett. J Pediatr Urol. 2016;12(4):198.e1–6. https://doi.org/10.1016/j.jpurol.2016.04.034.
5. Stanasel I, Le HK, Bilgutay A, et al. Complications following staged hypospadias repair using transposed preputial skin flaps. J Urol. 2015;194(2):512–6. https://doi.org/10.1016/j.juro.2015.02.044.
6. McNamara ER, Schaeffer AJ, Logvinenko T, et al. Management of proximal hypospadias with 2-stage repair: 20 year experience. J Urol. 2015;194(4):1080–5. https://doi.org/10.1016/j.juro.2015.04.105.

7. Misra D, Elbourne C, Vareli A, et al. Challenges in managing proximal hypospadias: a 17-year single-center experience. J Pediatr Surg. 2019;54(10):2125–9. https://doi.org/10.1016/j.jpedsurg.2019.04.019.
8. Catti M, Demède D, Valmalle AF, Mure PY, Hameury F, Mouriquand P. Management of severe hypospadias. Indian J Urol. 2008;24(2):233–40.
9. Catti M, Lottmann H, Babloyan S, Lortat-Jacob S, Mouriquand P. Original Koyanagi urethroplasty versus modified Hayashi technique: outcome in 57 patients. J Pediatr Urol. 2009;5(4):300–6. https://doi.org/10.1016/j.jpurol.2009.03.010.
10. Cousin I, Basmaison C, Cousin E, et al. Complication rates of proximal hypospadias: meta-analyses of four surgical repairs. J Pediatr Urol. 2022;18(5):587–97. https://doi.org/10.1016/j.jpurol.2022.08.005.
11. Koyanagi T, Matsuno T, Nonomura K, Sakakibara N. Complete repair of severe penoscrotal hypospadias in 1 stage: experience with urethral mobilization, wing flap-flipping urethroplasty and "glanulomeatoplasty". J Urol. 1983;130(6):1150–4. https://doi.org/10.1016/s0022-5347(17)51732-2.
12. Koyanagi T, Nonomura K, Yamashita T, Kanagawa K, Kakizaki H. One-stage repair of hypospadias: is there no simple method universally applicable to all types of hypospadias? J Urol. 1994;152(4):1232–7. https://doi.org/10.1016/s0022-5347(17)32556-9.
13. Hayashi Y, Kojima Y, Mizuno K, Nakane A, Kohri K. The modified Koyanagi repair for severe proximal hypospadias. BJU Int. 2001;87(3):235–8. https://doi.org/10.1046/j.1464-410x.2001.02029.x.
14. Kang L, Huang G, Zeng L, et al. A new modification of the Koyanagi technique for the one-stage repair of severe hypospadias. Urology. 2016;93:175–9. https://doi.org/10.1016/j.urology.2016.03.032.
15. Acimi S, Abderrahmane N, Debbous L, Acimi MA, Mansouri J. Koyanagi- snow-Hayashi urethroplasty in severe hypospadias repair: between hope and reality. Urology. 2021;152:129–35. https://doi.org/10.1016/j.urology.2020.11.058.
16. Emir H, Jayanthi VR, Nitahara K, Danismend N, Koff SA. Modification of the Koyanagi technique for the single stage repair of proximal hypospadias. J Urol. 2000;164(3 Pt 2):973–5; discussion 976. https://doi.org/10.1097/00005392-200009020-00013.
17. Sugita Y, Tanikaze S, Yoshino K, Yamamichi F. Severe hypospadias repair with meatal based paracoronal skin flap: the modified Koyanagi repair. J Urol. 2001;166(3):1051–3.
18. Madec FX, Desplanches M, Chabaud M, Irtan S, Suply E, Audry G. Koyanagi urethroplasty for proximal hypospadias: a stage procedure? Prog Urol. 2022;32(5):312–8. https://doi.org/10.1016/j.purol.2021.09.008.
19. Bracka A. Hypospadias repair: the two-stage alternative. Br J Urol. 1995;76(Suppl 3):31–41. https://doi.org/10.1111/j.1464-410x.1995.tb07815.x.
20. Chen Y, Zhang J, Ji C, Liang W, Pan S, Wu B. Modification of the Koyanagi technique for the single-stage repair of proximal hypospadias. Ann Plast Surg. 2016;76(6):693–6. https://doi.org/10.1097/SAP.0000000000000345.
21. Jorgensen B, Jorgensen TM, Olsen LH. Outcome of new surgical techniques in hypospadia repair. Scand J Urol Nephrol. 2003;37(2):134–8. https://doi.org/10.1080/00365590310008875.
22. Long CJ, Chu DI, Tenney RW, et al. Intermediate-term followup of proximal hypospadias repair reveals high complication rate. J Urol. 2017;197(3 Pt 2):852–8. https://doi.org/10.1016/j.juro.2016.11.054.
23. Shukla AK, Singh AP, Sharma P, Shukla J. Two stages repair of proximal hypospadias: review of 700 cases. J Indian Assoc Pediatr Surg. 2017;22(3):158–62. https://doi.org/10.4103/0971-9261.207627.
24. Zhu X, Huang L, Wang J, et al. Comparative study of one-stage and the novel two-stage urethroplasty using the transected urethral plate and transverse preputial island flap (TPIF) for severe hypospadias: a single-center experience. Transl Pediatr. 2021;10(4):843–50. https://doi.org/10.21037/tp-20-392.

25. Zhou G, Yin J, Sun J, Yang Z, Li S. Efficacy of one- and two-stage segment urethroplasty for severe chordee with congenital short urethra. Int J Urol. 2022;29(5):422–6. https://doi.org/10.1111/iju.14800.
26. Wang CX, Zhang WP, Song HC. Complications of proximal hypospadias repair with transverse preputial Island flap urethroplasty: a 15-year experience with long-term follow-up. Asian J Androl. 2019;21(3):300–3. https://doi.org/10.4103/aja.aja_115_18.
27. Elbakry A. Complications of the preputial island flap-tube urethroplasty. BJU Int. 1999;84(1):89–94. https://doi.org/10.1046/j.1464-410x.1999.00097.x.
28. Castagnetti M, Zhapa E, Rigamonti W. Primary severe hypospadias: comparison of reoperation rates and parental perception of urinary symptoms and cosmetic outcomes among 4 repairs. J Urol. 2013;189(4):1508–13. https://doi.org/10.1016/j.juro.2012.11.013.
29. Blanc T, Peycelon M, Siddiqui M, Muller C, Paye-Jaouen A, El-Ghoneimi A. Double-face preputial island flap revisited: is it a reliable one-stage repair for severe hypospadias? World J Urol. 2021;39(5):1613–24. https://doi.org/10.1007/s00345-020-03324-7.
30. Wiener JS, Sutherland RW, Roth DR, Gonzales ET. Comparison of onlay and tubularized island flaps of inner preputial skin for the repair of proximal hypospadias. J Urol. 1997;158(3 Pt 2):1172–4. https://doi.org/10.1097/00005392-199709000-00123.
31. Castagnetti M, El-Ghoneimi A. Surgical management of primary severe hypospadias in children: systematic 20-year review. J Urol. 2010;184(4):1469–75. https://doi.org/10.1016/j.juro.2010.06.044.

17 Proximal Hypospadias, One-Stage Reconstruction, Double-Face Preputial Island Flap

Alaa El-Ghoneimi, Aman-Allah Lachkar, Annabel Paye-Jaouen, and Matthieu Peycelon

Abstract

Proximal hypospadias poses challenges for surgical repair due to various anatomical factors, leading to high complication rates and the need for reoperations. Current approaches lack robust data, complicating treatment decisions. Surgical techniques can be broadly categorized into urethral plate preservation and transection procedures. Utilizing vascularized preputial flaps has been a key advancement in severe hypospadias repair, although concerns remain about dorsal penile skin ischemia post-surgery. Innovations such as the double-face preputial island flap procedure have improved single-stage treatment options. This summary highlights ongoing advancements in hypospadias repair, including our standardized approach to the double-face preputial island flap procedure.

Supplementary Information The online version contains supplementary material available at https://doi.org/10.1007/978-981-99-0795-3_17. The videos can be accessed individually by clicking the DOI link in the accompanying figure caption or by scanning this link with the SN More Media App.

A. El-Ghoneimi (✉) · A.-A. Lachkar · A. Paye-Jaouen · M. Peycelon
Department of Pediatric Surgery and Urology, University Hospital Robert Debré, Centre de référence, Malformations Rares des Voies Urinaires (MARVU), Centre de Référence Maladies Endocriniennes de la Croissance et du Développement (CRESCENDO), APHP, Université de Paris Cité, Paris, France
e-mail: alaa.elghoneimi@aphp.fr; amane-allah.lachkar@aphp.fr; annabel.paye-jaouen@aphp.fr; matthieu.peycelon@aphp.fr

T. O. Abbas (ed.), *Video Atlas of Hypospadias Surgery*, https://doi.org/10.1007/978-981-99-0795-3_17

Keywords

Proximal hypospadias · Urethral reconstruction · Vascularized preputial flap
Complications

Key Points

1. Preoperative explanation of the procedure, postoperative drainage modalities, complications rate are mandatory to have an optimal management of complex reconstruction.
2. Decision to make one-stage procedure is taken after degloving and correction of the penile curvature, the decision is taken according to the quality of the flaps (surface area and vitality).
3. The fundamental principles of hypospadias surgery should be followed: the flaps should be handled carefully throughout harvesting, the tourniquet should only be used during the erection test and never on the skin, micro-bipolar energy should be used exclusively, and micro-instruments should be handled with care on the skin in order to retain the flaps' viability.
4. Rigorous constructed follow-up is mandatory till puberty.
5. A detailed explanation of the procedure is given to the parents and to the child if his age allows, postoperative care, and complications rates and their management are obligations.

17.1 Introduction

The overall length of the urethroplasty, the curvature of the penile canal, and the presence of ventral penile hypoplasia make surgical care of proximal hypospadias challenging. The three goals of hypospadias restoration are penis straightening, urethral reconstruction, and ventral aspect of shaft coverage. The majority of surgeries for severe hypospadias end in a large number of complications and reoperations, which continues to be a challenge for pediatric urologists. There is still debate over the best method for addressing proximal hypospadias. Contemporary care of primary severe hypospadias is supported by little data, as shown in recent systematic reviews [1, 2].

We can classify the most popular primary repair techniques into three broad groups: firstly, urethral plate preservation procedures, such as onlay island flap urethroplasty [3] and tubularized incised plate (TIP) [4]; secondly, urethral plate transection procedures, such as Duckett tube [5], Koyanagi/Hayashi procedure and variants [6], and thirdly Cloutier-Bracka two-stage procedure [7].

There is a good intrinsic blood supply and an easily isolated pedicle, which justify the employing of a vascularized preputial flap [8, 9]. Duckett originally described the use of an island of skin with an axial blood supply for urethral reconstruction in his report on transverse preputial island flap urethroplasty, which he utilized to treat severe hypospadias [10].

Ischemia of the dorsal skin that covers the penile shaft following island flap harvesting is one negative outcome of the operation. A twin preputial flap procedure was suggested as a solution to this shortcoming, as it would allow the urethroplasty and the ventral skin to continue receiving the abundant preputial blood supply. In 1970, Hodgson published the initial account [11]. An important step forward in the single-stage treatment of hypospadias in the 1980s was the utilization of the double-island transverse preputial skin tube [12, 13]. The first method of full preputial double face is presented by Gonzalez et al. in 1996, and the most recent findings were published in 2018 [14].

With a few tweaks to the original method, we established a standard for the usage of the double-face preputial island flap (DFPIF) procedure.

17.2 Steps of the Procedure

17.2.1 Preoperative Preparation

- We routinely proceed for random urine analysis, and we do reconstruction surgery only on sterile urine.
- A detailed explanation of the procedure is given to the parents and to the child if his age allows. We focus specifically on the postoperative care of the urethral stent and the suprapubic drainage. These explanations are the key for accepting an early discharge with catheters. Complications rates and management of them are clearly explained, again the management of these complications is optimal and easier if the parents and or the patient are aware of them.
- We do not use routinely preoperative hormonal stimulation (as there is no evidence of positive impact on the surgical outcome). We keep this indication only for microphallus. The term is used to describe a penis whose flaccid length is stretched to less than or equal to 2 standard deviations. Microphallus patients received testosterone injections at a dosage of 100 mg/m^2 every two weeks for a duration of two months. Only in cases of 5 alpha-reductase deficiency was dihydrotestosterone (DHT) used topically.

17.2.2 Peroperative and Postoperative Pain Management

Children have routinely endotracheal intubation and general anesthesia associated with locoregional anesthesia (caudal or pudendal bloc). Anti-cholinergic treatment (Oxybutinine) is given routinely starting on the day of surgery and stopped on the day of stent removal.

17.2.3 Surgical Steps

- In a fully stretched flaccid status (Figs. 17.1, 17.2), the penis was determined by running a ruler down its dorsal surface, starting at the pubis and ending at the tip of the glans, all the while pressing down on the suprapubic fat pad, following the method outlined by Lee et al. [15].
- It is standard practice to inject 0.9% isotonic saline intramuscularly during erection tests in order to measure curvature. The surgeon visually assessed the extent of curvature and classified it as minor (<30°), medium (30–45°), or severe (> 45°).
- To fix the penile curvature, a methodical procedure was followed [1].

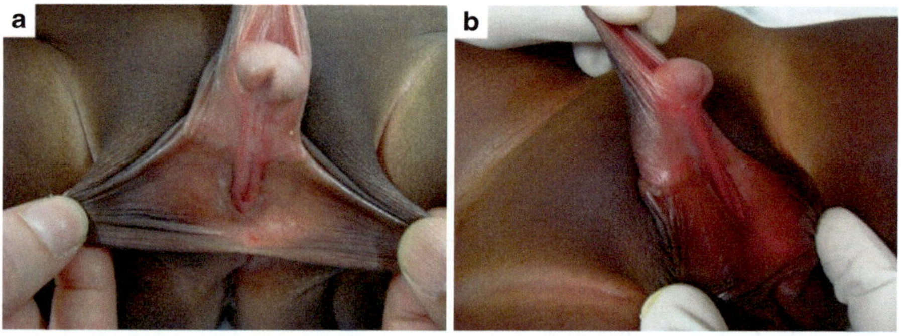

Fig. 17.1 (**a**–**b**) Scrotal hypospadias. (With permission from [17])

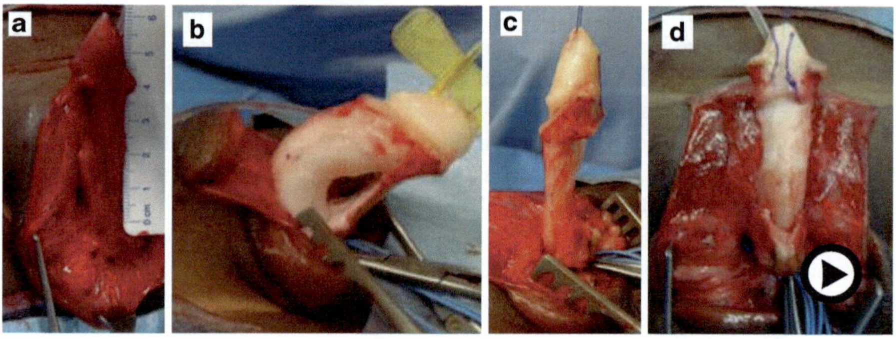

Fig. 17.2 (**a**) A thorough exploration of the corpora cavernosa's ventral side, reaching the bulbar urethra; urethroplasty length: 50 mm. (**b**) Test for an erection following detaching the urethral plate from the back of the body (**c** and **d**) show that the extreme curvature is still there. The urethral plate is transected halfway between the meatus and the tip of the glans in order to preserve both the proximal and distal plates. By carefully removing the distal spongiosum, the corpora on the penis's ventral side can be seen. (With permission from [17]). Tubularized island flap urethroplasty (https://doi.org/10.1007/000-cnd)

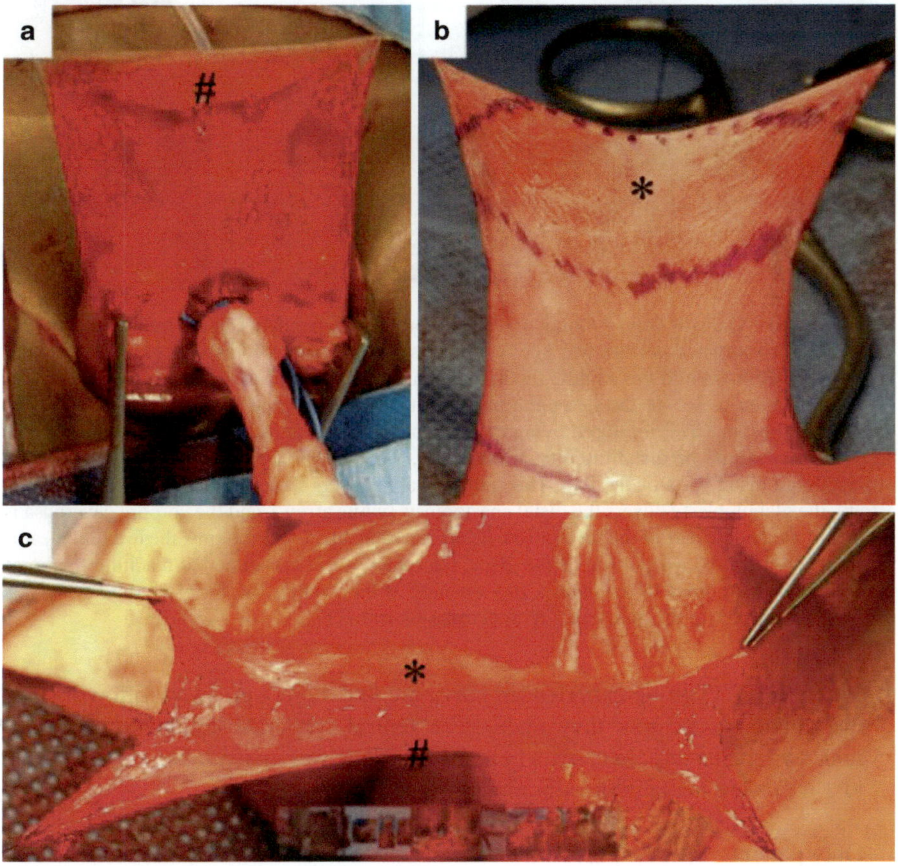

Fig. 17.3 (**a**) The preputial skin's inner surface. (**b**) A preputial skin flap that is supposed to be visible on the outside. (**c**) Getting the preputial flap ready. The inner and outer prepuce meet at the junction, and a transverse incision is performed there. In order to preserve their shared vascularity, the inner face was delicately separated from the outer face. Both the inner and outer surfaces of the preputial skin are used for uretroplasty and ventral skin covering, respectively. (With permission from [17])

- As an initial action in correcting curvature, we freed the external border of the corpus spongiosum, resected all fibrous attachments, and degloved the skin extensively for every patient.
- Since the urethral plate was not thought to be the cause of the curvature in the onlay group, it was left alone and dorsal plication was performed until 2013. Nobody has had a dorsal plication since 2013 because of worries about penile shortening [16].
- Fig. 17.3 from the film shows the surgical processes and flap harvesting.

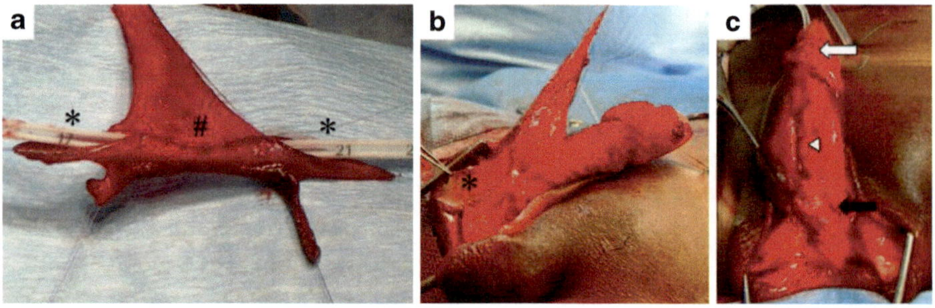

Fig. 17.4 (**a**) * Onlay # Tube * Onlay. In order to bridge the gap between the transected urethral plates, the reconstructed portion was kept as short as possible and used as a tube. Interrupted 7/0 vicryl was used to rebuild this middle section, which was then wrapped around an 8 or 10 French catheter. In order to secure the neo-urethra, two stitches were placed between the tube and the corpus cavernosum. (**b**) Prior to removing the extra parts of the flap, stitch the proximal onlay (*). To prevent proximal or distal circular anastomosis, we 7/0 vicryl anastomosed on the onlay's proximal and distal parts of the flap. The spongioplasty covers the proximal anastomosis (black arrow), the glanuloplasty covers the distal anastomosis (white arrow), and the corpora cavernosa is sutured to the middle part of the tube (arrow head) (**c**). If the glans was too tiny, the urethral meatus remained on the proximal portion of the glans, but otherwise, it was aimed at reaching the tip of the glans penis. In order to maintain a tiny opening at the meatus, the distal urethral plate was exclusively utilized for this purpose. (With permission from [17])

- When the OTO group experienced curvature that did not go away following urethral plate transection, they underwent ventral corporeal lengthening using a tunica vaginalis flap. In cases where the vaginalis was unavailable, tiny incisions of 1 mm were made in the albuginea (Fig. 17.4).

Only patients with a significant residual curvature greater than 30° were treated with ventral lengthening after thorough excision of the corpus spongiosum's lateral attachments and fibrous tissues on the ventral surface. The risk of penis shortening was lessened by using ventral lengthening rather than dorsal plication.

- The incision was made after each patient had an intravenous infusion of cephalosporin. Nobody was given antibiotics to prevent infection after the surgery.

17.2.4 Postoperative Care

- A collecting bag was used to drain the suprapubic catheter, and one diaper was left free with the urethral stent.
- Following the removal of the dressing and the absence of new dressing on the skin, children were discharged from the hospital 48 hours following surgery (Figs. 17.5, 17.6).

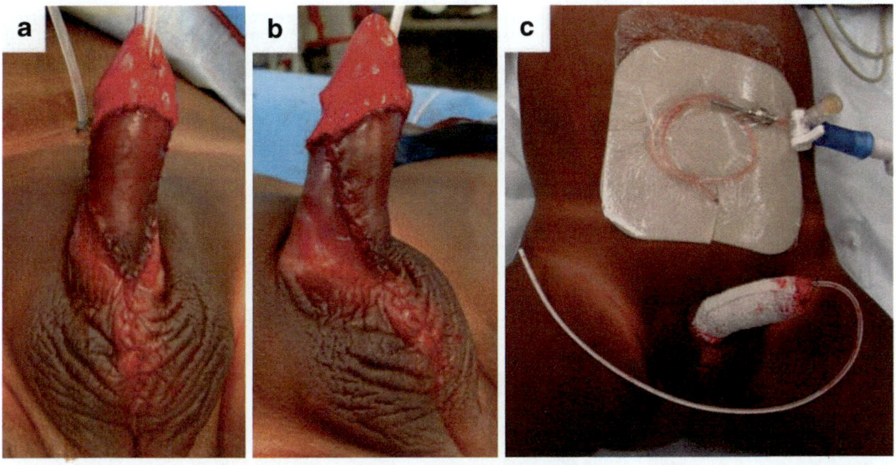

Fig. 17.5 (**a**–**b**) In the end, the remaining penile skin was employed in conjunction with the outer prepuce, which is now ventral skin coverage, to complete the skin coverage. To accommodate the ventral skin defect and eliminate ventral bulkiness, the skin of the pedicle flap was cut correctly. (**c**) Dressing A 6–8 Fr catheter was used to drain the bladder, and a suprapubic catheter was utilized on a regular basis. The penis was placed immediately on a semi-occlusive dressing (NexcareTM CobanTM Self-Adhering Wrap) without the use of topical ointment. (With permission from [17])

- If the child had no voids without urine diffusion in the scrotal area, the suprapubic catheter was closed and removed after the removal of the urethral stent on day 10, provided that healing was optimal.
- In case there was any uncertainty, the suprapubic catheter was left in place for an extra week to redirect urine.
- One month later, every three months for a year, and then once a year after that, there will be a follow-up. Uroflowmetry was performed six months subsequent to potty training. A comprehensive cosmetic and functional sheet was filled up by the surgeon at each clinic [17].
- The urine stream and uroflowmetry investigations were used to objectively evaluate voiding function (Fig. 17.7).
- The goal was to achieve an anatomically and cosmetically appealing penis that could direct a strong urine stream with no further surgery. This meant a straight penis with the urethral meatus at the tip.
- The child or parent's subjective report was used to evaluate the residual curvature. We specifically inquire as to whether or not the parents observed their child experiencing an erection, the kind of the erection, and the severity of the penis's curvature during the clinical examination, or if the child experienced an erection spontaneously. Patients who reached puberty were the only ones instructed to take photos. The purpose of the erection test was to determine whether the youngster would later require general anesthesia (Fig. 17.8).

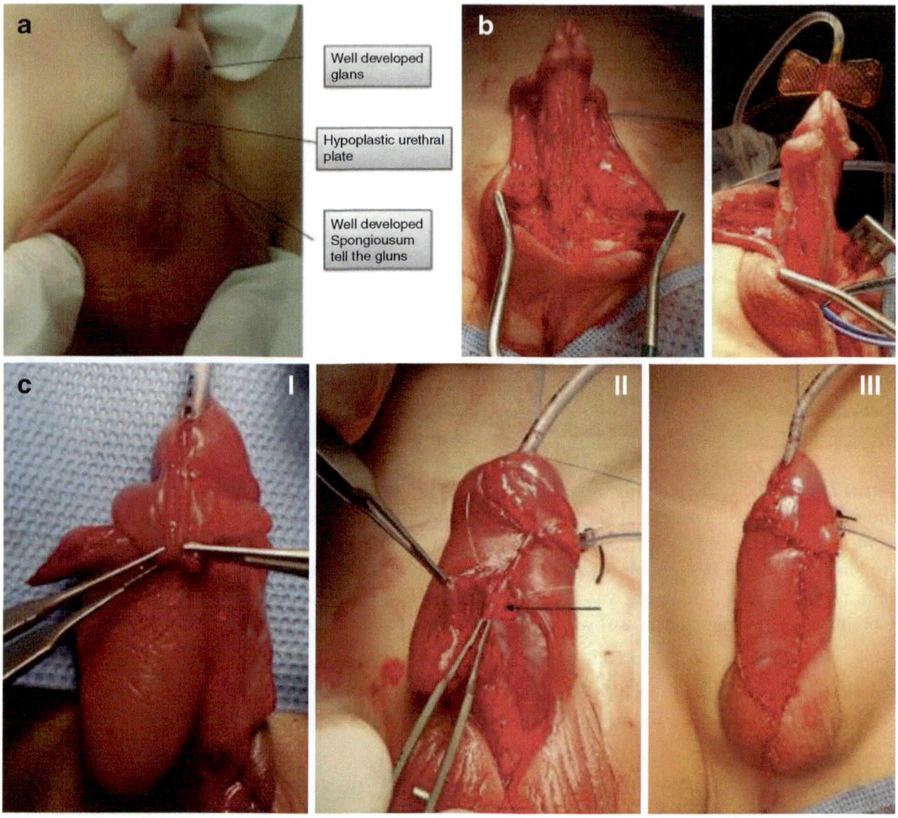

Fig. 17.6 Double-face urethroplasty procedure reconstruction without removing the urethral plate. (**a**) The thoroughly mature corpus spongiosum and glans are shown in the photograph. (**b**) An erection test reveals that scrotal hypospadias is not a common reason to remove the spongiosum. (**c**) I-A complete rebuilding with an apical wide meatus can be reasonably accomplished when the glans is in its ideal state. II In order to cover the left border of the urethroplasty—the source of the fistula—and to ancre the double face ventral skin, a well-preserved spongiosum was used (arrow). The procedure was completed in aspect III. (With permission from [17])

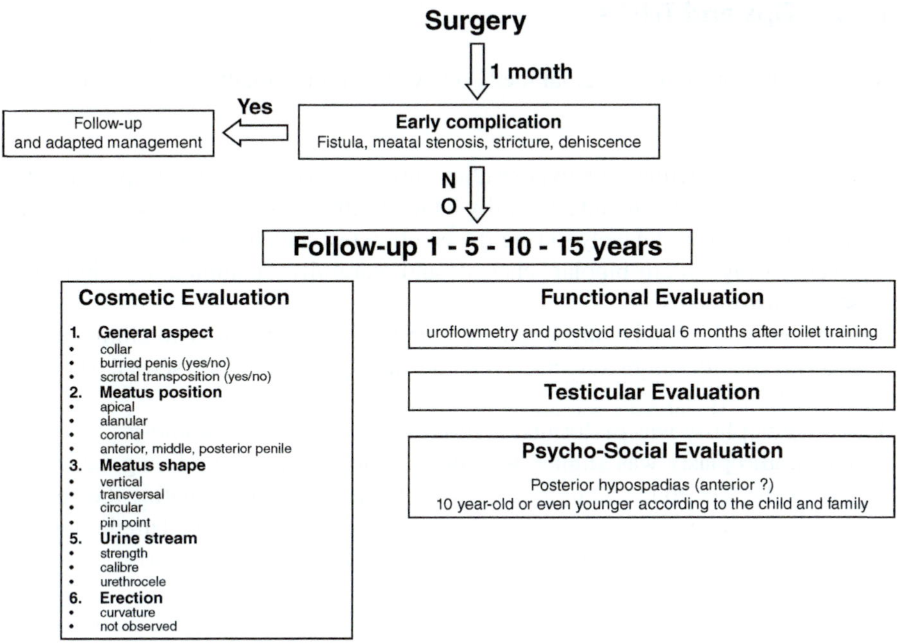

Fig. 17.7 Detailed cosmetic and functional sheet used for follow-up in outpatient clinic. (With permission from [17])

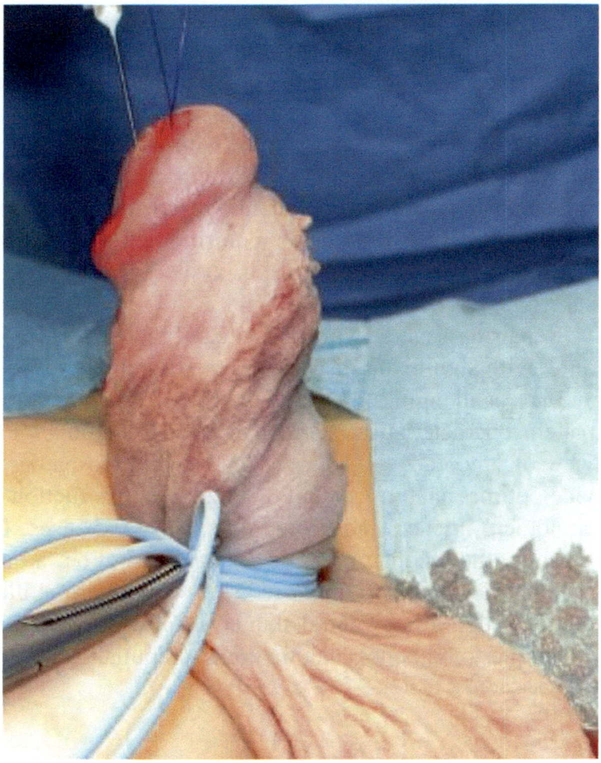

Fig. 17.8 Findings four years following a single-stage ventral lengthening using cavernoplasty and a double-face onlay-tube-onlay procedure for scrotal hypospadias. Evaluation of inguinal hernia repair erection under general anesthesia. (With permission from [17])

17.3 Tips and Tricks

A few adaptations to the original method have been implemented to lessen the likelihood of problems:

1. Follow all guidelines for hypospadias surgery: Essential steps to preserve the vitality of the flaps include carefully handling the flaps during harvesting, using the tourniquet exclusively during the erection test and never on the skin, exclusively using micro-bipolar energy, and carefully manipulating skin with micro-instruments.
2. The area immediately surrounding the urethral plate: in order to eliminate hair growth and to suture directly with the healthy urethra, all scrotal skin was excised.
3. A spongioplasty was performed to protect the proximal anastomosis.
4. The urethroplasty was aligned with the corpora cavernosa by fixing the middle part of the tube to the albuginea. This could be useful in preventing the neourethra from becoming twisted and kinked, as is the case when tubed urethral reconstruction "floats" under the skin. This kind of problem did not arise for any of our patients.
5. The part of the plate that was farther down was left alone and not cut off so that the onlay could be sutured.

17.4 Results and Conclusions

We published our experience a few years ago [17]. We have demonstrated the successful correction of the most intricate type of hypospadias in a single procedure. We conducted a study with the biggest group of patients treated using a single approach for severe hypospadias, with a uniform follow-up at one center. Over a decade of adopting a standardized approach, we have found that utilizing the one-stage DFPIF technique consistently results in maintaining a healthy skin covering in all instances. Out of 34 cases requiring redo surgery, only one procedure was successful in 24 cases, resulting in a success rate of 96% after an average of 1.8 surgeries.

Repairing severe hypospadias can be done with a single or multi-stage procedure, with significant discussion regarding the preferred approach. Outcomes vary and are challenging to evaluate because of significant differences in pre-operative patient characteristics, surgical methods, length of follow-up, and the surgeon's view of outcomes [1, 18, 19]. One-stage hypospadias restoration attempts to provide optimal anatomical and functional reconstruction of the urethra, minimal psychological impact, and decreased societal expenses. In addition to the benefit of finishing the reconstruction in a single operation, a one-stage operation offers the advantage of utilizing unscarred skin with a normal blood supply. The double-face preputial flap offers ventral skin covering with well-vascularized skin. We find this technique to be better than the inner preputial transverse island skin tube or onlay island flap, as it avoids separating the two layers of prepuce and prevents compromising the blood supply to the penile dorsal skin utilized for ventral covering.

Multiple authors have observed a decrease in problems after onlay repair [20, 21]. Wiener et al. found a complication risk of 36% with tube repairs compared to 31% with onlay repairs for proximal hypospadias [21].

The complication rates of the onlay island flap procedure in our series (44%) are comparable to rates of 22% [22] and 45% [23] reported in other studies. In our study, the occurrence of fistula following the onlay surgery was 12%, a rate consistent with earlier published studies [24, 25].

The second most prevalent complication was diverticulum, occurring in 14% of cases. The flap in onlay repair is narrower and secured to the urethral plate on both sides, unlike tubularized flaps, which lack the support of the urethral plate and may be more susceptible to diverticular development. No difference was observed between the onlay and OTO. All diverticula were successfully treated with a single procedure to decrease them without any additional complications based on our experience. Gonzales et al. proposed that utilizing the dorsal skin of the prepuce could prevent this problem [14]. We encountered just three instances of strictures among a group of 41 severe hypospadias individuals (7%), indicating a low stenosis rate in this population. Rigamonti et al. described the technique of Onlay on albuginea to decrease the rate of stenosis [26].

There is a paucity of long-term outcomes for the double-face approach. The published series includes various surgical procedures for distal and proximal hypospadias. Only a small percentage of patients (22%) have had surgery for proximal hypospadias using the double-face technique.

Curvature correction is a topic of debate. Ventral lengthening offers enhanced penile shaft length and avoids dorsal nerve damage, unlike dorsal plication. Braga et al. [27] found that dorsal plication was more commonly linked to recurrent ventral curvature than ventral penile lengthening.

Multiple studies have highlighted that the primary concern among adolescents and adults who have undergone hypospadias surgery is the short length of the penis and the persistent curvature [28–30]. Since 2013, we stopped using dorsal plication for proximal hypospadias to prevent surgical shortening of the penis. One stage remained viable even after ventral extension procedures based on our experience.

The Cloutier-Bracka two-stage repair is a popular procedure utilized by many, but we only view it as a viable alternative for salvage surgery or in rare instances involving older children with minimal preputial skin surface [7, 31].

Some people think that when circumferential urethroplasty is necessary, Bracka's method is the best option. Transecting the urethral plate did not significantly affect the complication rate. However, the OTO group had more severe curvature and included cases of scrotal and perineal hypospadias.

A recent study on surgical outcomes for posterior hypospadias in large North American hospitals found concerning [2]. Complication rates for one-stage or two-stage urethroplasty ranged from 32% to 68%. Performing phased urethroplasty can lead to a considerable amount of difficulties, even in specialized medical facilities.

Various perioperative factors can impact the outcome in proximal hypospadias [32]. Our institution follows standardized perioperative treatment and operational technical specifications for all cases.

Proving the factors that affect the success of surgery in hypospadias surgery is challenging. None of the 75 individuals in our experience exhibited skin sloughing or necrosis of the flaps. It is crucial to handle the flaps carefully during harvesting, only apply the tourniquet during the erection test and never on the skin, exclusively employ micro-bipolar energy, and handle the skin cautiously with micro-instruments to maintain the life of the flaps.

Overall, the double-face preputial island flap approach for one-stage surgical hypospadias treatment yields favorable outcomes. This treatment is our favored approach for repairing severe hypospadias. Having healthy and well-vascularized skin on the front part of the body enables safe repeat surgery if necessary.

References

1. Castagnetti M, El-Ghoneimi A. Surgical management of primary severe hypospadias in children: systematic 20-year review. J Urol. 2010;184(4):1469–74.
2. Long CJ, Canning DA. Hypospadias: are we as good as we think when we correct proximal hypospadias? J Pediatr Urol 2016 Aug;12(4):196.e1–196.e5.
3. Elder JS, Duckett JW, Snyder HM. Onlay island flap in the repair of mid and distal penile hypospadias without chordee. J Urol. 1987;138(2):376–9.
4. Snodgrass WT. Snodgrass technique for hypospadias repair. BJU Int. 2005;95(4):683–93.
5. Duckett JW. The island flap technique for hypospadias repair. Urol Clin North Am. 1981;8(3):503–11.
6. Hayashi Y, Sasaki S, Mogami T, Yamada Y, Tsugaya M, Kohri K. One-stage urethroplasty with the modified OUPF IV for proximal hypospadias. Nihon Hinyokika Gakkai Zasshi. 1996;87(1):56–60.
7. Bracka A. Hypospadias repair: the two-stage alternative. Br J Urol. 1995;76(Suppl 3):31–41.
8. Hinman F Jr. The blood supply to preputial island flaps. J Urol. 1991;145(6):1232–5.
9. Jordan GH. Penile reconstruction, phallic construction, and urethral reconstruction. Urol Clin North Am. 1999;26(1):1–13. vii
10. Duckett JW Jr. Transverse preputial island flap technique for repair of severe hypospadias. Urol Clin North Am. 1980;7(2):423–30.
11. Hodgson NB. A one-stage hypospadias repair. J Urol. 1970;104(2):281–3.
12. Asopa R, Asopa HS. One stage repair of hypospadias using double island preputial skin tube. Indian J Urol. 1984;1(1):41–3.
13. Standoli L. One-stage repair of hypospadias: preputial island flap technique. Ann Plast Surg. 1982;9(1):81–8.
14. Gonzalez R, Lingnau A, Ludwikowski BM. Results of onlay preputial flap urethroplasty for the single-stage repair of mid- and proximal hypospadias. Front Pediatr. 2018;6:19.
15. Lee PA, Mazur T, Danish R, Amrhein J, Blizzard RM, Money J, et al. Micropenis. I. Criteria, etiologies and classification. Johns Hopkins Med J. 1980;146(4):156–63.
16. Castagnetti M, El-Ghoneimi A. Surgical management of primary severe hypospadias in children: an update focusing on penile curvature. Nat Rev Urol. 2022;19(3):147–60.
17. Blanc T, Peycelon M, Siddiqui M, Muller C, Paye-Jaouen A, El-Ghoneimi A. Double-face preputial island flap revisited: is it a reliable one-stage repair for severe hypospadias? World J Urol. 2021;39(5):1613–24.

18. Kiss A, Sulya B, Szasz AM, Romics I, Kelemen Z, Toth J, et al. Long-term psychological and sexual outcomes of severe penile hypospadias repair. J Sex Med. 2011;8(5):1529–39.
19. Prasad MM, Marks A, Vasquez E, Yerkes EB, Cheng EY. Published surgical success rates in pediatric urology – fact or fiction? J Urol. 2012;188(4 Suppl):1643–7.
20. Patel RP, Shukla AR, Snyder HM 3rd. The island tube and island onlay hypospadias repairs offer excellent long-term outcomes: a 14-year followup. J Urol. 2004;172(4 Pt 2):1717–9. discussion 9
21. Wiener JS, Sutherland RW, Roth DR, Gonzales ET Jr. Comparison of onlay and tubularized island flaps of inner preputial skin for the repair of proximal hypospadias. J Urol. 1997;158(3 Pt 2):1172–4.
22. Sedberry-Ross S, Stisser BC, Henderson CG, Rushton HG, Belman AB. Split prepuce in situ onlay hypospadias repair: 17 years of experience. J Urol. 2007;178(4 Pt 2):1663–7.
23. Baskin LS, Duckett JW, Ueoka K, Seibold J, Snyder HM 3rd. Changing concepts of hypospadias curvature lead to more onlay island flap procedures. J Urol. 1994;151(1):191–6.
24. de Mattos e Silva E, Gorduza DB, Catti M, Valmalle AF, Demede D, Hameury F, et al. Outcome of severe hypospadias repair using three different techniques. J Pediatr Urol. 2009;5(3):205–11. discussion 12-4
25. Wallis MC, Braga L, Khoury A. The role of flaps and grafts in modern hypospadiology. Indian J Urol. 2008;24(2):200–5.
26. Rigamonti W, Castagnetti M. Onlay on albuginea: modified onlay preputial island flap urethroplasty for single-stage repair of primary severe hypospadias requiring urethral plate division. Urology. 2011;77(6):1498–502.
27. Braga LH, Lorenzo AJ, Bagli DJ, Dave S, Eeg K, Farhat WA, et al. Ventral penile lengthening versus dorsal plication for severe ventral curvature in children with proximal hypospadias. J Urol. 2008;180(4 Suppl):1743–7. discussion 7-8
28. Benson CR, Hoang L, Clavell-Hernandez J, Wang R. Sexual dysfunction in urethral reconstruction: a review of the literature. Sex Med Rev. 2018;6(3):492–503.
29. Moriya K, Kakizaki H, Tanaka H, Furuno T, Higashiyama H, Sano H, et al. Long-term cosmetic and sexual outcome of hypospadias surgery: norm related study in adolescence. J Urol. 2006;176(4 Pt 2):1889–92. discussion 92-3
30. Blanc T, Ayedi A, El-Ghoneimi A, Abdoul H, Aigrain Y, Paris F, et al. Testicular function and physical outcome in young adult males diagnosed with idiopathic 46 XY disorders of sex development during childhood. Eur J Endocrinol. 2011;165(6):907–15.
31. Badawy H, Orabi S, Hanno A, Abdelhamid H. Posterior hypospadias: evaluation of a paradigm shift from single to staged repair. J Pediatr Urol. 2018;14(1):28.e1–8.
32. Castagnetti M, El-Ghoneimi A. The influence of perioperative factors on primary severe hypospadias repair. Nat Rev Urol. 2011;8(4):198–206.

Chordee Excision and Distal Urethroplasty (CEDU) for Perineal Hypospadias

18

Michael Sennert and Ahmed T. Hadidi

Abstract

Perineal hypospadias correction has swung from two-stage repair in the 1960s to one-stage repair in the 1980s and back to two-stage repair in the 2000s. Here, we present our experience with a technique where Chordee Excision and Distal Urethroplasty (CEDU) are performed at the first operation leaving a 1–2 cm segment as perineal urethrotomy to be reconstructed at the second operation. The principle is to excise the hypoplastic urethral plate, atretic corpus spongiosum and longitudinal layer of tunica albuginea, (the TALE technique) split the glans in the midline and reconstruct a healthy urethral plate using preputial and lateral skin flaps to the tip of the glans. Distal urethroplasty was performed leaving 1 cm at the proximal end to be reconstructed 3–6 months later. Follow-up period ranged from 17 to 84 months (mean 60). Satisfactory results were obtained in 114 patients (90%). The CEDU technique diverts urine away from the urethroplasty for 3 months without a catheter. It reduces the hospital stay and patient discomfort. It produces satisfactory results and has become the standard technique for perineal hypospadias in the hypospadias center, Frankfurt since 2013.

Supplementary Information The online version contains supplementary material available at https://doi.org/10.1007/978-981-99-0795-3_18. The videos can be accessed individually by clicking the DOI link in the accompanying figure caption or by scanning this link with the SN More Media App.

M. Sennert · A. T. Hadidi (✉)
Hypospadias Center, Sana Klinikum Offenbach, Offenbach am Main, Germany
e-mail: michael.sennert@uke.de

T. O. Abbas (ed.), *Video Atlas of Hypospadias Surgery*,
https://doi.org/10.1007/978-981-99-0795-3_18

Keywords

Hypospadias · Chordee · Urethroplasty · Proximal Hypospadias · Perineal Hypospadias · Tunica Albuginea · Staged Hypospadias Repair

18.1 Introduction

Perineal hypospadias or Grade IV hypospadias [1] is a complex deformity or syndrome consisting of; a perineal urethral orifice, hypoplastic ventral penile structures resulting in severe chordee, small-sized glans & penis, bifid scrotum and often undescended testis and occasionally penoscrotal transposition [2]. It remains a major challenge for the experienced hypospadias surgeon. The bilateral based flap [2], Koyanagi technique [3], Duckett Island flap [4] and Cloutier/Bracka two stage repair [5] and Chordee Excision and Distal Urethroplasty (CEDU) [6] are the current techniques used for perineal hypospadias [1].

Recent reports demonstrated that one stage repairs of "severe" proximal and perineal hypospadias often produce unsatisfactory results and the majority of patients require further surgery [2, 7–13]. The principle of the *Chordee Excision & Distal Urethroplasty (CEDU)* technique is to excise the severe chordee, mobilize the foreskin from both sides ventrally to create a "Urethral Plate" and reconstruct distal new urethra during the first operation leaving the perineal orifice intact as a "natural perineal fistula" [6]. Three to six months later, proximal urethroplasty is performed together with the correction of bifid scrotum.

18.2 Patient's Selection

The CEDU technique is suitable for patients with grade IV hypospadias. For the purpose of the study, grade IV hypospadias is a severe form of hypospadias defined when the urethral opening lies at or proximal to the penoscrotal junction, associated with severe deep chordee that requires division of the urethral plate (curvature of 30 degrees or more during erection) and usually associated with bifid scrotum and occasionally with penoscrotal transposition and undescended testis.

18.3 Video Demonstration

Factors	Findings
Age at surgery (months)	18 m
Gestational age (weeks)	38w
Birth weight (g)	2820
Family history	none
Testosterone	no
Undescended testis	Right side high
Penile dimensions ()	Shown on the video

18.3.1 Stage 1 Surgical Technique (Figs. 18.1, 18.2)

- Under general anesthesia and caudal block, a traction suture of 4/0 Prolene is placed through the tip of the glans. An artificial erection test is performed. Careful assessment of the penis and both testes is performed. If the child has undescended testis, orchidopexy is performed as the first step.
- A transverse subcoronal incision is performed 3 mm below the coronal sulcus.
- All the hypoplastic tissues are excised including the longitudinal layer of tunica albuginea (Tunica Albuginea Longitudinal Excision or TALE technique).
- The glans is split in the midline like an open book.
- The proximal skin edge usually retracts to the proximal penis and a transverse lateral skin incision in the preputial skin separates the outer skin from the inner mucosal layer in both sides.
- Both medial edges are fixed together in the midline to the tip of the penis creating a new "urethral plate" that is well fixed to the tunica albuginea in the midline as well as laterally.
- A catheter size F12 is inserted into the bladder. Two longitudinal incisions are made that stop 1 cm before the meatus.
- Distal urethroplasty is performed using Vicryl® 6/0 around a catheter size F12.
- Two protective layers are mobilized from both sides.
- The remaining skin is tailored to cover the glans and penis. The catheter is replaced with a silastic catheter size 10 F at the end of the procedure. The glans is fixed to the abdominal wall to stretch the penis and provide stability for 2–3 weeks after surgery.
- *Urine drainage.* The Nelaton catheter size F12 is replaced with silastic Tiemann balloon catheter 10F at the end of the operation for 4 days into a urine bag. Urethral stents can also be used with the same result. After 4 days, no stent or catheter is needed as urine is diverted away from the new urethra through the original orifice.
- *Abdominal Wall fixation:* The glans penis is fixed to the anterior abdominal wall with one Prolene 4/0 stay suture for 2–3 weeks (Figs. 18.3, 18.4).
- *Dressing*

All patients had a standard dressing in the form of gentamycin local ointment, gauze, and adhesive tape that compresses the penis, gauze and catheter against the lower abdominal wall and allows free mobility of the patient [8, 9, 14, 15]. The dressing is removed at the time of removal of the transurethral catheter and the penis is left exposed. If the dressing became wet with urine or blood, the dressing was changed using a similar standard dressing. Broad-spectrum antibiotics (second-generation cephalosporin) were administered for one week. Paracetamol and ibuprofen suppositories and syrup were routinely used for pain relief as required.

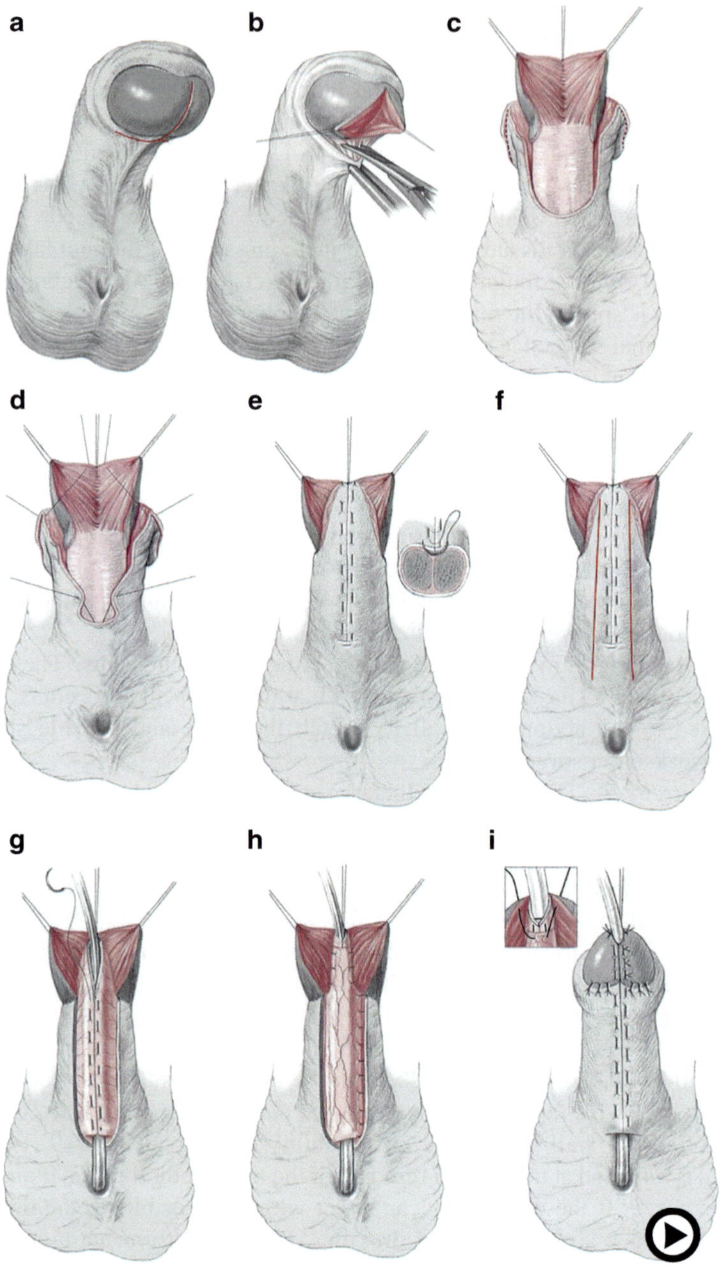

Fig. 18.1 The CEDU technique. After excision of severe chordee (**a**–**c**), the two lateral skin edges are brought to the midline and fixed to the underlying corpora cavernosa to create a "urethral plate" (**d**, **e**). At the same first stage, distal urethroplasty is performed leaving a "perineal urethrotomy" for urinary diversion (**f**–**i**). During the second stage, the perineal urethrotomy is closed (). CEDU procedure [6] (https://doi.org/10.1007/000-cne)

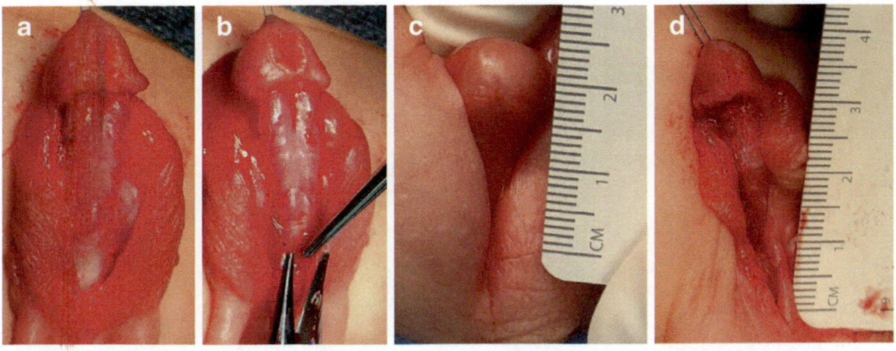

Fig. 18.2 *The technique of severe chordee excision* (TALE: *T*unica *A*lbuginea *L*ongitudinal *E*xcision): In order to correct severe chordee in perineal hypospadias, we excise all the ventral hypoplastic tissues as well as the outer longitudinal Tunica Albuginea layer. (**a**) Shows after the subcoronal incision, the hypoplastic tissues were excised as well as the Tunica Albuginea Longitudinal distally. Proximally, you can still see the white fibrous longitudinal layer. (**b**) Shows the approach to excise the Tunica Albuginea Longitudinale using sharp scissors and cutting along the longitudinal axis of the penis. No skin was excised at all, the skin simply retracted very proximally. (**c**) Shows the length of the penis of a child with perineal hypospadias (2.5 cm). (**d**) Shows the length of the same penis after TALE (4 cm). (©Ahmed T. Hadidi 2022. All Rights Reserved)

18.3.2 Stage II: Perineal (Proximal) Urethroplasty

Proximal urethroplasty was routinely performed 3-4 months after CEDU after edema subsides and healing is adequate. Adherent scar (if present) was excised and artificial erection was performed as the first step to ensure that the penis is adequately straight. Care is taken to avoid hair-bearing scrotal skin. Usually, the perineal mucosa is wide enough to close over a catheter size 12F using the Thiersch principle. In 14 children, the perineal mucosa was not wide enough and a skin flap from the penis was mobilized laterally or distally to ensure a wide healthy proximal urethra. *It is important to have 2 thick protective layers from scrotal fascia on both sides to reduce the chances of diverticulum formation.* A Z-Plasty at the penoscrotal junction was often required to create an angle between the penis and scrotum (87 patients). Again, the F12 Nelaton catheter is replaced with a F10 silicon Foley catheter that drains into a urine bag for 7 days. The glans penis is fixed to the abdominal wall with 4/0 Prolene suture for 2–3 weeks. A drain in the scrotum was needed in 4 patients after mobilization of the scrotal fascia as a protective layer to avoid development of scrotal hematoma.

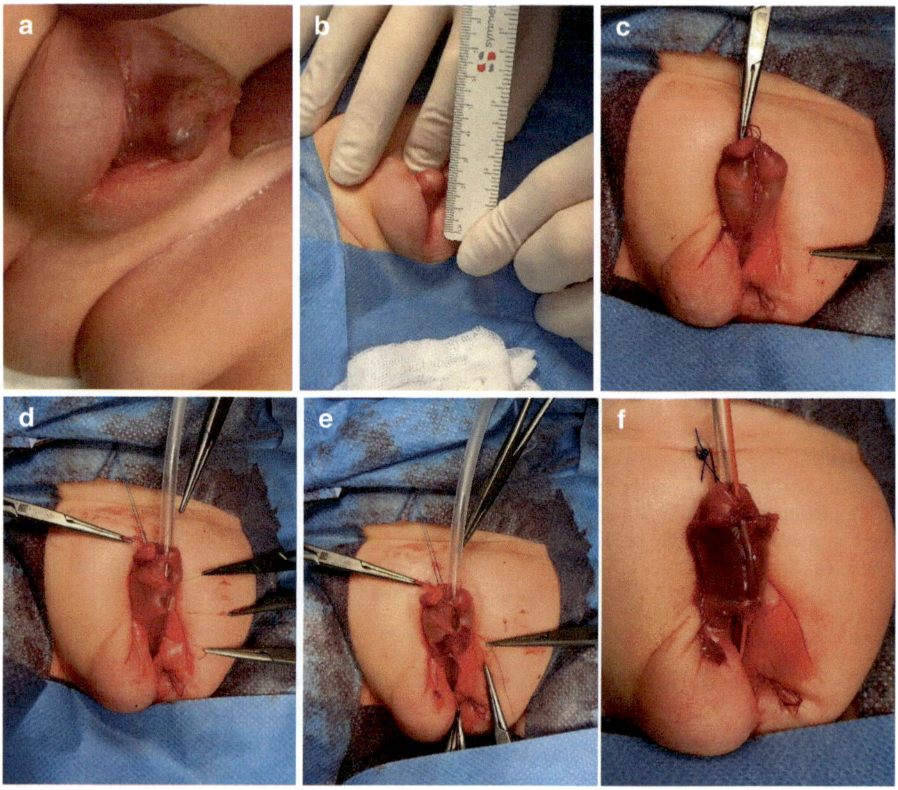

Fig. 18.3 *Perineal hypospadias*. (**a**) A 6-month-old child with perineal hypospadias, severe chordee, and bifid scrotum. (**b**) The penis measured 2 cm in length. The child had a left undescended testis and was fixed at the same operation. (**c**) After total chordee excision using the TALE technique and the foreskin was mobilized ventrally and medially a new urethral plate was reconstructed. (**d**) A catheter size F12 was inserted and 3 stay sutures were put to accurately determine the exact width need. (**e**) The skin was incised in a step manner. (**f**) At the end of the operation, notice that the penis was fixed with proline 4/0 to help straighten the penis, allow proper healing, and avoid coiling of the penis

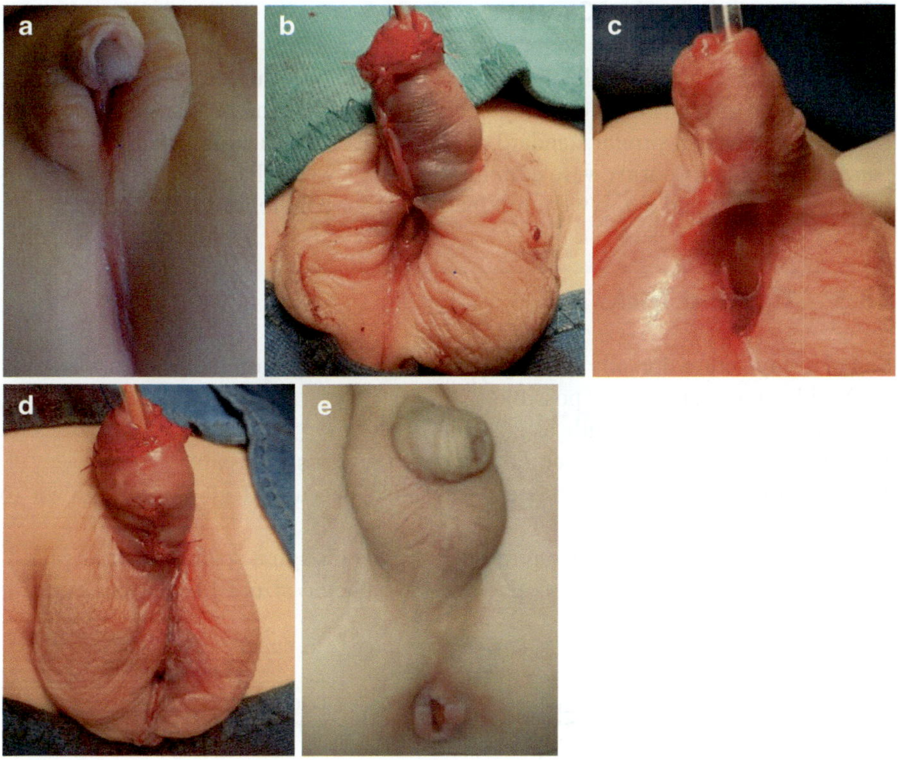

Fig. 18.4 Perineal hypospadias with severe chordee, bifid scrotum, penoscrotal transposition, and high imperforate anus. (**a**) Before surgery. (**b**) At the end of operation of Chordee Excision and Distal Urethroplasty (CEDU); (**c**) 3 months after CEDU. Notice that although the penis looks nice, the scrotum is still bifid and the child still passes urine from the perineum. (**d**) At the end of proximal urethroplasty operation. Notice the little Z-Plasty performed at the penoscrotal junction. (**e**) One year after closure of the perineal orifice and correction of bifid scrotum. Notice how the scrotum has healed with minimal scarring and one can hardly see the Z-plasty at the peno-scrotal junction. The penoscrotal transposition has corrected itself as the bifid scrotum was corrected). (©Ahmed T. Hadidi 2022. All Rights Reserved)

18.4 Postoperative Care

The dressing is removed at the time of removal of the transurethral catheter, and the penis is left exposed. If the dressing became wet with urine or blood, the dressing was changed using a similar standard dressing. Broad-spectrum antibiotics (second-generation cephalosporin) were administered for 1 week. Paracetamol and ibuprofen suppositories and syrup were routinely used for pain relief as required.

18.5 Tips and Tricks

- Put a stay suture dorsally in the glans to ensure tension on the penis.
- Avoid using tourniquet if possible.
- Handle the tissues as gentle as possible.
- Limit the operation to the ventral aspect of the penis if possible.
- Sometimes excision of chordee tissue must be carried all the way down to the anus.
- Use the F12 catheter for the urethroplasty even though it seems rather large.
- In children over 3 years of age even a catheter size F14 can be used for urethroplasty.

18.6 Results and Conclusions

The CEDU technique has been our standard technique for patients with perineal hypospadias or patients with severe chordee >30 degrees since 2013. Between January 2013 and December 2016, the CEDU technique was performed in 126 patients with perineal hypospadias including 14 patients from other countries. It is preferred to operate on patients with perineal hypospadias as early as 6 months because it increases the chance to correct the severe chordee using the TALE technique without the need to incise the corpora cavernosa. Patients who had persistent chordee after the TALE procedure underwent tunica vaginalis flap or dermal graft, and the first operation ends as a two-stage BILAB technique. Patient age ranged from 6 months to 2 years (mean 8 months). On presentation, all the patients had perineal hypospadias (meatus proximal to penoscrotal junction) with severe deep chordee and bifid scrotum. At operation, all patients had severe chordee excision, splitting of the glans, and distal urethroplasty performed in the first operation. Patients with unilateral or bilateral undescended testis had the testis fixed during the first operation.

References

1. Hadidi AT. History of hypospadias; lost in translation. J Pediatr Surg. 2017;52:211–7.
2. Hadidi AT. Perineal hypospadias; the bilateral (BILAB) skin flap technique. J Pediatr Surg. 2014;49:218–23.

3. Koyanagi T, Matsuno T, Nonomura K, et al. Complete repair of severe penoscrotal hypospadias in 1 stage: experience with urethral mobilization, wing-flap-flipping urethropasty and'glanulomeatoplasty'. J Urol. 1983;130:1150–4.
4. Duckett JW, Baskin LS. Hypospadias. In: Gillenwater JY, Grayback JT, Howards SS, Duckett JW, editors. Adult and pediatric urology. 3rd ed. St. Louis: Mosby-Year Book; 1996. p. 2549–89.
5. Bracka A. Hypospadias repair: the two-stage alternative. Br J Urol. 1995;76(Suppl. 3):31–41.
6. Hadidi AT. Perineal hypospadias: Back to the future; Chordee Excision and Distal Urethroplasty (CEDU). J Pediatr Urol. 2018;14:424:e1–e9.
7. Long CJ, Chu DI, Tenney RW. Intermediate term follow up of proximal hypospadias reveals high complication rate. J Urol. 2017;197:852–8.
8. Weber DM, Schönbucher VB, Landolt MA, et al. The pediatric perception score: an instrument for patient self assessment and surgeon evaluation after hypospadias repair. J Urol. 2008;180:1080–8.
9. Castagnetti M, El-Ghoneimi A. Surgical management of primary severe hypospadias in children: systematic 20-year review. J Urol. 2010;184:1469–75.
10. de Mattos e Silva E, Gorduza DB, Catti M, et al. Outcome of severe hypospadias repair using three different techniques. J Pediatr Urol. 2009;5:205–11.
11. Castagnetti M, Zhapa E, Rigamonti W. Primary severe hypospadias: comparison of reoperation rates and parental perception of urinary symptoms and cosmetic outcomes among 4 repairs. J Urol. 2013;189:1508–13.
12. Braga LH, Lorenzo AJ, Bägli DJ, et al. Ventral penile lengthening versus dorsal plication for severe ventral curvature in children with proximal hypospadias. J Urol. 2008;180:1743–8. [Suppl]
13. Long CJ, Canning DA. Hypospadias; are we as good as we think when we correct proximal hypospadias? J Pediatr Urol. 2016;12(196):1e–5e.
14. Hadidi AT. Double Y glanuloplasty for glanuar hypospadias. J Pediatr Surg. 2010;45:655–60.
15. Hadidi AT. The Slit-Like adjusted Mathieu (SLAM) technique for distal hypospadias. J Ped Surg. 2012;47:797–801.

Single-Stage Primary Proximal Hypospadias Repair with Penile Curvature Correction

19

Pankaj M. Joshi and Tariq O. Abbas

Abstract

The management of severe penoscrotal hypospadias with penile curvature is challenging and demands professional rectification. Various correction methods for severe hypospadias have been described. With severe penile curvature, stage procedures are recommended in children. However, when an adult presents with severe untreated hypospadias, a single-stage correction is often preferred. This stimulated us to standardize our penile curvature correction with corpus augmentation via a pedicled preputial tube for hypospadias.

Keywords

Hypospadias · Corporal augmentation · Penile curvature · Pedicled preputial flap

---

Supplementary Information The online version contains supplementary material available at https://doi.org/10.1007/978-981-99-0795-3_19. The videos can be accessed individually by clicking the DOI link in the accompanying figure caption or by scanning this link with the SN More Media App.

P. M. Joshi (✉)
UROKUL, Pune, India

T. O. Abbas
Urology Division, Surgery Department, Sidra Medicine, Doha, Qatar
e-mail: tabbas@sidra.org

T. O. Abbas (ed.), *Video Atlas of Hypospadias Surgery*,
https://doi.org/10.1007/978-981-99-0795-3_19

19.1 Introduction

Hypospadias is characterized by four phenotypic abnormalities: urethral deficiency, penile curvature, preputial hood, and, in certain cases, peno-scrotal transposition [1, 2]. The severity of hypospadias correlates with the likelihood of sexual differentiation abnormalities [3, 4]. Penoscrotal hypospadias in adults who were raised by parents who sought multiple perspectives, were confused, and denied correction is common. Few of these individuals have access to trained specialists. Adults of marriageable age desire a penis that is straight, pee from the tip, and a single-stage repair. Experts in the subject have published algorithms on how to do a two-stage repair on patients with severe penile curvature [5–8]. Reparations in stages might cause grafts to contract, necessitating revision surgery [9] and still no assurance of total success. We describe a strategy for the single-stage management of penile curvature, hypospadias, and cosmesis.

19.2 Indications

19.2.1 Penoscrotal Hypospadias

Patients with penoscrotal hypospadias should use our technique [10]. We carry out pedicled preputial grafts. The length of the harvestable pedicled preputial flap is equal to the width of the prepuce. In 1971, Asopa [11] presented his findings about the single-stage pedicled preputial tube.

19.2.2 Severe Penile Curvature

Penile curvature more than 60% is usually repaired by two-stage urethroplasty [12–16]. We perform a single-stage surgery even if penile curvature is more than 60%.

19.2.3 Availability of Prepuce Tissue

Availability of prepuce is important for performing this surgery. In case prepuce is absent distal penile skin flap can be used.

19.3 Steps of the Procedure

- The patient is placed in supine position under general anesthesia.
- Perineum is painted with betadine solution and draped.

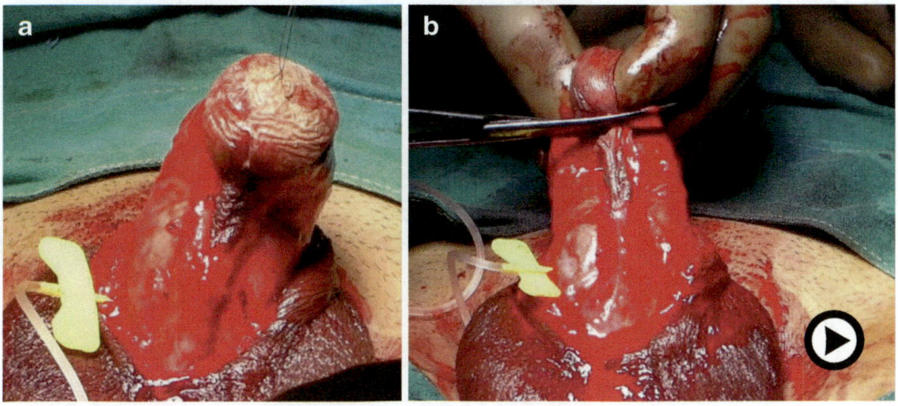

Fig. 19.1 (**a**) Severe penile curvature. (**b**) Transection of urethral plate. Single stage repair with severe curvature (https://doi.org/10.1007/000-cnf)

19.3.1 Penile Degloving

- A 5-0 a 4-0 non-absorbable suture is taken on the glans.
- Penis is placed under stretch.
- Look for the natural lines of fusion of penile skin, preputial skin, and scrotal skin.
- It is often easy to look for the wide divergent spongiosa underneath the skin.
- Incision is made around the urethral plate and then circumferentially close to the glans groove (Fig. 19.1a).

19.3.2 Dissection of Spongiosa

- The spongiosa is identified and traced upwards till it enters on to the glans.
- Careful dissection is done to lift the widely divergent spongiosa.
- Urethra is lifted from the corpora.
- Multiple corporotomies are done along with excision of scar tissue.

19.3.3 Transection of Urethral Plate

- Gitte's test is performed by injecting warm saline through a needle in corpora.
- The degree of penile curvature is assessed.
- Any remaining fibrous tissue leading to curvature is excised.
- Once all this does not resolve penile curvature, the urethra is transected at the level of corona (Fig. 19.1).
- Gitte's test is performed again to see for penile curvature resolution.

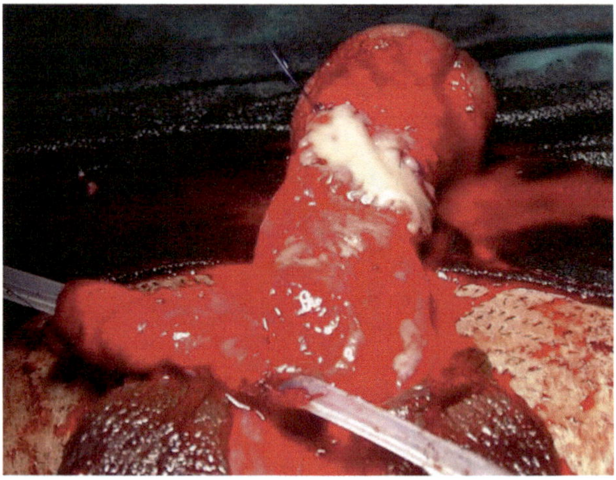

Fig. 19.2 Corporal augmentation with buccal graft along with urethral tubularization with pedicled preputial tube

19.3.4 Penile Curvature Correction

- A transverse incision is made on the ventral corpora.
- An elliptical defect results on the corporal wall.
- Buccal graft of appropriate length and width is harvested.
- BMG is sutured in the ventral corpora to correct the penile curvature (Fig. 19.2).

19.3.5 Urethroplasty

- Traction suture is taken on the prepuce.
- Incision is made at junction of inner and outer prepuce.
- The width of the tube should be 25 French.
- The penile skin is dissected from the underlying dartos.
- The prepuce is now a flap based on the dartos Fig. 19.2.
- The pedicled preputial flap is rotated on the ventral aspect of penis. Fig. 19.3.
- The flap is tubularized over 14 Fr Silicone catheter.
- The distal extent of the native urethral plate is fixed to corpora.
- Anastomosis is performed between urethral plate and preputial tube.
- Wide glans wings are made.
- The distal urethra is sutured inside the glans to form a wide meatus.
- Overlying dartos acts as second layer cover.

19.3.6 Skin Closure

- Skin is closed using interrupted sutures.
- The penis is coated with a Tegaderm and Coban® in a slightly compressed manner.

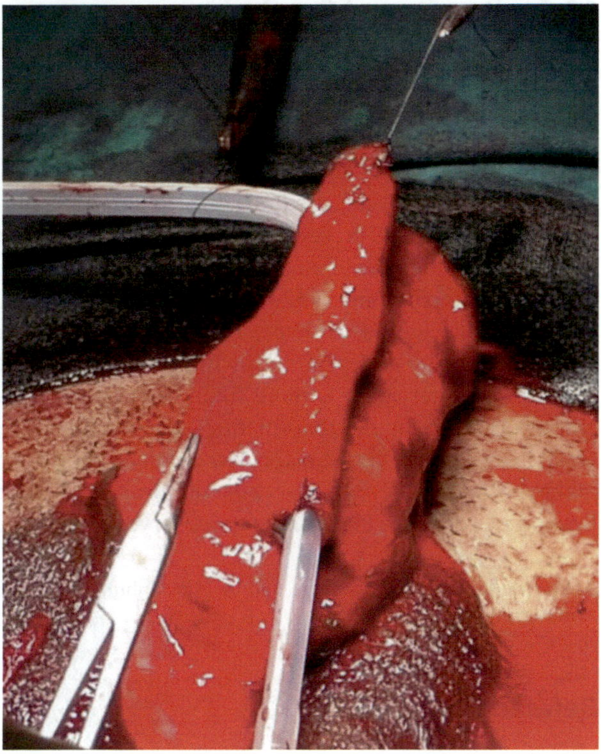

Fig. 19.3 Pedicled preputial tube

19.4 Post-operative Care

- To keep the Coban dressing for 24 hours.
- The urethral catheter/stent to be removed after 21 days.
- Antibiotic prophylaxis while the urethral catheter in place.

19.5 Tips and Tricks

- Initial degloving must be in the avascular plane just superficial to the Buck's fascia.
- Transection of urethra must be done as distal as possible.
- BMG applied on corpora must be wide and long enough.
- Check for corporeal anastomotic leaks while suturing BMG to corporotomy.
- Careful dissection between penile skin and underlying dartos during making the penciled flap.
- The suture line of preputial tube lies dorsally reducing the risk for fistulas formation.
- Wide anastomosis between the native urethra and pedicled preputial tube.

19.6 Results and Conclusion

Between 2015 and 2016, four studies from high-volume pediatric urology centers in North America revealed overall complication rates following proximal hypospadias surgery ranging between 32% and 68% [17–20]. Glans dehiscence is an early consequence that can be detected in as little as two months, whereas fistulae, meatal stenosis/strictures, and urethral diverticula typically become visible after six months. Spinoit et al. presented a big series that encompassed all forms of hypospadias treated at their center and noted that only 47% of problems occurred within the first year following surgery [21]. Others have demonstrated that substantially longer follow-up is required to detect recurrence of penile curvature as a child enters puberty and has rapid penile growth [22]. Several studies have demonstrated that recurrence of curvature is more likely if simply degloving +/− dorsal plication is employed to fix initial abnormalities greater than 30 degrees [23]. It is safe and feasible to perform single-stage correction of penile curvature and urethra in proximal hypospadias. If you transect the urethra, avoid surgery on dorsal side like mobilization of neurovascular bundle to preserve glans blood supply.

Acknowledgments The authors thanks Mrs. Subimol Abhilash, Nurse for helping to edit the manuscript.

References

1. Abbas T, McCarthy L. Foreskin and penile problems in childhood. Surg (United Kingdom). 2016;34(5):221.
2. Abbas TO, editor. HYPOSPADIOLOGY: current challenges and future perspectives. 2023. 190 p.
3. Kulkarni SB, Joglekar O, Alkandari MH, Joshi PM. Redo hypospadias surgery: current and novel techniques. Res Rep Urol. 2018;10:117–26.
4. Abbas T, Vallasciani S. Toward an ecosystem model of hypospadiology. In: Abbas TO, editor. Hypospadiology; 2023. p. 1–23.
5. Joshi PM, Barbagli G, Batra V, Surana S, Hamouda A, Sansalone S, et al. A novel composite two-stage urethroplasty for complex penile strictures: a multicenter experience. Indian J Urol. 2017;33(2):155–8.
6. Bethell GS, Chhabra S, Shalaby MS, Corbett H, Kenny SE, BAPS NOAH Contributors. Parental decisional satisfaction after hypospadias repair in the United Kingdom. J Pediatr Urol. 2020;16(2):164.e1–7.
7. Gopal M, Abbas T, Salle JLP. Management of proximal hypospadias: current challenges and future directions. In: Abbas TO, editor. Hypospadiology; 2023. p. 81–91.
8. Villanueva C, Abbas T. Penile curvature assessment in hypospadias. In: Abbas TO, editor. Hypospadiology; 2023. p. 93–102.
9. Spinoit A-F, Waterschoot M, Sinatti C, Abbas T, Callens N, Cools M, et al. Fertility and sexuality issues in congenital lifelong urology patients: male aspects. World J Urol. 2020;39:1013.
10. Abbas TO, editor. An objective hypospadias classification system. J Pediatr Urol. 2022;18(4):481.e1–8.
11. Asopa HS, Elhence IP, Atri SP, Bansal NK. One stage correction of penile hypospadias using a foreskin tube. A preliminary report. Int Surg. 1971;55(6):435–40.

12. Abbas TO. Evaluation of penile curvature in patients with hypospadias; gaps in the current practice and future perspectives. J Pediatr Urol 2021;
13. Abbas TO, Hatem M, Chandra P. Plate objective scoring tool: a new preoperative indicator of penile curvature degree in children with distal hypospadias. Int J Urol 202229, 511;
14. Abbas TO, AbdelMoniem M, Chowdhury M. Automated quantification of penile curvature using artificial intelligence. Front Artif Intell. 1AD.;0:188.
15. Abbas TO. The rising need for preoperative objective quantification of curvature in patients with hypospadias. J Pediatr Urol. 2021;17(4):599–600.
16. Abbas T. The need to optimize measurement of penile curvature in cases of hypospadias. J Pediatr Urol. 2023;0(0):577.
17. Stanasel I, Le H-K, Bilgutay A, Roth DR, Gonzales ET, Janzen N, et al. Complications following staged hypospadias repair using transposed preputial skin flaps. J Urol. 2015;194(2):512–6.
18. McNamara ER, Schaeffer AJ, Logvinenko T, Seager C, Rosoklija I, Nelson CP, et al. Management of proximal hypospadias with 2-stage repair: 20-year experience. J Urol. 2015;194(4):1080–5.
19. Pippi Salle JL, Sayed S, Salle A, Bagli D, Farhat W, Koyle M, et al. Proximal hypospadias: a persistent challenge. Single institution outcome analysis of three surgical techniques over a 10-year period. J Pediatr Urol. 2016;12(1):28.e1–7.
20. Long CJ, Canning DA. Hypospadias: are we as good as we think when we correct proximal hypospadias? J Pediatr Urol. 2016;12(4):196.e1–5.
21. Spinoit A-F, Poelaert F, Groen L-A, Van Laecke E, Hoebeke P. Hypospadias repair at a tertiary care center: long-term Followup is mandatory to determine the real complication rate. J Urol. 2013;189(6):2276–81.
22. Golomb D, Sivan B, Livne PM, Nevo A, Ben-Meir D. Long-term results of ventral penile curvature repair in childhood. Urology. 2018;112:161–3.
23. Braga LHP, Lorenzo AJ, Bägli DJ, Dave S, Eeg K, Farhat WA, et al. Ventral penile lengthening versus dorsal plication for severe ventral curvature in children with proximal hypospadias. J Urol. 2008;180(4):1743–8.

Part IV

Procedures to Correct Penile Curvature

Penile Curvature Correction Using Dorsal Plication

20

Martin Kaefer

Abstract

Achieving complete and lasting penile straightening is paramount in hypospadias correction, as untreated curvature can lead to significant psychological distress for patients. Inadequately addressing chordee during initial repair may necessitate complex revision surgeries, increasing the risk of complications. Effective correction relies on accurately assessing the underlying causes, including skin tethering, dartos/Buck's fascia dysplasia, corporal disproportion, and urethral foreshortening. Accurate characterization is crucial for comparing success rates among different repair methods.

Keywords

Hypospadias correction · Chordee assessment · Penile straightening · Curvature severity

Supplementary Information The online version contains supplementary material available at https://doi.org/10.1007/978-981-99-0795-3_20. The videos can be accessed individually by clicking the DOI link in the accompanying figure caption or by scanning this link with the SN More Media App.

M. Kaefer (✉)
Indiana University, Indianapolis, IN, USA
e-mail: mkaefer@iupui.edu

T. O. Abbas (ed.), *Video Atlas of Hypospadias Surgery*,
https://doi.org/10.1007/978-981-99-0795-3_20

Key Points

- Chordee has four potential etiologies. These are a) asymmetric skin distribution resulting in skin tethering, b) dysplastic periurethral tissue that restricts corporal lengthening, c) corporal disproportion, and d) a short urethra. These etiologies can exist either alone or in combination.
- Lesser degrees of chordee (typically less than or equal to 30 degrees) are amenable to a variety of plication techniques.

20.1 Introduction

Complete and lasting straightening of the penis is crucial for treating isolated curvature and is the primary and essential element in any hypospadias correction. Inadequate attention to this issue could lead to substantial psychological suffering for the patient. Men with untreated congenital chordee or Peyronie's disease with a curvature above 20–30 degrees might encounter challenges during intercourse and negative effects on body image [1, 2]. If chordee is not fully addressed during the initial repair, it may necessitate a more complex revision surgery, which could lead to higher risks of problems.

Correcting chordee effectively relies on accurately evaluating the cause and seriousness of the condition. There are four acknowledged causes for chordee [3]. The factors are skin tethering, dysplasia of the dartos and/or Buck's fascia, corporal disproportion, and foreshortened urethra. These can manifest independently but are more commonly observed in varying degrees of combination. It is crucial to recognize each of these elements and address them accordingly.

Different assessment procedures have been used. Compression of the corporal bodies at the base of the penis can trap venous blood in the penis and help determine curvature. Applying pressure might be particularly beneficial before removing the skin from the penis. However, this may not provide the level of rigidity that is indicative of what might be anticipated during sexual function. Most experts recommend inducing an artificial response by injecting normal saline into the corporal bodies after the penis has been exposed. To do this, a tourniquet is placed at the base of the penis, and a needle is inserted either through the side of one corpora or deeper through the glans until it reaches the cavernosum [4]. Some experts believe that using a tourniquet at the base of a degloved penis restricts the evaluation of more proximal forms of curvature. They suggest administering saline injections without using a tourniquet instead. We recommend using a sterile rubber band at the base of the penis during the initial assessment. Subsequently, we release the tourniquet while continuing to inject fluid into the penis to rule out a more proximal component.

Curvature severity can be assessed using visual inspection, a goniometer, or an electronic application [5, 6]. A replicable measurement of the angle is recommended above visual description to establish a reliable intra-observer method for characterizing severity. Abbas and colleagues have recently proposed using artificial intelligence to evaluate chordee more accurately and reliably [7]. Accurate description is essential for precise comparison of success rates in different repair methods. The degree of curvature is commonly categorized as minor (< 30 degrees), moderate (30–45 degrees), and severe (>45 degrees).

20.2 Indications

- Chordee correction is indicated at the time of hypospadias repair and elective circumcision. This is the most ideal time to address this issue. However, the surgical correction of isolated chordee in patients not already undergoing elective penile surgery is less well defined. In general, isolated chordee correction, as a child should be considered when it is expected that the degree of curvature is likely to effect sexual function. Many experts feel that with curvature less than 30 degrees in this specific cohort of patients (i.e., isolated chordee not undergoing elective circumcision), that it is reasonable to offer the parents the option of delaying surgical intervention until the time at which the patient themselves voices a concern that the curvature may be detrimental. As with all surgical intervention the individual risks and benefits should be considered and discussed thoroughly with the family in order to prove the correct environment for shared decision-making. Residual chordee following the excision of the paraspongiosal tissues can be addressed in two ways: dorsal plication or ventral corporal lengthening.
- There are concerns that utilizing dorsal plication for curvatures over 30 degrees may have a notable drawback. One issue is that it can shorten the penis and may not be strong enough to preserve straightness over time. Extensive folds can lead to significant compression of the tunica albuginea, perhaps restricting proper expansion of the corporal tissue during erection. Therefore, it is believed that having two little folds would be more beneficial than having a single larger one.

20.3 Surgical Technique

- The correction of chordee always initiates with the total degloving of the penis.
- Next, carefully remove dysplastic components from the underside of the corpora Fig. 20.1.
- Dorsal plication is carried out by first shifting the neurovascular complex away from the intended site of plication. This can be achieved by lifting the complete neurovascular complex or by separating the components at the 12 o'clock position [8]. The author favors the traditional strategy of lifting the complete neurovascular bundle from the dorsal part of the penis in cases of chordee nearing 30

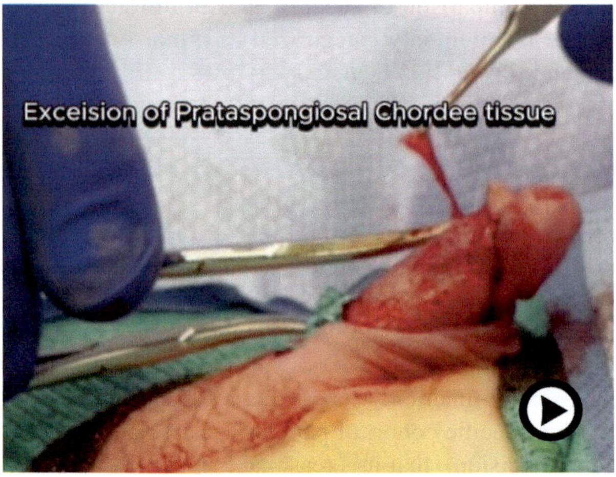

Fig. 20.1 Excision of the paraspongiosal chordee tissues. Dorsal plication (https://doi.org/10.1007/000-cng)

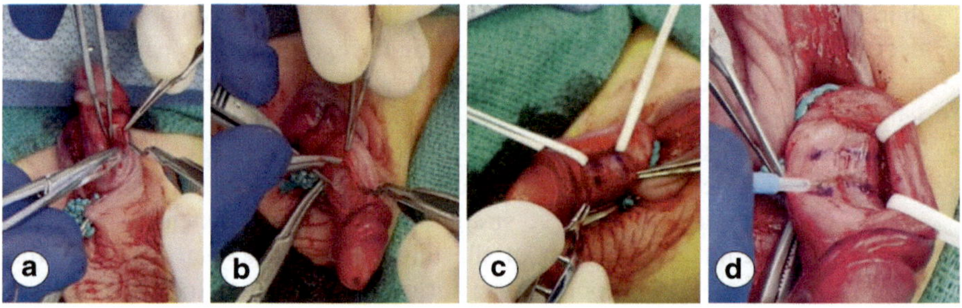

Fig. 20.2 Steps of the dorsal plication. Elevation of the neurovascular bundles starts from the ventral aspect lateral to urethra dissecting at the level of the tunica albuginea (**a**) and completed mobilization dorsally (**b**). The neurovascular bundles are then elevated using two vessel loops (**c**) to mark and incise the tunica albuginea (**d**)

degrees since it offers superior exposure. Begin this process on the ventral side of the penis (Fig. 20.2a) to precisely identify the outermost part of the neurovascular bundle and prevent any harm to it. The dissection is moved to the dorsal side of the penis (Fig. 20.2b) to fully raise the bundles and then surround them with vascular loops (Fig. 20.2c).

- Dorsal plications aim at shortening the dorsum of the penis and can be done in various ways, such as using absorbable or permanent sutures, with or without corporal incisions, and with or without excision of a segment of tunica albuginea (the technique initially described by Nesbit) [9]. The different techniques used for dorsal plication make it difficult to compare success rates among groups. The author favors using permanent sutures and corporal incisions (Fig. 20.2d) to promote a more robust healing response between two cut edges. The sutures are inserted in an inverted manner to reduce the likelihood of the knots being noticeable to the patient.

- An artificial erection is then induced after plication to confirm that full straightened has been accomplished.
- Dorsal skin flaps can then be used to provide adequate ventral penile skin coverage.
- The author utilizes a conforming dressing to provide adequate hemostasis and minimize postoperative swelling.

20.4 Tips and Tricks

1. Be aware of proximal bends. These can be overlooked if one simply uses the standard placement of a tourniquet for creation of an artificial erection. It is therefore useful to fill the penis both with and without a tourniquet applied. In order to exclude a more proximal component, we recommend putting a sterile rubber band at the base of the penis for the initial examination and then relaxing the tourniquet while continuing to inject fluid into the penis.
2. Prior to mobilizing the neurovascular bundles away from the proposed site of corporal plication, it is useful to release a tourniquet (if one is used) in order to allow penile structures to refill with blood. This refilling allows the surgeon to more readily identify the plane between the neurovascular bundles and the tunica albuginea.
3. For greater degrees of chordee, two small plications may prove more beneficial than one large plication. Larger plications carry the risk of creating a significant indentation of the corporal body with the greater potential for impingement of the underlying erectile tissue.

20.5 Results and Outcomes

Dorsal plication is considered the gold standard for treating ventral curvature <30 degrees, with ventral corporal lengthening reserved for the most severe cases, according to most practitioners [10]. Patients with moderate to severe curvature who have dorsal plication as opposed to ventral lengthening operations have a higher risk of experiencing recurrent post-surgical curvature, according to multiple studies published in the pediatric literature [11]. The recurrence rate of curvature was significantly higher in boys who underwent dorsal plication compared to corporal grafting (28% vs. 9%), according to Braga et al. [12].

The proper identification of the location and degree of chordee is critical to developing an appropriate strategy for its correction. With lesser degrees of chordee, typically less than 30 degrees, the use of one or two plications can completely correct the curvature and obviate the need for exposing the corporal erectile tissue (as with ventral grafting). Long-term follow-up is required to assure that any form of chordee correction has provided a durable and satisfactory result.

References

1. Menon V, Breyer B, Copp HL, Baskin L, Disandro M, Schlomer BJ. Do adult men with untreated ventral penile curvature have adverse outcomes? J Pediatr Urol. 2016;12:e1–7.
2. Walsh TJ, Hotaling JM, Lue TF, Smith JF. How curved is too curved? The severity of penile deformity may predict sexual disability among men with Peyronie's disease. Int J Impot Res. 2013;25:109–12.
3. Donnahoo KK, Cain MP, Pope JC, et al. Etiology, management and surgical complications of congenital chordee without hypospadias. J Urol. 1998;160:1120–2.
4. Gittes RF, McLaughlin AP. Injection technique to induce penile erection. Urology. 1974;4:473–4.
5. Villanueva CA. Goniometer not better than unaided visual inspection at estimating ventral penile curvature on plastic models. J Pediatr Urol. 2019;15:628–33.
6. Villanueva CA. Ventral penile curvature estimation using an app. J Pediatr Urol. 2020;16:e1–3.
7. Baray SB, Abdelmoniem M, Chowdhury M, Abbas TO. Machine-learning based opitmized measurement of penile curvature. Presented at the 33rd Congress of the European Society of Pediatric Urology. Lisbon, Portugal. April, 2023.
8. Mingin G, Baskin LS. Management of chordee in children and young adults. Urol Clin North Am. 2002;29:277–84.
9. Nesbit RM. The surgical treatment of congenital chordee without hypospadias. J Urol. 1954;72:1178–80.
10. Springer A, Krois W, Horcher E. Trends in hypospadias surgery: results of a worldwide survey. Eur Urol. 2011;60:1184–9.
11. Gershbaum MD, Stock JA, Hanna MK. A case for 2-stage repair of perineoscrotal hypospadias with severe chordee. J Urol. 2002;168:1727–8. discussion 9
12. Braga LH, Lorenzo AJ, Bagli DJ, et al. Ventral penile lengthening versus dorsal plication for severe ventral curvature in children with proximal hypospadias. J Urol. 2008;180:7–8. 1743-7; discussion

Deep Transverse Incisions of Tunica Albuginea (DTITA) Repair for Severe Ventral Penile Curvature

21

Tariq O. Abbas and J. L. Pippi Salle

Abstract

Severe ventral penile curvature continues to be challenging to treat. The objective of this chapter is to demonstrate ventral transverse incisions of the external shell of tunica albuginea repair. In cases of proximal hypospadias in which the spongiosa bifurcation is below the pubic bone or the penile curvature is greater than 45 degrees, a staged preputial graft repairs (SPG) may be used. Deep transverse incisions in the tunica albuginea at the penis's maximal curvature (DTITA) is an efficient treatment for moderate to severe chordee.

Keywords

Proximal hypospadias · Corporotomy · Curvature · Staged repair

21.1 Introduction

Twenty percent of all primary hypospadias cases are of proximal hypospadias, and since it is still challenging to treat, it compounds the complexity of penile curvature (PC) management [1–6]. Since different inclusion criteria are used to define

Supplementary Information The online version contains supplementary material available at https://doi.org/10.1007/978-981-99-0795-3_21. The videos can be accessed individually by clicking the DOI link in the accompanying figure caption or by scanning this link with the SN More Media App.

T. O. Abbas (✉)
Weil-Cornell Medical College-Qatar, Sidra Medicine, Doha, Qatar
e-mail: tabbas@sidra.org

J. L. P. Salle
Pediatric Urology Section, Sidra Medicine, Doha, Qatar

T. O. Abbas (ed.), *Video Atlas of Hypospadias Surgery*,
https://doi.org/10.1007/978-981-99-0795-3_21

case severity and associated chordee, it is challenging to compare the various repair techniques described to date [7, 8]. This results in procedure selection being heavily reliant on subjective judgments and the personal preferences of surgeons. Therefore, objective evaluation of the degree of penile curvature [9] could potentially help communication between the surgeons and researchers and help standardize the cutoff for the selection between the different PC management approaches. Not many studies have reported on the long-term effects, especially in terms of how satisfied patients were with their treatment [10, 11]. Various PC repair methods have been described. In general, they can be broken down into two categories: methods that lengthen the ventral aspect at the point of greatest curvature and procedures that shorten the convex (dorsal) side of the penis (dorsal plications). We advocate doing a ventral lengthening operation as the primary method of repairing severe PC because many patients with proximal hypospadias also come with a small penis size. After a graft of synthetic or organic material is used to cover the created corporal defect, no further grafting can be performed on the area. As a result, skin flap with a good blood supply is required for these procedures, and Byar's flaps are commonly used for ventral covering. When the meatus is properly placed in orthotopic position, flaps tend to produce diverticulae, so we prefer employing preputial grafts, which connect to the corpora, during the first step. In order to lengthen and widen the penis's ventral aspect and allow using skin grafts at the same time, we make three deep transverse incisions in the tunica albuginea at the penis's maximal curvature (DTITA). This method allows for the graft to be placed immediately over the incisions, allowing for fast correction of chordee [12].

21.2 Indications

1. The penile curvature is >45 degrees [13, 14].
2. Staged preputial graft can be employed in proximal hypospadias cases where the spongiosa bifurcation is below the pubic bone (hypospadias severity Grade 3 in Urethral defect ratio classification) [4].

21.3 Video Demonstration

Factors	Findings
Age at surgery (months)	13
Gestational age (weeks)	36
Birth weight (g)	1850
Gestational risks	IVF
Family history	None
Testosterone	Glans 11 mm, 2 mg/kg/dose 12, 8, and 4 weeks prior to surgery
Any features of DSD	None

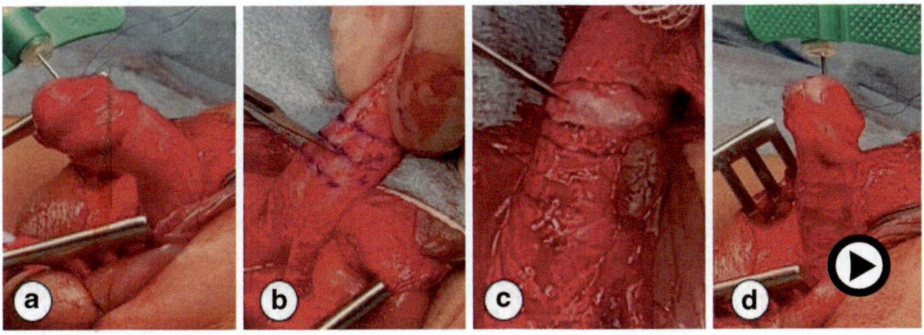

Fig. 21.1 Correction of ventral penile curvature >45 degrees. (**a**) Erection test after division of the urethral plate (70 degrees); (**b**, **c**) Ventral deep transverse incisions of tunica albuginea (DTITA); (**d**) Erection test after penile curvature correction with DTITA. DTITA procedure. (https://doi.org/10.1007/000-cnh)

21.4 Steps of the Procedure

1.1 During the first stage of SPG approach, a test for curvature is performed after totally degloving the penis, removing the ventral tethering tissue, and using an artificial erection.

1.2 The urethral plate is separated and mobilized, and any fibrous/dysplastic ventral tissue is excised, if the penile curvature is still greater than 45 degrees [15–17].

1.3 Three ventral transverse incisions of the external shell of tunica albuginea are made at the level of maximal curvature, from 3 to 9 o'clock, without the use of a tourniquet, if the penile curvature is greater than 45 degrees during the initial erection test. Care is taken to not cut into the corporal erectile tissue (the albuginea is incised, but the thin outer layer protecting the erectile tissue is left intact). After that, another erection test is performed (Fig. 21.1).

1.4 The graft or the mobilized proximal urethral plate covers the ventral bare region, including the DTITA.

21.5 Post-operative Care After the First Stage

- Vacuum physiotherapy starts in the third week postoperatively, 10 pumps holding vacuum for 3 seconds, twice a day, for 4–6 months.

21.6 Tips and Tricks

1. One should not use a tourniquet when performing DTITA, allowing bleeding to occur if the incision is too deep.
2. If modest residual penile curvature remains after DTITA, a midline dorsal plication stitch is used to correct it.

3. Evaluation of penile curvature should always occur after penile degloving, as the degree of curvature frequently improves after such dissection [18].

21.7 Outcomes

Pippi Salle et al. reported a 10-year analysis of 3 different techniques in 140 boys with proximal hypospadias; 60 underwent SGR and 75% had ventral lengthening with DTITA, achieving a success rate of 72%, despite being the most severe cases [19]. In another study, patients who did not use vacuum physiotherapy (VP) post first stage displayed a significantly higher rate of complications and VP appears to promote and expedite graft suppleness and significantly improves patient outcomes. (Ref).

References

1. Spinoit A-F, Waterschoot M, Sinatti C, Abbas T, Callens N, Cools M, et al. Fertility and sexuality issues in congenital lifelong urology patients: male aspects. World J Urol. 2020;
2. Abbas T, McCarthy L. Foreskin and penile problems in childhood. Surg (United Kingdom). 2016;34(5)
3. Wani SA, Baba AA, Mufti GN, Rashid KA, Bhat NA, Buch M, et al. Bracka verses Byar's two-stage repair in proximal hypospadias associated with severe chordee: a randomized comparative study. Pediatr Surg Int. 2020;36(8):965–70.
4. Abbas TO. An objective hypospadias classification system. J Pediatr Urol. 2022;18(4):481.e1–8.
5. Abbas TO, AlSalihi M, El-Hout Y, Ali M, AbdAlla E. General perioperative considerations. In: Abbas TO, editor. Hypospadiology; 2023. p. 53–65.
6. Abbas T, Vallasciani S. Toward an ecosystem model of hypospadiology. In: Abbas TO, editor. Hypospadiology. 2023. p. 1–23.
7. Bethell GS, Chhabra S, Shalaby MS, Corbett H, Kenny SE, BAPS NOAH Contributors. Parental decisional satisfaction after hypospadias repair in the United Kingdom. J Pediatr Urol. 2020;16(2):164.e1–7.
8. Abbas TO. The rising need for preoperative objective quantification of curvature in patients with hypospadias. J Pediatr Urol. 2021;17(4):599–600.
9. Abbas TO, Hatem M, Chandra P. Plate objective scoring tool: a new preoperative indicator of penile curvature degree in children with distal hypospadias. Int J Urol. 2022;
10. Mureau MAM, Slijper FME, Slob AK, Verhulst FC, Nijman RJM. Satisfaction with penile appearance after hypospadias surgery: the patient and surgeon view. J Urol. 1996;155(2):703–6.
11. Gopal M, Abbas TO, Salle JLP. Management of proximal hypospadias: current challenges and future directions. In: Abbas TO, editor. Hypospadiology; 2023. p. 81–91.
12. Leslie B, Weber B, Romao R, Farhat W, Bagli D, Lorenzo A, et al. 546 alternative for ventral lengthening in children with severe penile curvature that allows graft coverage during staged hypospadias repair. J Urol. 2011;
13. Villanueva C, Abbas T. Penile curvature assessment in hypospadias. In: Abbas TO, editor. Hypospadiology; 2023. p. 93–102.
14. AbdulMoniem M, Abbas T, Khandakar A, Shuzan MNI, Chowdhury MH, Chowdhury MEH. Artificial intelligence in hypospadiology: role, applications, and benefits. In: Abbas TO, editor. Hypospadiology; 2023. p. 137–65.

15. Abbas TO. Evaluation of penile curvature in patients with hypospadias; gaps in the current practice and future perspectives. J Pediatr Urol. 2021;
16. Abbas TO, AbdelMoniem M, Chowdhury M. Automated quantification of penile curvature using artificial intelligence. Front Artif Intell. 1AD. 0:188
17. Baray SB, Abdelmoniem M, Mahmud S, Kabir S, Faisal MAA, Chowdhury MEH, et al. Automated measurement of penile curvature using deep learning-based novel quantification method. Front Pediatr. 2023;11:438.
18. Weber BA, Braga LHP, Patel P, Pippi Salle JL, Bägli DJ, Khoury AE, et al. Impact of penile degloving and proximal ventral dissection on curvature correction in children with proximal hypospadias. Can Urol Assoc J. 2014;8(11–12):424–7.
19. Pippi Salle JL, Sayed S, Salle A, Bagli D, Farhat W, Koyle M, et al. Proximal hypospadias: a persistent challenge. Single institution outcome analysis of three surgical techniques over a 10-year period. J Pediatr Urol. 2016;12(1):28.e1–7.

22 The Corporotomy and Dermal Graft Procedure: The Case for Severe Curvature

Antonio Macedo and Emanuelle Lima Macedo

Abstract

The Corporotomy and Dermal Graft Procedure technique is suggested for complex hypospadias forms associated with severe curvature. In cases with more than 30 degrees of ventral curvature, we believe that the disproportionate ventral/dorsal length of corpora cavernosa is a major limiting factor for more conservative procedures, such as dorsal plication, including Baskin and classical Nesbit procedures lifting the neurovascular bundle. The so-called "fairy cuts" procedure, which is based on more superficial parallel transverse ventral corporal incisions, has not passed the test of time and the fear of retraction and recurrence of curvature limits its spread as a widely acceptable alternative technique. The corporotomy and the use of a dermal graft to restore corporal integrity is based on the concept of ventral corporal lengthening and mimics the strategy in Peyronie's disease. It has the advantage of being versatile enough to treat all forms of severe curvature but normally requires a two-stage strategy for urethral reconstruction. In young children and babies, a tunica vaginalis flap is also acceptable to replace the dermal graft and correct the corporal defect, but for adolescents and teenagers, our preference is the use of dermal grafts obtained from the groin.

Supplementary Information The online version contains supplementary material available at https://doi.org/10.1007/978-981-99-0795-3_22. The videos can be accessed individually by clicking the DOI link in the accompanying figure caption or by scanning this link with the SN More Media App.

A. Macedo
NUPEP/CACAU Pediatric Urology Department, Federal University of São Paulo, São Paulo, Brazil

E. L. Macedo (✉)
Albert Einstein Medical School, São Paulo, Brazil

T. O. Abbas (ed.), *Video Atlas of Hypospadias Surgery*,
https://doi.org/10.1007/978-981-99-0795-3_22

Keywords

Hypospadias · Proximal hypospadias · Penile curvature · Corporotomy Corporoplasty and dermal graft

22.1 Introduction

Normally, a corporotomy is preceded by a decision of correcting hypospadias in one or two stages. The grade of curvature is the main challenge whenever treating complex primary hypospadias forms or cripple hypospadias with residual curvature. The division of the urethral plate by primary forms is the initial decision to be taken and an initial U-shape incision defining the urethral plate should be a regular step in all primary forms. Thereafter, the degloving of the penile skin and detaching of all fibrotic tissue and chordee is performed until an honest artificial erection with a tourniquet can provide the final grade of curvature pre-division of the urethral plate. If indicated, the urethral plate is divided and a second artificial erection test performed. If the grade of curvature is higher than 30 degrees we proceed with the lengthening procedure.

22.2 Indications

Proximal hypospadias with severe ventral curvature (> 30 degrees) after all steps to treat curvature: chordee excision and division of the urethral plate.

22.3 Steps of the Procedure

- We initially deglove the penis and perform an artificial erection.
- If corporal disproportion causing curvature is clearly confirmed and the degree of ventral curvature is higher than 30 degrees after urethral plate division, the indication for corporotomy is established (Fig. 22.1a, b, c).
- The landmark to incise transversely the corpora is opposite to the most convex point at the dorsal surface outlining the curvature.
- The incision of tunica albuginea is done from 4 to 8 o'clock, creating an elliptical defect and elongating the ventral surface of the penis (Fig. 22.1d).
- We perform an elliptical incision in the groin and a de-epithelialized dermal graft is obtained. The dermal graft is sutured to the corpora with a running suture with polyglycolic acid 4.0 (Fig. 22.1e, f).

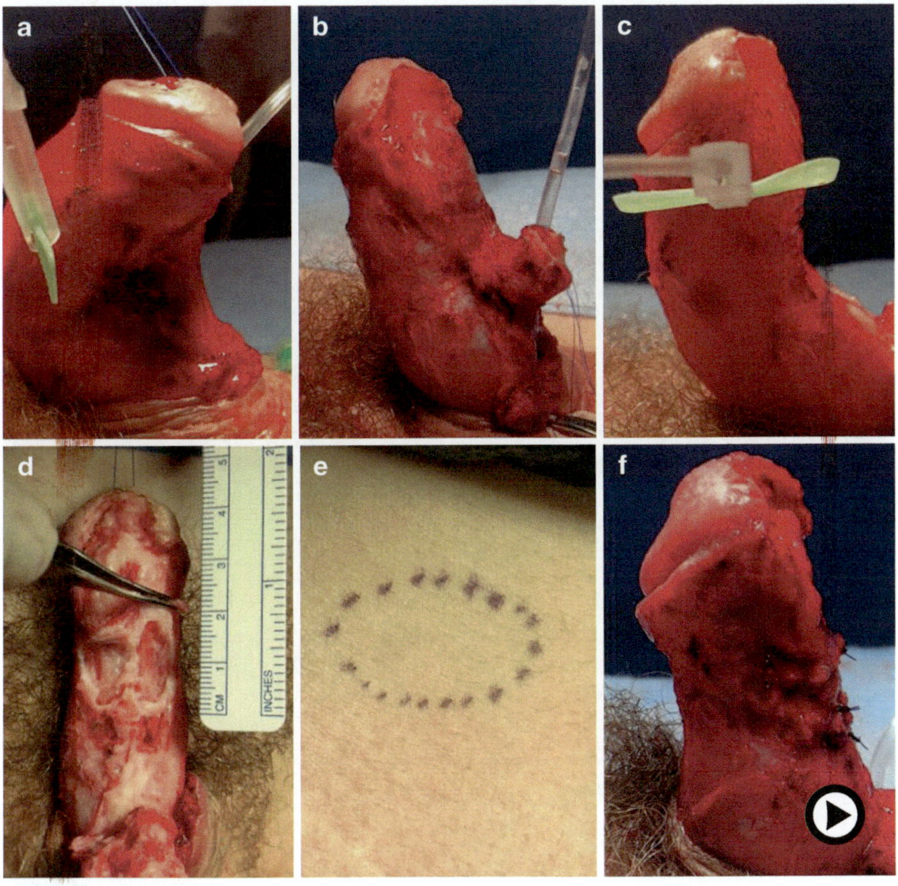

Fig. 22.1 Steps of the procedure: (**a**) Artificial erection test with urethra in situ, (**b**) Urethra detached from the corpora to improve curvature, (**c**) Curvature persisted, ventral length of the corpora inferior to the dorsal one, (**d**) Ventral corporotomy and dissection enlarged the length of corpora in 2 cm, (**e**) Donor area of the graft from the groin, (**f**) Dermal graft anastomosed to the corpora. The corporotomy and dermal graft procedure (https://doi.org/10.1007/000-cnj)

- After concluding the corporoplasty, the penile skin is restored to cover the penile shaft. In our case, the patient was multi-operated, had a cripple proximal hypospadias and paucity of skin. Therefore, we gained a buccal mucosa to complete the ventral penile defect and planned a two-stage urethroplasty (Fig. 22.2a).

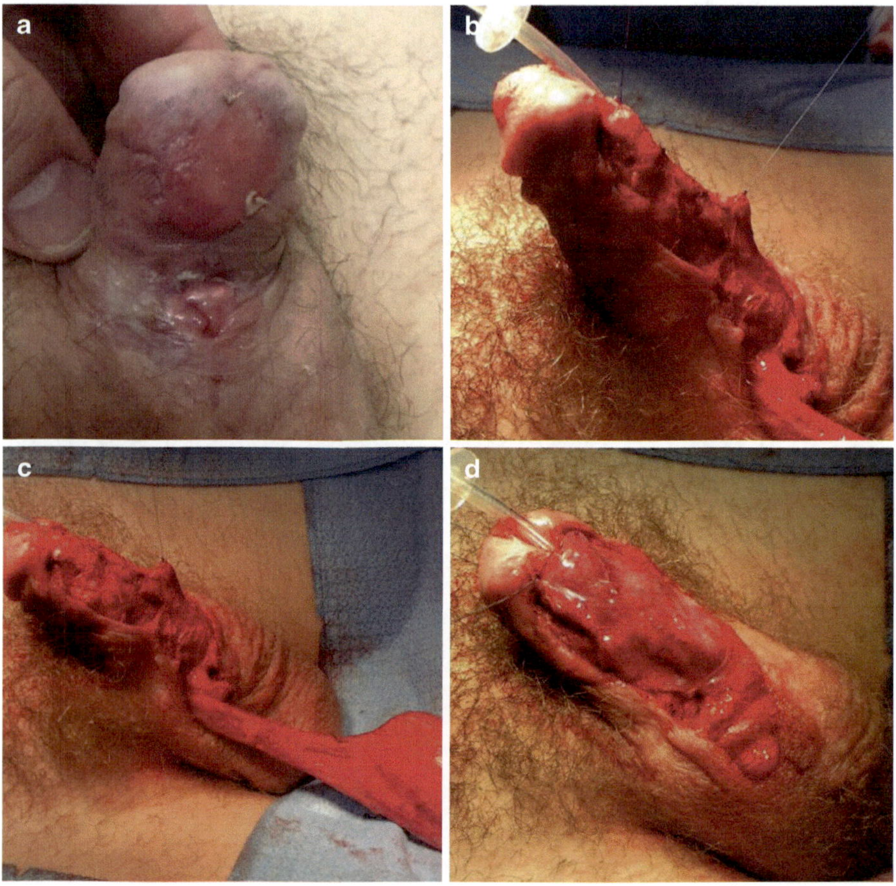

Fig. 22.2 Second-stage urethroplasty, (**a**) Initial aspect of the penis without curvature and good uptake of buccal mucosa to repair the skin defect, (**b**) Tubularization of the urethra completed, (**c**) Right testis exposed to gain access to a tunica vaginalis flap, (**d**) Tunica vaginalis flap covering the neourethra

22.4 Tips and Tricks

1. The indication for corporoplasty can only be confirmed after all steps to treat curvature and division of the urethral plate proved to be insufficient.
2. Incise the ventral surface of Buck's fascia of the corpora in the opposite level of maximal convexity dorsally under artificial erection.
3. Incisions should go from 4 to 8 o'clock and expose the trabeculae of the corpora cavernosa of the penis.
4. Measure the defect created in the corpora to incise the groin and gain an equivalent dermal graft in size, that will be transposed to the surgical site.
5. The dermal graft is sutured to the corpora with a running suture with polyglycolic acid 4.0.

22.5 Results and Conclusion

The patient had an excellent clinical evolution, we have used a buccal mucosa graft additionally to replace ventral skin (two grafts used at the same time) and came back 6 months after to reconstruct the urethra (tubularization and barrier layer with a tunica vaginal flap) (Fig. 22.2b, c, d). The patient has no residual curvature and voids straight; without any complaint.

Corporoplasty with dermal grafts is a surgical technique that aims to correct penile curvature in individuals with hypospadias. The procedure involves reinforcing the tunica albuginea using dermal grafts to achieve improved penile alignment and functional outcomes. By adding structural support to the tunica albuginea on the concave side of the curvature, the graft helps straighten the penis, resulting in improved penile alignment [1–7]. Other alternatives to dermal graft in corporoplasty are SIS and tunica vaginalis (flap or graft). Some authors who have used the TV and SIS still recognize the efficacy and durability of the dermal graft and even consider the DG as the gold standard to recreate the corpus cavernosum

Hendren and Keating [8] corrected the chordee with dermal graft and performed the urethroplasty with bladder mucosa-free graft in one stage in 10 patients. Kajbafzadeh performed the repair on his 16 patients in one stage with 1 urethrocutaneous fistula and 2 others in two stages with 1 meatal stenosis [9]. Hendren and Keating reported that the correction of chordee with DG and urethroplasty could be performed simultaneously, presumably because the DG obtained blood supply from the corpora cavernosa. They decided to repair in one stage on the basis of the quality of the penile skin. If, after degloving, the skin had enough dartos to cover the neourethra, they applied the two grafts simultaneously [10].

We, in our case, used two grafts (dermal graft and buccal mucosa), and we prepared the urethroplasty for a two-stage procedure. We conclude that all efforts for correcting the curvature are worthwhile and that dermal graft has demonstrated long-term efficacy for lengthening of the ventral corporal body for repair of severe chordee with hypospadias.

References

1. Barroso U Jr, Macedo A Jr. Initial experience with 'inverted U' staged buccal mucosa graft (Bracka) for hypospadias repair. J Pediatr Urol. 2009;5:90–2.
2. Snodgrass W, Bush NC. Persistent or recurrent ventral curvature after failed proximal hypospadias repair. J Pediatr Urol. 2019;15:344.e1–6.
3. Nesbit RM. Operation for correction of distal penile ventral curvature with or without hypospadias. J Urol. 1967;97:720–2.
4. Hoebeke P, Weyne E. Hypospadias repair: an overview of the actual techniques. Semin Plast Surg. 2011;25(3):206–12.
5. Snodgrass W. Tubularized incised plate hypospadias repair: indications, technique, and complications. Urol Clin North Am. 2002;29(2):397–404.
6. Castagnetti M, El-Ghoneimi A. Management of severe hypospadias in children: an update. Nat Rev Urol. 2012;9(11):678–88.

7. Park JM, Hwang EC, Kim SO, et al. Corporoplasty with porcine small intestine submucosa graft for penile curvature in Peyronie's disease: a preliminary report. Int J Impot Res. 200.
8. Devine CJ Jr, Horton CE. Use of dermal graft to correct chordee. J Urol. 1975;113(56):3.
9. Kajbafzadeh AM, Arshadi H, Payabvash S, Salmasi AH, Tousi VN, Sahebpor ARA. Proximal hypospadias with severe chordee: single stage repair using corporeal tunica vaginalis free graft. J Urol. 2007;178:1036–42.
10. Hardy H, Michael K. Use of dermal graft and free urethral graft in penile reconstruction. J Urol. 1988;140:1265–9.

Part V

Surgical Harvest for Intervening Coverage Layers

Harvest of Ventral Dartos Flap for Second Coverage of Urethroplasty

23

Tariq O. Abbas

Abstract

Neourethra dartos flap coverage is frequently employed as a protective layer for improved postoperative problems, particularly fistula development. Although several forms of dartos flaps have been developed, only the dorsal and ventral dartos flaps (VDF) have gained widespread recognition for use in distal and mid-shaft hypospadias correction. Concerning the most appropriate covering flap approach in terms of complication rates in distal hypospadias treatment, there is still some dispute. We here show the key steps to harvest and fix the ventral dartos flap.

Keywords

Dartos flap · Ventral · Hypospadias · Coverage

23.1 Introduction

The adoption of the dorsal dartos flap for the second layer is a globally accepted technique due to its efficacy [1–3]. The harvesting of dorsal dartos, on the other hand, can harm the vascularity of the skin and has detrimental repercussions. The

Supplementary Information The online version contains supplementary material available at https://doi.org/10.1007/978-981-99-0795-3_23. The videos can be accessed individually by clicking the DOI link in the accompanying figure caption or by scanning this link with the SN More Media App.

T. O. Abbas (✉)
Weil-Cornell Medical College-Qata, Sidra Medicine, Doha, Qatar
e-mail: tabbas@sidra.org

T. O. Abbas (ed.), *Video Atlas of Hypospadias Surgery*,
https://doi.org/10.1007/978-981-99-0795-3_23

dorsal dartos flap has a problem with penile rotation, which ranges between 5% and 10% [4, 5]. This reflected tissue not only provides a vascularized tissue barrier between the urethroplasty suture line and skin, but also isolates urethral repair to the distal glandular area [6–8]. If accomplished successfully, the VDF can be harvested intraoperatively in a short time frame with a robust vascular component.

23.2 Indication

(a) VDF should be employed in distal hypospadias repairs objectively characterized as grade one per urethral defect ratio according to Abbas's classification [9]. According to this classification, VDF is to be used when the spongiosa bifurcation is at or distal to the midpenile shaft (Grade 1).
(b) Based on a recent systematic study, tunica vaginalis flap should be the primary option for proximal, repeat, and fistula repairs [10].
(c) Penile curvature should be <45 degrees [11–13].

23.3 Key Steps of the Procedure

1. The distance needed to be covered, which is equal to the urethra defect, [9] from the spongiosa bifurcation to the distal extent of the urethroplasty, is measured (Fig. 23.1).
2. The proximal part of the dartos dascia was harvested by perpendicular dissecting to the level of the Buck's fascia just superficial to urethral spongiosa (Fig. 23.2).
3. The VDF was turned up continuing dissection in the same bloodless plane.
4. After being released from the proximal shaft, the vascularized pedicle is fanning out to reduce bulk before being sutured into the lateral recesses of the elevated glans wings with fine absorbable suture (Fig. 23.3).

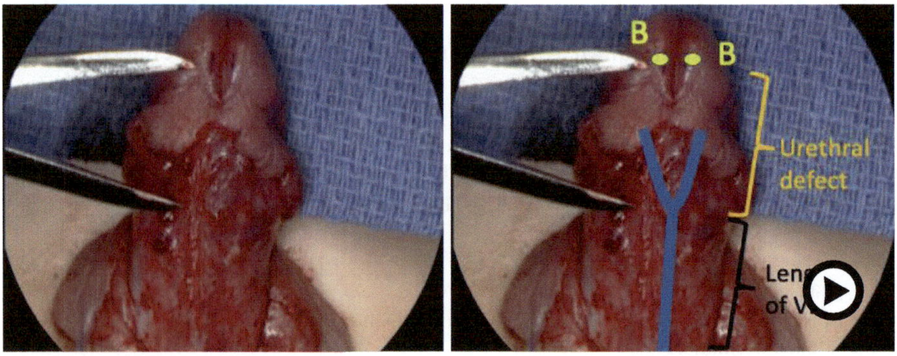

Fig. 23.1 Measurement of the needed length of the ventral dartos flap (VDF). Ventral dartos flap (https://doi.org/10.1007/000-cnk)

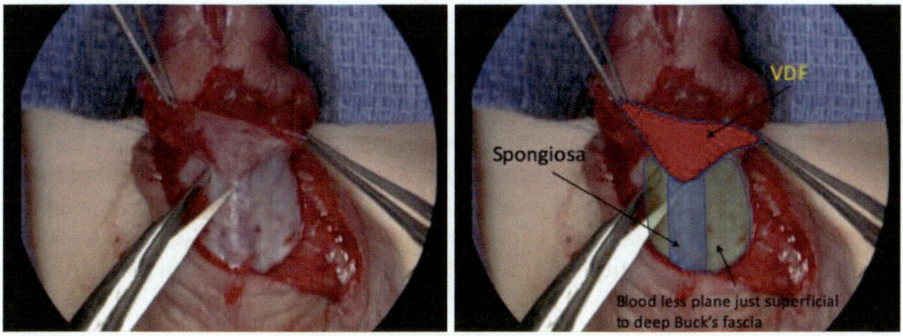

Fig. 23.2 Releasing the VDF all the way deep to the level of the Buck's fascia

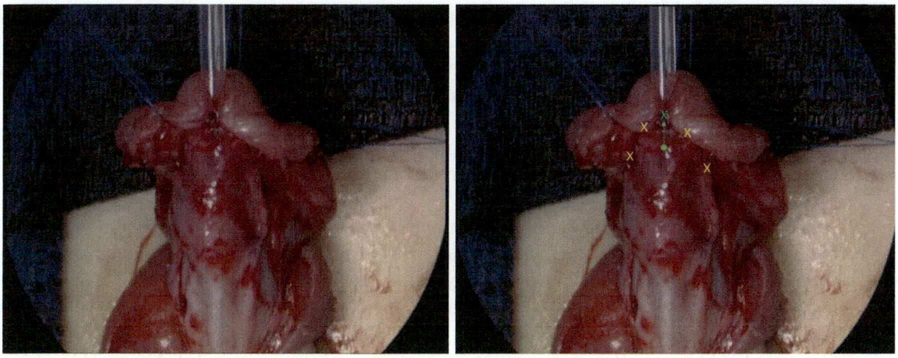

Fig. 23.3 Attachment of the prepped ventral dartos flap. To fix the VDF, several lateral sutures (orange crosses) are performed beginning distally to the grooves of the dissected glanular wings and proceeding laterally to the corpora. A midline extra-fixation suture (green cross) at the most distal glanuloplasty suture to anchor the distal end of the VDF (green dot) to embrace the entire urethroplasty zone

23.4 Tips and Tricks

(a) The dissection on the right plane just superficial to the deep Buck's fascia surrounding the spongiosa.
(b) No tension to exist during the fixation of the VDF around the neourethra.
(c) To excise any excess of the VDF at the territory of the glanuloplasty to avoid glanular and dehiscence.
(d) Distal pedicle dissection should be performed with caution to avoid urethral damage and preserve the vascular supply.
(e) To prevent injury to the primary arterial supply or severing of the pedicle, dissection must cease before reaching the hypoplastic urethral that is marked by the site of the spongiosa bifurcation.

23.5 Outcomes

The restoration of hypospadias has been the subject of numerous surgical approaches and alterations, leading to a wide range of problems, the most common of which is urethrocutaneous fistula [14]. Urethral covering is now routinely performed by most surgeons to minimize the risk of fistula formation. Furness advised a method to use a ventral dartos flap with a success rate of 98.2% [15]. Savanelli et al. compared two randomized groups of patients with distal hypospadias treated with and without ventral dartos coverage after TIPU repair, and found better results in fistula rate.

References

1. Chatterjee US, Mandal MK, Basu S, Das R, Majhi T. Comparative study of dartos fascia and tunica vaginalis pedicle wrap for the tubularized incised plate in primary hypospadias repair. BJU Int. 2004;94(7):1102–4.
2. Soygur T, Arikan N, Zumrutbas AE, Gulpinar O. Snodgrass hypospadias repair with ventral based dartos flap in combination with mucosal collars. Eur Urol. 2005;47(6):879–84. discussion 884
3. Abbas T, McCarthy L. Foreskin and penile problems in childhood. Surg. 2016;34(5):221–5.
4. Kamal BA. Double dartos flaps in tubularized incised plate hypospadias repair. Urology. 2005;66(5):1095–8.
5. Hypospadiology: current challenges and future perspectives. 2023. 190 p.
6. Abbas T. Management of distal hypospadias: new insights and stepwise management algorithm. In: Abbas TO, editor. Hypospadiology; 2023. p. 67–80.
7. Abbas T, Vallasciani S. Toward an ecosystem model of hypospadiology. In: Abbas TO, editor. Hypospadiology; 2023. p. 1–23.
8. Villanueva C, Abbas T. Penile curvature assessment in hypospadias. In: Abbas TO, editor. Hypospadiology; 2023. p. 93–102.
9. Abbas TO. An objective hypospadias classification system. J Pediatr Urol. 2022;18(4):481.e1–8.
10. Fahmy O, Khairul-Asri MG, Schwentner C, Schubert T, Stenzl A, Zahran MH, et al. Algorithm for optimal urethral coverage in hypospadias and fistula repair: a systematic review. Eur Urol. 2016;70(2):293–8.
11. Abbas TO. Evaluation of penile curvature in patients with hypospadias; gaps in the current practice and future perspectives. J Pediatr Urol. 2021;
12. Baray SB, Abdelmoniem M, Mahmud S, Kabir S, Faisal MAA, Chowdhury MEH, et al. Automated measurement of penile curvature using deep learning-based novel quantification method. Front Pediatr. 2023;11:438.
13. Abbas TO. The rising need for preoperative objective quantification of curvature in patients with hypospadias. J Pediatr Urol. 2021;17(4):599–600.
14. Dokter EM, Mouës CM, van Rooij IALM, van der Biezen JJ. Complications after hypospadias correction: prognostic factors and impact on final clinical outcome. Eur J Pediatr Surg. 2018;28(2):200–6.
15. Furness PD, Hutcheson J. Successful hypospadias repair with ventral based vascular dartos pedicle for urethral coverage. J Urol. 2003;169(5):1825–7. discussion 1827

Dorsal Dartos Flap Covering of the Neourethra for Fistula Prevention in Hypospadias Repair

24

Borko Stojanovic, Marko Bencic, Slavica Pusica, Marta Bizic, and Miroslav L. Djordjevic

Abstract

Distal hypospadias repair has become a relatively safe surgical procedure with tubularized incised plate urethroplasty. However, fistula formation still represents the most common complication, in various rates. Covering of the neourethra with vascularized tissue has proven effective in reducing urethrocutaneous fistula rate. We present our technique based on using dorsal dartos flap for neourethra covering.

Keywords

Hypospadias · Reconstruction · Longitudinal dartos flap · Urethroplasty Urethrocutaneous fistula

---

Supplementary Information The online version contains supplementary material available at https://doi.org/10.1007/978-981-99-0795-3_24. The videos can be accessed individually by clicking the DOI link in the accompanying figure caption or by scanning this link with the SN More Media App.

B. Stojanovic · M. Bencic · M. Bizic · M. L. Djordjevic (✉)
School of Medicine, Department of Urology, University of Belgrade, Belgrade, Serbia

Belgrade Center for Urogenital Reconstructive Surgery, Belgrade, Serbia
e-mail: stojanovic@uromiros.com; bencic@uromiros.com; martabizic@uromiros.com; djordjevic@uromiros.com

S. Pusica
Belgrade Center for Urogenital Reconstructive Surgery, Belgrade, Serbia

T. O. Abbas (ed.), *Video Atlas of Hypospadias Surgery*,
https://doi.org/10.1007/978-981-99-0795-3_24

24.1 Introduction

Hypospadias repair is one of the most common surgical procedures in pediatric surgery. Although a variety of techniques have been described, tubularized incised plate (TIP) urethroplasty is nowadays a mostly performed technique for primary distal hypospadias repair [1, 2]. In general, urethrocutaneous fistula is the most common complication. To prevent fistula formation, plenty of techniques have been described, but none proved superior [3, 4]. Overall, tissue interposition between two suture lines is essential for good outcome. Different tissues and techniques have been described to solve this problem: spongioplasty [5]; asymmetrical, rotational, subcutaneous dartos tissue flap harvested from the dorsal preputial and shaft skin [6]; Y-to-I wrap of spongiosum for neourethral reinforcement [7]; lateral-based de-epithelialized flap in previous hypospadias failures [8]. We proposed dorsal dartos flap, with excellent results [9].

24.2 Indications

(a) *Distal hypospadias (glanular, subcoronal, penile)*
(b) *Proximal hypospadias with well-developed and elastic urethral plate*

Reconstruction of distal or midshaft hypospadias with well-developed urethral plate, which is used for TIP urethroplasty. Also, some cases of proximal (penoscrotal) hypospadias can present with wide and elastic urethral plate, which is suitable for TIP urethroplasty (extended Snodgrass). Dartos flap can be a good solution in those cases as well.

24.3 Video Demonstration

Factors	Findings
Age at surgery (months)	32
Gestational age (weeks)	39
Birth weight (gm	3300
Gestational risk:	None
Family history	None
Testosterone	None
Any features of DSD	None

24.4 Steps of the Procedure

24.4.1 Suprapubic Catheter

- A 6Fr Nelaton catheter is introduced, and bladder is filled with saline. Suprapubic tube 9Fr is placed into the bladder and fixed to the skin with 3–0 Nylon suture.

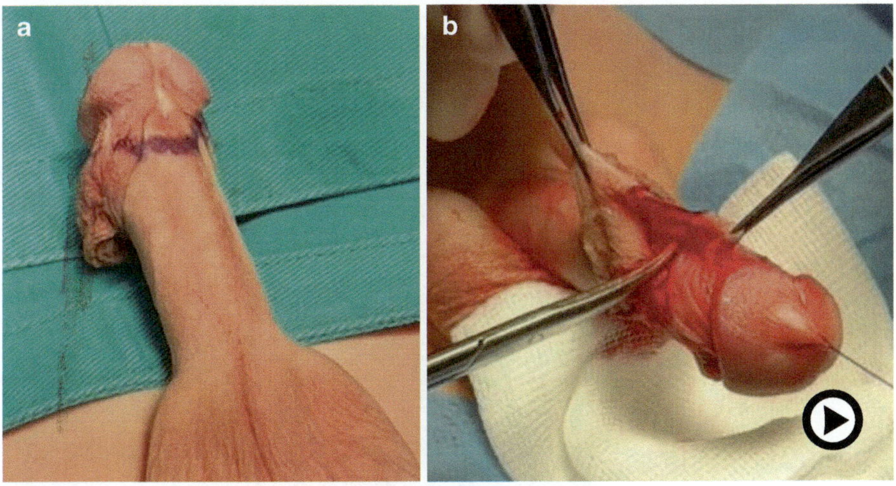

Fig. 24.1 (**a**) Incision line is marked on the border with healthy penile skin under the ectopic meatus. (**b**) Dissection above Buck's fascia is performed (https://doi.org/10.1007/000-cnm)

24.4.2 Penile Degloving

- A 4-0 Vycril stay suture is placed through the glans for traction.
- Incision line is marked on the ventral side transversely under hypospadic meatus, on the border with healthy skin (Fig. 24.1).
- Transversal incision is made ventrally and degloving is started.
- Blunt and sharp dissection is done just above Buck's fascia dorsally, to prevent thinning of dartos layer.
- Meticulous dissection around divergent spongiosal tissue ventrally is performed to avoid injury and possible excessive bleeding. Dissection is done ventrally to the scrotal fat and dorsally to the penile suspensor ligament.
- After complete degloving, artificial erection is done to check for associated curvature (Fig. 24.2).
- In cases where significant curvature is revealed, correction should be done.

24.4.3 Preparation of Longitudinal Dorsal Dartos Flap

- A longitudinal dorsal dartos flap is marked on the dorsal distal penile skin (Fig. 24.3a).
- Blood supply of the flap is identified with transillumination.
- De-epithelialization is started proximally in the region where subcutaneous tissue is well-developed (Fig. 24.3b).
- Meticulous dissection is performed to avoid devascularization of created flap (Fig. 24.3c).
- Button-hole maneuver is used to transpose flap on the ventral side (Fig. 24.3d-f).

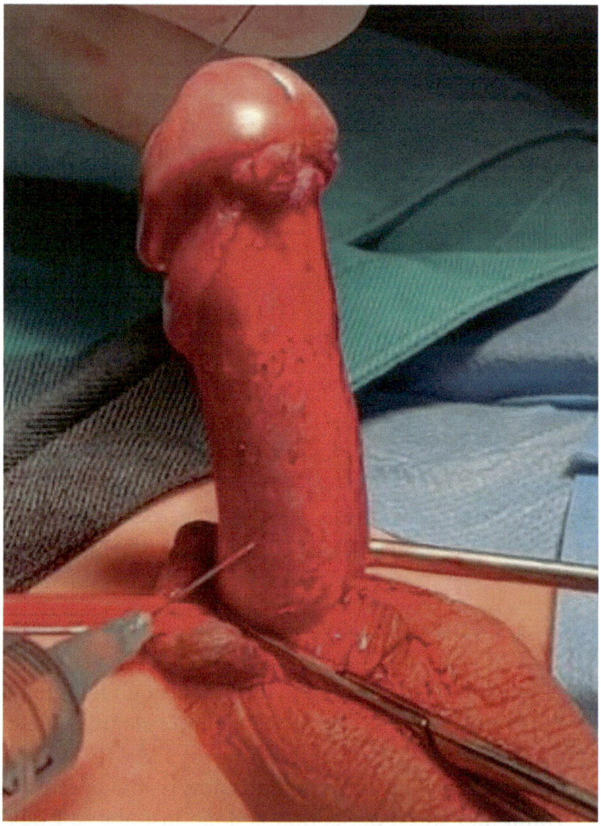

Fig. 24.2 Degloving is done. Artificial erection demonstrates completely straight penis

24.4.4 Urethroplasty

- Excessive bleeding after glans incision should be avoided with tourniquet placement.
- Glans wings are created by using two longitudinal incisions to the tip of corpora cavernosa (Fig. 24.4a).
- The urethral plate is opened in the midline from the ectopic meatus toward tip of the glans (Fig. 24.4b).
- One interrupted suture 6-0 Monocryl is placed to define the oval-shaped neometus.
- Tubularization is performed over a 6-8 Fr stent with a one-layer running suture of 6-0 Monocryl.
- Urethral stent is fixed to the glans on 12-o'clock position, with one interrupted suture 5-0 Monocryl.

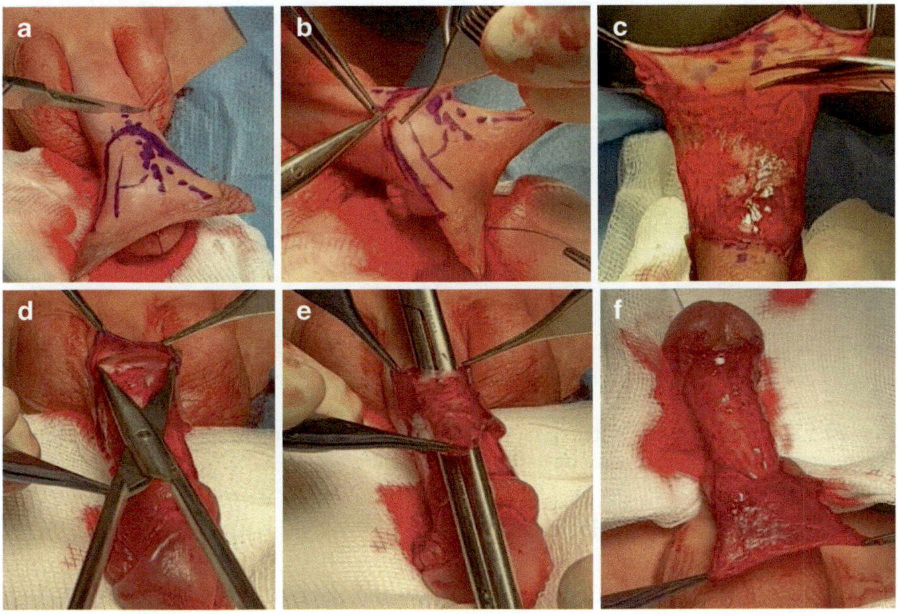

Fig. 24.3 (**a**) Longitudinal dorsal dartos flap is marked at the dorsal distal penile skin. (**b**) De-epithelialization is started proximally. (**c**) Dissection is performed towards the border of inner and outer prepuce. (**d**) Base of the flap is mobilized from the skin. (**e**) Hole is created at the flap base. (**f**) Dartos flap is transposed ventrally using button-hole maneuver

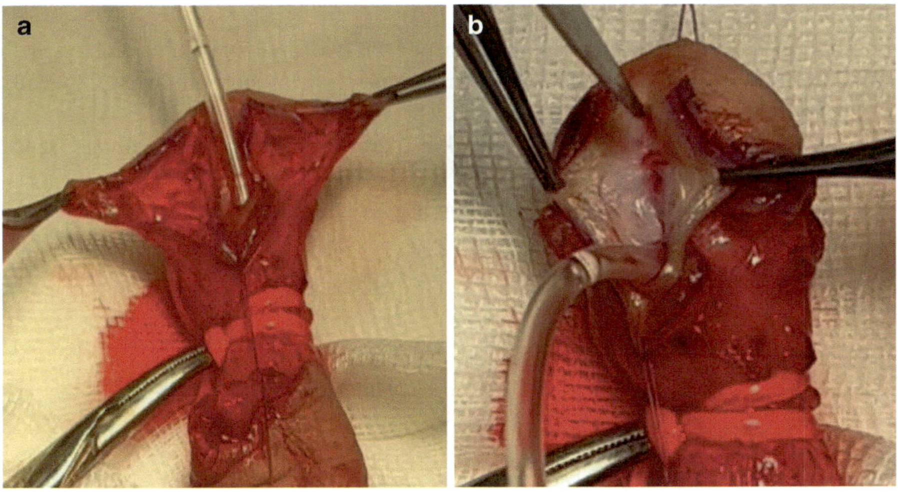

Fig. 24.4 (**a**) Glans wings with good mobility are created. (**b**) Midline incision of urethral plate

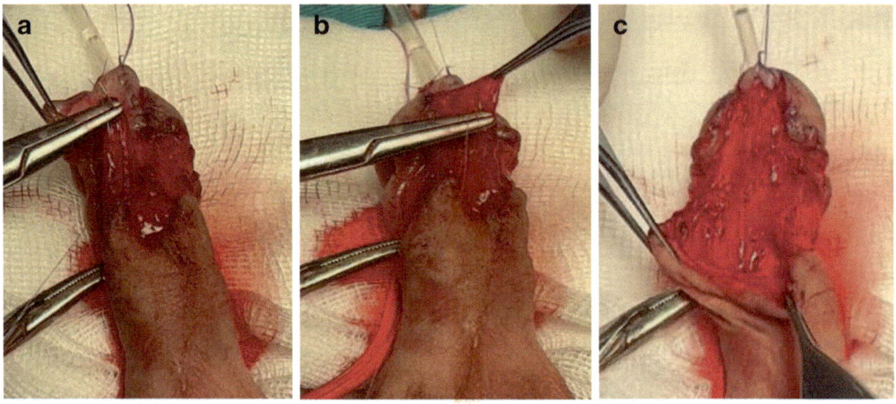

Fig. 24.5 (**a**, **b**, **c**) Fixation of the distal part of dartos flap to the tip of glans wings around neomeatus and to the corporal bodies up to the healthy urethra

24.4.5 Fixation of the Dartos Flap

- The flap is wrapped around the neourethra and fixed to both tips of glans wings with two interrupted sutures 6-0 Monocryl.
- This method allows all suture lines to be covered with a well-vascularized onlay dartos flap (Fig. 24.5).

24.4.6 Glansplasty and Penile Skin Reconstruction

- The glans wings are approximated in one or two layers without tension with several interrupted sutures 6-0 Monocryl, starting from coronal level. Conically shaped glans is created.
- Special care is taken during penile skin reconstruction prevent damage of the blood supply of the dartos flap.
- Coban dressing (3 M Inc., USA) is applied around the penis in a stretched position (Fig. 24.6).

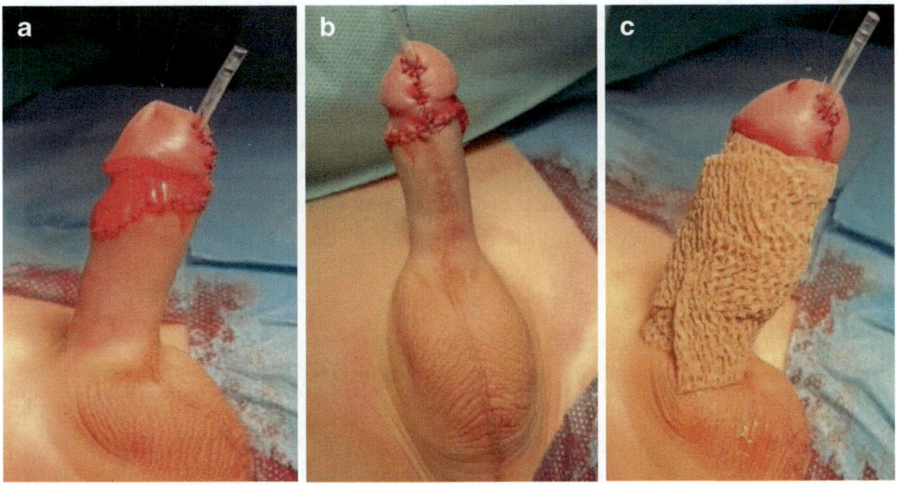

Fig. 24.6 (**a**) Final appearance from lateral aspect. (**b**) Final appearance from ventral aspect. (**c**) Coban dressing is placed

24.5 Post-operative Care

- The Coban dressing is replaced on the third postoperative day and removed 7 days after surgery.
- Urethral stent is removed 7 days after surgery.
- The suprapubic urinary catheter is removed 10–12 days after surgery.
- Antibiotic prophylaxis is prescribed while the suprapubic catheter is in place.

24.6 Tips and Tricks

- Penile degloving should be performed properly to avoid thinning of dartos layer.
- Artificial erection is mandatory after complete penile shaft release from cutaneous chordee to exclude concomitant curvature.
- De-epithelialization is started proximally in the region where subcutaneous tissue is well-developed toward inner and outer prepuce junction.
- Button-hole maneuver is used to transpose flap on the ventral side.
- After urethra is created, dartos flap should be fixed with interrupted sutures to tip of the glans on both sides, over the meatus.

24.7 Results and Conclusion

According to our experience and results after hypospadias repair with using dartos flap for fistula prevention, we suggest that the neourethral covering should be performed as part of a Snodgrass procedure. A longitudinal, well-vascularized dartos flap, harvested dorsally and buttonholed ventrally, represents a good option for fistula prevention. The flap's redundancy and excellent vascularization is essential and depends on the harvesting technique [9, 10].

References

1. Snodgrass W. Tubularized, incised plate urethroplasty for distal hypospadias. J Urol. 1994;151:464–5.
2. Snodgrass WT. Snodgrass technique for hypospadias repair. BJU Int. 2005;95:683–93.
3. Choudhury P, Saroya KK, Jain V, Yadav DK, Dhua AK, Anand S, Mawar S, Verma V, Kapahtia S, Acharya SK, Shah R, Bajpai M, Goel P. 'Waterproofing layers' for urethrocutaneous fistula repair after hypospadias surgery: evidence synthesis with systematic review and meta-analysis. Pediatr Surg Int. 2023;39(1):165.
4. Joshi PM, Bandini M, Kulkarni SB. Common flaps in genitourinary reconstruction. Urol Clin North Am. 2022;49(3):361–9.
5. Verma A, Murtaza S, Kundal VK, Sen A, Gali D. Comparison of Dartos flap and spongioplasty in Snodgrass urethroplasty in distal penile hypospadias. World J Pediatr Surg. 2021;4(3):e000294.
6. Retik AB, Borer JG. Primary and reoperative hypospadias repair with the Snodgrass technique. World J Urol. 1998;16:186–91.
7. Yerkes EB, Adams MC, Miller DA, Pope JC IV, Rink RC, Brock JW III. Y-to-I wrap: use of distal spongiosum for hypospadias repair. J Urol. 2000;163:1536–9.
8. Shanberg AM, Sanderson K, Duel B. Re-operative hypospadias repair using Snodgrass incised plate urethroplasty. BJU Int. 2000;87:544–7.
9. Djordjevic ML, Perovic SV, Slavkovic Z, Djakovic N. Longitudinal dorsal dartos flap for prevention of fistula after a Snodgrass hypospadias procedure. Eur Urol. 2006;50:53–7.
10. Djordjevic ML, Stojanovic B, Agrawal K. Hypospadias. In: Agrawal K, Mahajan RK, editors. Textbook of plastic, reconstructive, and aesthetic surgery volume IV: reconstruction of trunk, genitalia, lower limb, and maxillofacial trauma. Noida: Thieme Medical and Scientific Publishers Pvt. Ltd; 2019. p. 167–92.

Harvest of Tunica Vaginalis Flap for Second Coverage of Urethroplasty

25

Tariq O. Abbas

Abstract

To prevent surgical complications, most notably fistula formation, surgeons typically use a neourethral dartos flap covering. The neourethra requires an intermediary layer for optimal functional and aesthetic results. We here show the key steps to harvest and fix the tunica vaginalis flap (TVF) which is considered a viable other option particularly in proximal hypospadias variants and redo procedures.

Keywords

Tunica vaginalis flap · Hypospadias · Coverage · Staged

25.1 Introduction

There are insufficient reports in the scientific literature about the selection of an intermediate layer to cover the neourethra in cases of staged repair [1, 2]. Tunica vaginalis flap (TVF) covering of the neourethra is beneficial in proximal hypospadias and posturethroplasty-associated recurrent urethrocutaneous fistulas (UCF) [3,

Supplementary Information The online version contains supplementary material available at https://doi.org/10.1007/978-981-99-0795-3_25. The videos can be accessed individually by clicking the DOI link in the accompanying figure caption or by scanning this link with the SN More Media App.

T. O. Abbas (✉)
Weil-Cornell Medical College-Qata, Sidra Medicine, Doha, Qatar
e-mail: tabbas@sidra.org

T. O. Abbas (ed.), *Video Atlas of Hypospadias Surgery*,
https://doi.org/10.1007/978-981-99-0795-3_25

4]. The procedure is simple and quick, and rarely encounters any complications. TVF repair is particularly useful as the tissue of choice for repairing UCF following a failed initial TIP urethroplasty, yielding excellent long-term results [5–7].

25.2 Indications

(a) Based on a recent systematic study, TVF should be the primary option for proximal, repeat, and fistula repairs [8].
(b) TVF can be employed in proximal hypospadias repairs objectively characterized as grades two or three per urethral defect ratio according to Abbas's classification [9] when the spongiosa bifurcation is proximal to the mid-penile shaft (Fig. 25.1).

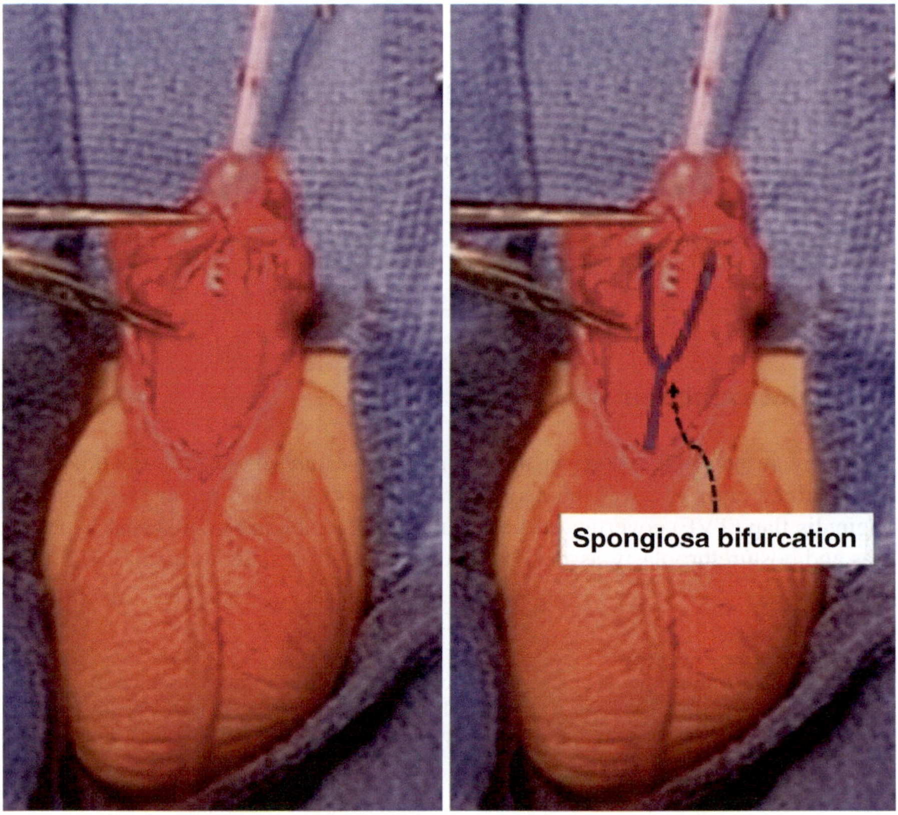

Fig. 25.1 Spongiosa bifurcation is located proximal to the mid-penile shaft the reason why TVF is selected rather than ventral dartos flap

25.3 Key Steps of the Procedure

1. The hemi-scrotum was explored by retracting the degloved skin at the root of penis.
2. After layer-by-layer dissection of the scrotum, the tunica vaginalis was exposed and testis was delivered into the wound.
3. A rectangular flap of tunica vaginalis was harvested with a vascular pedicle of adequate length so as to reach the site of insertion, that is, the neourethral tube (Fig. 25.2).
4. To increase the portion of the TVF that can be harvested, posterior dissection and release of the tunica vaginalis from the adjacent vas and vessels of the spermatic cord is carried out while traction is applied (Fig. 25.3).
5. The flap was spread over the neourethral tube and fixed with 6-0 polyglactin.
6. In most cases, the length and width of the flap were sufficient to cover from the apex of the shaft to the penile urethra and nearly half of the circumference of the penile shaft (Fig. 25.4).

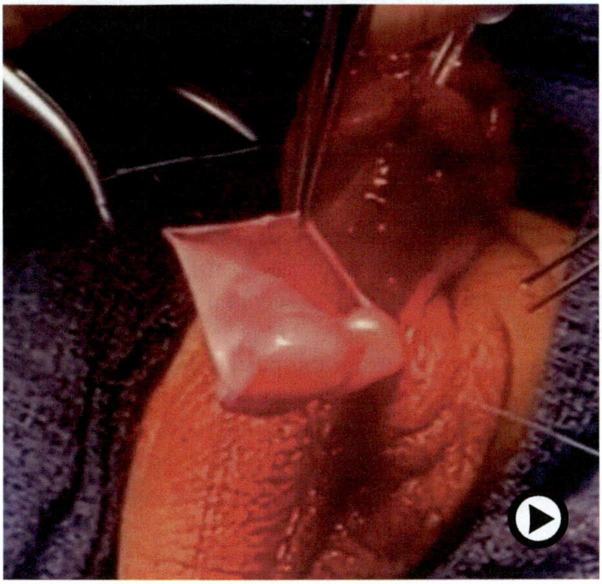

Fig. 25.2 Several traction points are implemented to expose the margins and allow safe release of the TVF. Tunica vaginalis flap (https://doi.org/10.1007/000-cnn)

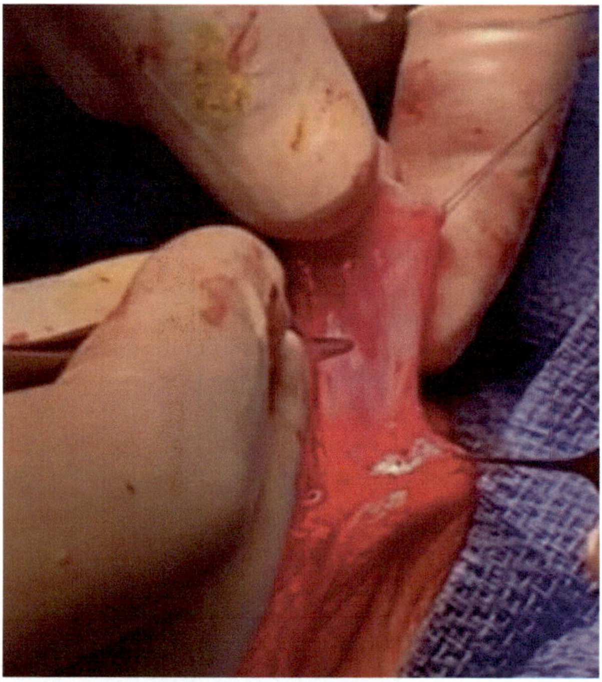

Fig. 25.3 Posterior dissection of the TVF from the vas and vessels

25.4 Tips and Tricks

- There should be no tension during the fixation of the TVF around the neourethra.
- If, after urethral reconstruction, there was insufficient space between the reconstructed urethra and glanular tissue to accommodate an additional tunica flap, it was sutured just above the corona.
- Attempt to unwrap the TVF from the posterior portion of the spermatic cord contents.
- To excise any excess TVF at the glanuloplasty site in order to prevent glanular and dehiscence.
- Dissection of the TVF to the external inguinal ring in order to achieve maximum mobility.
- It is of utmost importance to avoid twisting the pedicle during mobilization.

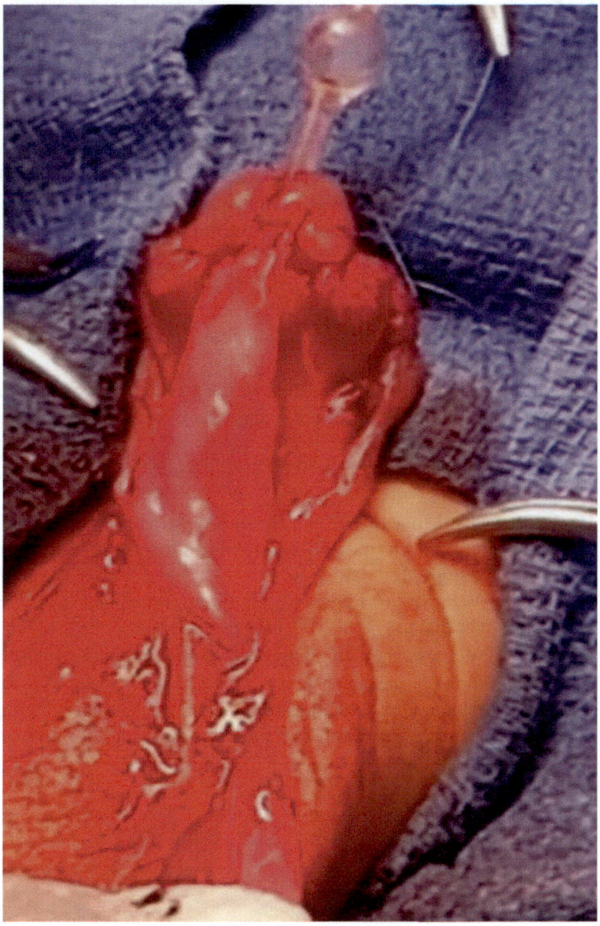

Fig. 25.4 The released TVF is positioned to cover the neourethra

25.5 Outcomes

The repair of hypospadias has been the target of several surgical techniques and modifications, resulting in a wide spectrum of complications, with urethrocutaneous fistula being the most prevalent [10]. TVF is an alternative tissue that can be utilized in hypospadias repair. This flap's accessibility and superior vascularity are its primary benefits. In addition, the use of the TVF for urethrocutaneous fistula repair has produced satisfactory results. In a research, the TVF had a 100% success rate without any noteworthy complications [11]. In a study conducted by Snow and colleagues, the majority of post-TVF complications were related to scrotal hematoma and abscess, whereas the rate of urethrocutaneous fistula was found to be 5% [12]. It has been demonstrated that the TVF is a suitable buttress for severe hypospadias correction. It is widely available, simple to harvest, and its excellent vascularity greatly reduces the incidence of postoperative fistula to less than 2% [13].

References

1. Castagnetti M, El-Ghoneimi A. Surgical Management of Primary Severe Hypospadias in children: systematic 20-year review. J Urol. 2010;184(4):1469–75.
2. Baaklini GT, Abbas T, Hofer MD. Urethral anatomy, physiology, and regeneration. In: Abbas TO, editor. Hypospadiology; 2023. p. 25–35.
3. Abbas T, McCarthy L. Foreskin and penile problems in childhood. Surg. 2016;34(5):221–5.
4. Gopal M, Abbas T, Salle JLP. Management of proximal hypospadias: current challenges and future directions. In: Abbas TO, editor. Hypospadiology; 2023. p. 81–91.
5. Routh JC, Wolpert JJ, Reinberg Y. Tunneled tunica vaginalis flap for recurrent urethrocutaneous fistulae. Adv Urol. 2008;2008:615928.
6. Abbas TO, editor. Hypospadiology: current challenges and future perspectives. 2023. 190 p.
7. Abbas T, Vallasciani S. Toward an ecosystem model of hypospadiology. In: Abbas TO, editor. Hypospadiology; 2023. p. 1–23.
8. Fahmy O, Khairul-Asri MG, Schwentner C, Schubert T, Stenzl A, Zahran MH, et al. Algorithm for optimal urethral coverage in hypospadias and fistula repair: a systematic review. Eur Urol. 2016;70(2):293–8.
9. Abbas TO. An objective hypospadias classification system. J Pediatr Urol. 2022;18(4):481.e1–8.
10. Dokter EM, Mouës CM, van Rooij IALM, van der Biezen JJ. Complications after hypospadias correction: prognostic factors and impact on final clinical outcome. Eur J Pediatr Surg. 2018;28(2):200–6.
11. Snow BW. Use of tunica vaginalis to prevent fistulas in hypospadias surgery. J Urol. 1986;136(4):861–3.
12. Snow BW, Cartwright PC, Unger K. Tunica vaginalis blanket wrap to prevent urethrocutaneous fistula: an 8-year experience. J Urol. 1995;153(2):472–3.
13. Radhakrishnan CN, Radhakrishna V. The tunica-vaginalis flap to prevent postoperative fistula following severe hypospadias repair: has the search for holy grail ended? Actas Urol Esp. 2021;

Part VI

Harvest of Grafts from Non-preputial Sources

Upper Lip Mucosal Graft for Hypospadias Cases

26

Tariq O. Abbas, Santiago Vallasciani, and J. L. Pippi Salle

Abstract

The restoration of hypospadias remains challenging. Despite all advancements in technology, a significant proportion of cases develop complications (Cimador et al. Nat Rev Urol 10:657–666, 2013). Oral mucosa is harvested from various donor sites, including the inner cheek, lower lip, and, on occasion, the lower surface of the tongue. We have been utilizing the upper lip graft (ULG) in recent years.

Keywords

Buccal graft · Urethroplasty · Upper lip

Supplementary Information The online version contains supplementary material available at https://doi.org/10.1007/978-981-99-0795-3_26. The videos can be accessed individually by clicking the DOI link in the accompanying figure caption or by scanning this link with the SN More Media App.

T. O. Abbas (✉)
Weil-Cornell Medical College-Qata, Sidra Medicine, Doha, Qatar
e-mail: tabbas@sidra.org

S. Vallasciani · J. L. P. Salle
Pediatric Urology Section, Sidra Medicine, Doha, Qatar
e-mail: svallaciani@sidra.org

T. O. Abbas (ed.), *Video Atlas of Hypospadias Surgery*,
https://doi.org/10.1007/978-981-99-0795-3_26

26.1 Introduction

When evaluating the efficacy of extragenital tissue retrieval, complications at the donor site are among the most crucial variables to consider. Bleeding is not a typical complication following buccal graft harvest from the lower lip or inner cheek, but oral numbness, tightness of the mouth, and discomfort are common in the early postoperative period [2]. The thickness of inner cheek mucosa can make it difficult to graft the glanular region. In contrast, lower lip grafts provide a thin and soft graft material, but in some instances the donor site can contract [3, 4].

26.2 Steps of the Procedure

- To expose the inner mucosa, two stay sutures were applied in the mid and lateral aspects of the upper lip (Fig. 26.1a).
- The area to be extracted is marked with a marking pen and injected with lidocaine 1% and epinephrine 1/200,00 (Fig. 26.1b).

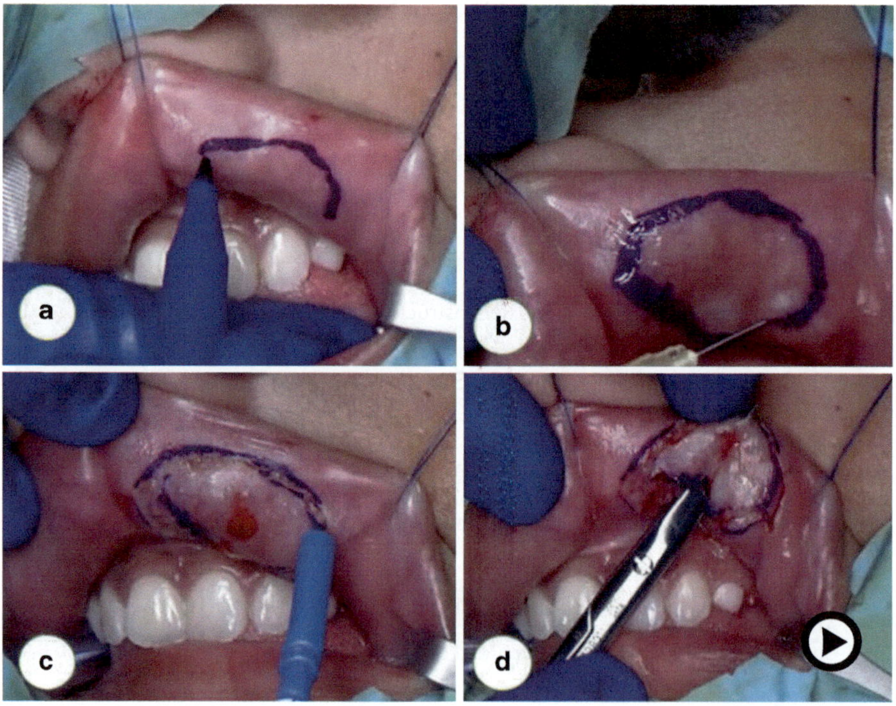

Fig. 26.1 Steps of harvesting upper lip graft. (**a**) Two stay sutures were applied in the mid and lateral aspect of the upper lip and the area to be harvested is marked with a marking pen and injected with lidocaine 1% and epinephrine 1/200,00 (**b**). The edges are incised using monopolar cautery (**c**), and a plane of submucosa is created using scissors. (**d**) Upper lip mucosal graft (https://doi.org/10.1007/000-cnp)

- The edges are incised using monopolar cautery (Fig. 26.1c), and a plane of submucosa is created using scissors (Fig. 26.1d).
- Using the standard technique, the graft is detached, de-fatted, and then applied to the recipient site.
- Hemostasis is maintained using cautery, while the donor site is left exposed.

26.3 Post-operative Care

- The patient promptly resumed a normal diet as tolerated.
- Non-steroidal anti-inflammatories were used to treat oral discomfort.

26.4 Results and Outcomes

From 2015 to 2018, a retrospective study was conducted on patients who underwent urethral augmentation with ULG. The donor site variables included demographics, pain, and morbidity. The perioral area was cleansed and draped prior to surgery. 25 ULG harvests were done in 24 patients. Minimum follow-up duration was two months [5]. There were no signs of hemorrhage or infection observed. In the first 24 hours, only one patient (5%) reported significant local pain associated with the procedure, and none reported perioral numbness, difficulty with mouth opening, donor site contraction, or alterations in salivation. The ULG is safe and straightforward to acquire, with a low complication rate (one case in our series). It is essential to note that ULG only provides a small quantity of tissue for urethral augmentation, so it cannot be used for long urethroplasties [6].

References

1. Cimador M, Vallasciani S, Manzoni G, Rigamonti W, De Grazia E, Castagnetti M. Failed hypospadias in paediatric patients. Nat Rev Urol. 2013;10(11):657–66.
2. Kamp S, Knoll T, Osman M, Hacker A, Michel MS, Alken P. Donor-site morbidity in buccal mucosa urethroplasty: lower lip or inner cheek? BJU Int. 2005;96(4):619–23.
3. Leslie B, Lorenzo AJ, Figueroa V, Moore K, Farhat WA, Bägli DJ, et al. Critical outcome analysis of staged buccal mucosa graft urethroplasty for prior failed hypospadias repair in children. J Urol. 2011;185(3):1077–82.
4. Baaklini GT, Abbas T, Hofer MD. Urethral anatomy, physiology, and regeneration. In: Abbas TO, editor. Hypospadiology; 2023. p. 25–35.
5. Abbas TO, Pippi Salle JL. Dorsal Inlay TIP (DTIP). In: Hypospadias surgery; 2022. p. 451–60.
6. Abbas T. Management of distal hypospadias: new insights and stepwise management algorithm. In: Abbas TO, editor. Hypospadiology; 2023. p. 67–80.

Buccal (Cheek) Mucosa Graft

27

Pankaj M. Joshi, Sanjay B. Kulkarni, and Tariq O. Abbas

Abstract

Buccal mucosa is an excellent option for urethroplasty for urethral stricture repair due to its harvestability, pliability, and low donor site morbidity. We discuss here harvesting the buccal mucosa and elaborate on preoperative patient evaluation, postoperative course, and complications.

Keywords

Hypospadias · Buccal graft · Lingual mucosa

27.1 Introduction

Buccal mucosa is valuable for repeat urethroplasty due to the simplicity of harvesting, the pliability of the graft, and the minimal donor site morbidity, which can be accomplished with a proper harvesting procedure [1–3]. Due to limited oral cavity access and a reduced harvesting area, obtaining these grafts from younger patients is more difficult from a technical standpoint [4].

Supplementary Information The online version contains supplementary material available at https://doi.org/10.1007/978-981-99-0795-3_27. The videos can be accessed individually by clicking the DOI link in the accompanying figure caption or by scanning this link with the SN More Media App.

P. M. Joshi (✉) · S. B. Kulkarni
UROKUL, Pune, India

T. O. Abbas
Urology Division, Surgery Department, Doha, Qatar

T. O. Abbas (ed.), *Video Atlas of Hypospadias Surgery*,
https://doi.org/10.1007/978-981-99-0795-3_27

27.2 Preoperative Assessment and Preparation

- Before harvesting buccal mucosa from the cheek, the patient should be thoroughly evaluated to determine the size of the mouth opening, the quantity of tissue on both cheeks, and the presence of scars caused by chronic cheek-biting or previous surgeries. The following groups of patients are not optimal candidates for oral mucosa cheek harvesting:
  - Patients currently suffering from an infectious disease of the mouth (candida, lichen, varicella-virus, and others).
  - Patients who have had mandibular arch surgery in the past, preventing a broad mouth opening.
  - Patients who perform with acoustic instruments.
  - Adult patients who consume areca nut products are at risk for developing oral submucosa fibrosis, a disease characterized by severe progressive fibrosis of the oral cavity resulting in dysphagia and a diminished ability to open the mouth [5].
  - Patients functioning as speakers.
- The patient should begin using chlorhexidine mouthwash twice daily for oral cleansing 3 days prior to surgery. The patient is given prophylactic antibiotics through an IV the day before surgery.

27.3 Steps of the Procedure

1. The external and internal mucosal surfaces of the cheek are sterilized and draped prior to preparation.
2. The placement of a retractor and the placement of three stay sutures along the border of the mouth to stretch the oral mucosa.
3. The Stensen's duct in close proximity to the second molar (Fig. 27.1).

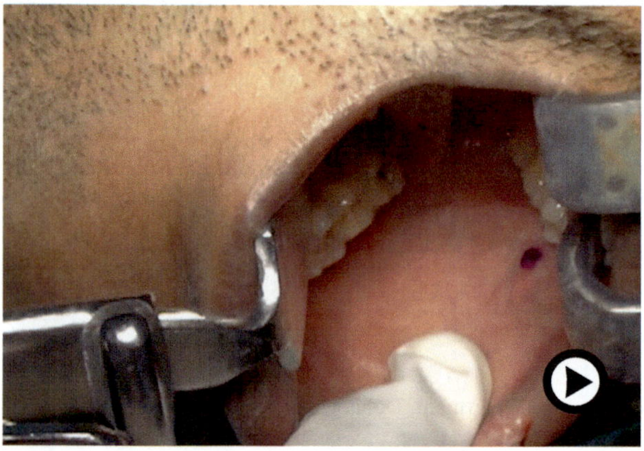

Fig. 27.1 The Stensen's duct in proximity of the second molar is marked. Buccal (cheek) mucosa graft (https://doi.org/10.1007/000-cnq)

4. Along the margins of the graft, a solution containing Lidocaine 1% with 1:100,000 epinephrine is injected to facilitate hemostasis and dissection (Fig. 27.2).
5. The graft is dissected in the plane between the mucosa and the muscle. The mucosa and submucosa were incised with a #15 blade, and the submucosa was dissected from the buccinator muscle at the anterior edge using sharp scissors. Once the graft was released, 3-0 silk stay sutures were used to help retract the anterior margin (Fig. 27.3).
6. The donor site is thoroughly examined, and the hemorrhage is stopped using bipolar electrocautery (Fig. 27.4).
7. The graft is stabilized to extract the submucosal tissue (Fig. 27.5).

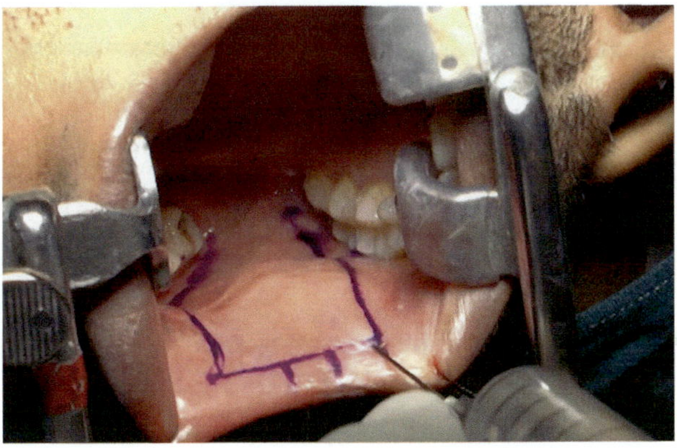

Fig. 27.2 The graft is designed in a rectangular shape and submucosal injection of Lidocaine 1% with 1:100,000 epinephrine is injected to facilitate hemostasis and dissection

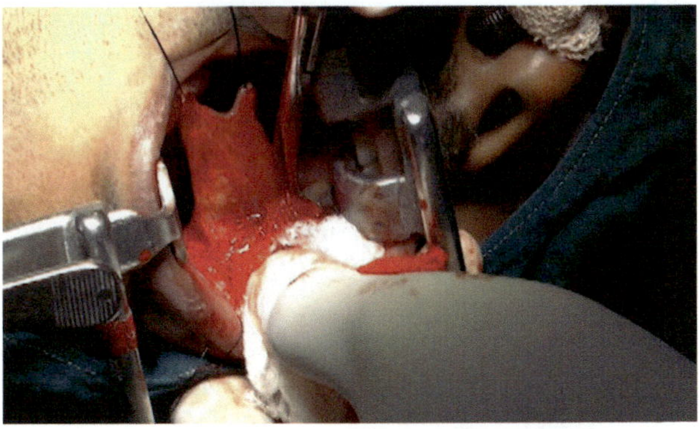

Fig. 27.3 The graft is dissected in the plane between the mucosa and the muscle

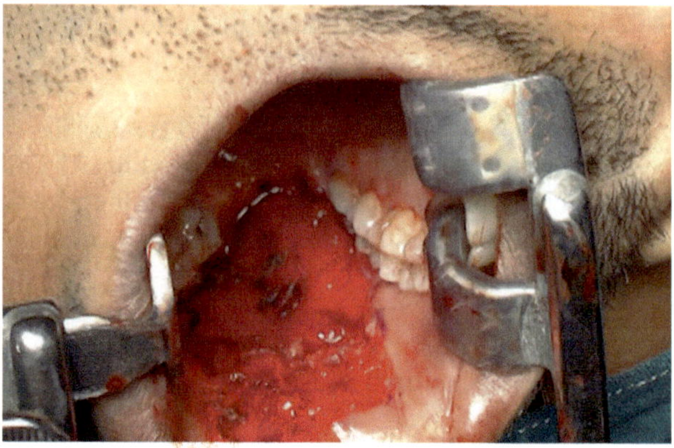

Fig. 27.4 The harvesting site is left opened

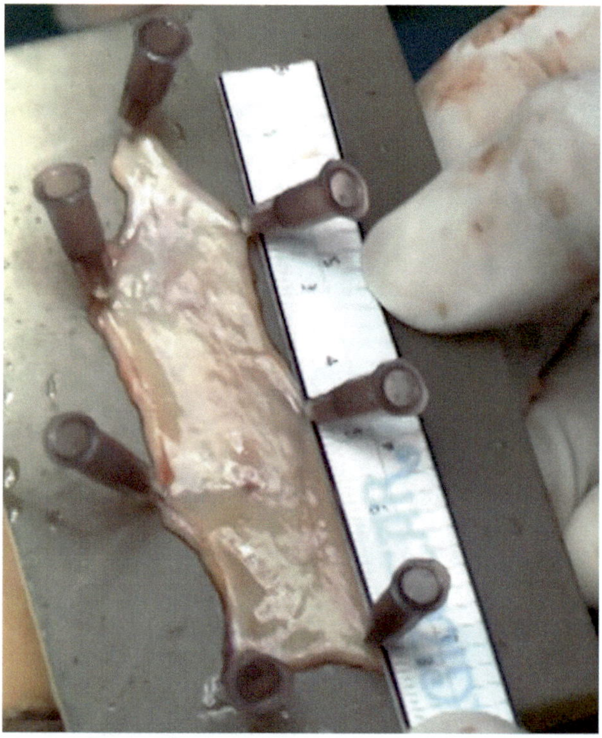

Fig. 27.5 Fixation of the graft to remove ant muscle of subcutaneous tissues

27.4 Tips and Tricks

- If the Stensen's duct cannot be identified, stimulating parotid gland secretion with a few droplets of lemon juice may be possible. The Stensen's duct must be readily apparent during the dissection of the graft.

- It is recommended to close an ovoid-shaped donor site but not a rectangular-shaped donor site because of the potential associated post-operative pain [6].
- Although not essential, nasal intubation can be helpful for patients who have a limited mouth opening or small mouth, as well as for those who need two grafts.
- It is conceivable, though slightly more challenging, to harvest a new graft from the cheek of a patient who has already had one done in the past. This is because of fibrosis and the fact that the new graft will need to be smaller than the old one. When bilateral buccal mucosa transplant harvesting is in the works, it's important to let the patient and anesthesiologist know well in advance of operation.

27.5 Postoperative Care

- The patient consumes a clear liquid diet on the first postoperative day before progressing to a regular diet the following day
- The patient continues to use chlorhexidine mouthwash twice daily for 3 days after surgery and is maintained on oral antibiotics until the catheter is removed.

27.6 Results and Outcomes

The buccal mucosa graft exhibited excellent uptake within 5 days and was well-vascularized and flexible at 6 months [7, 8]. The incidence of early (during the first 10 postoperative days) complications was observed in a series of 553 patients: bruising (3.4%), discomfort (1%), mouth swelling (1.1%), and bleeding (3.4%). Three days after surgery, 57% of patients have returned to a normal diet [9]. The incidence of late complications (4 months after surgery) was reported as follows: Extreme or moderate numbness as a result of the oral sutures (1.1%); extreme or moderate numbness as a result of the oral scar (0.2%); oral infection (1.8%); extreme or moderate difficulty opening the mouth (0%); difficulties smiling (0%).

References

1. Nerli RB, Neelagund SE, Guntaka A, Patil S, Hiremath SC, Jali SM, et al. Staged buccal mucosa urethroplasty in reoperative hypospadias. Indian J Urol [Internet]. 2011;27(2):196–9.
2. Abbas TO, Pippi Salle JL. When to graft the incised plate during TIP repair? A suggested algorithm that may help in the decision-making process. Front Pediatr [Internet]. 2018;6:326.
3. Abbas T, McCarthy L. Foreskin and penile problems in childhood. Surg [Internet]. 2016;34(5):221–5.
4. Abbas TO, editor. Hypospadiology: current challenges and future perspectives. Singapore: Springer; 2023. 190 p.
5. Manoj B, Sanjeev N, Pandurang PN, Jaideep M, Ravi M. Postauricular skin as an alternative to oral mucosa for anterior onlay graft urethroplasty: a preliminary experience in patients with oral mucosa changes. Urology [Internet]. 2009;74(2):345.
6. Barbagli G, Balò S, Sansalone S, Lazzeri M. How to harvest buccal mucosa from the cheek. African J Urol [Internet]. 2016;22(1):18–23.

7. Mokhless IA, Kader MA, Fahmy N, Youssef M. The multistage use of buccal mucosa grafts for complex hypospadias: histological changes. J Urol [Internet]. 2007;177(4):1496.
8. Baaklini GT, Abbas T, Hofer MD. Urethral anatomy, physiology, and regeneration. In: Abbas TO, editor. Hypospadiology [Internet]. Singapore: Springer; 2023. pp. 25–35.
9. Barbagli G, Fossati N, Sansalone S, Larcher A, Romano G, Dell'Acqua V, et al. Prediction of early and late complications after oral mucosal graft harvesting: multivariable analysis from a cohort of 553 consecutive patients. J Urol [Internet]. 2014;191(3):688–93.

Buccal (Lingual) Mucosa Graft

28

Pankaj M. Joshi, Sanjay B. Kulkarni, and Tariq O. Abbas

Abstract

Tongue mucosa, which is comparable to oral mucosa, is a safe and effective graft material for urethral repair, with little potential risks associated with the donor area. Procedures for harvesting lingual mucosa and fixing the donor site are discussed. This chapter explores more into the evaluation of patients before surgery, their recovery, and any complications that may arise.

Keywords

Hypospadias · Buccal musosa · Graft · Redo surgery

28.1 Introduction

Urethroplasty has made use of a wide range of free extragenital graft tissues [1]. Oral mucosal grafts are currently regarded as the best tissue delivering great clinical results when free extragenital tissue is required for urethroplasty [2, 3]. Oral mucosal grafts eliminate cosmetic issues including penile/glans torsion, subcutaneous

Supplementary Information The online version contains supplementary material available at https://doi.org/10.1007/978-981-99-0795-3_28. The videos can be accessed individually by clicking the DOI link in the accompanying figure caption or by scanning this link with the SN More Media App.

P. M. Joshi (✉) · S. B. Kulkarni
UROKUL, Baner, Pune, India

T. O. Abbas
Urology Division, Surgery Department, Sidra Medicine, Doha, Qatar

T. O. Abbas (ed.), *Video Atlas of Hypospadias Surgery*,
https://doi.org/10.1007/978-981-99-0795-3_28

abnormalities, and chordee that can arise from using local genital skin. Oral mucosa (buccal mucosa graft, BMG) for substitute urethroplasty is typically harvested from the patient's cheek at present [4]. Perioral numbness, difficulties opening the mouth, scarring, and dry mouth are just some of the donor site morbidities that have been linked to its harvesting [5]. On the other hand, tissue characteristics (thick epithelium, high content of elastic fibers, thin lamina propria, rich vascularization) and immunologic properties (resistance to infection) of lingual mucosa are similar to those of buccal mucosa, making it an ideal graft material for imbibition, inosculation, and re-vascularization [6]. Moreover, there is no long-term morbidity associated with LMG harvesting in children and only a small risk of short-term problems at the donor location. The buccal mucosa requires a mouth retractor for harvesting, whereas the tongue is easily accessible for the LMG [7].

28.2 Indications

- Because of its high success rate, LMG urethroplasty is often recommended as a first-line option for repeat hypospadias surgery. Temporary and mildly debilitating oral problems are rather uncommon compared to BMG and are largely attributable to the size of the graft [8].
- Patients who regularly use products made from areca nuts may develop oral submucosa fibrosis, a condition characterized by severe increasing fibrosis of the oral cavity that can lead to dysphagia and a reduced capacity to open the mouth [9]. Such patients are not optimal candidates for oral mucosa cheek harvesting but lingual mucosa (Fig. 28.1).

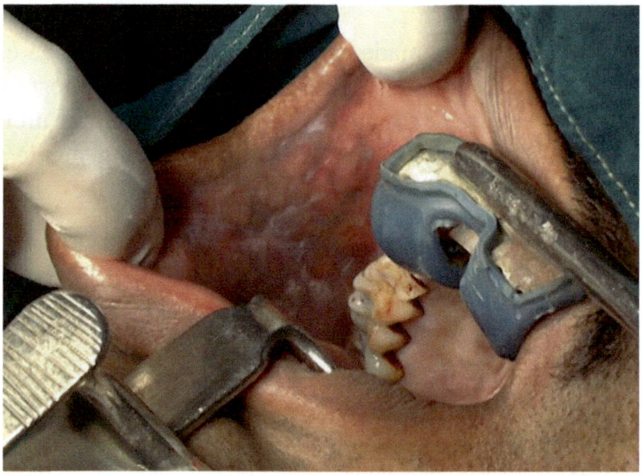

Fig. 28.1 Oral mucosa in a patient who chews tobacco

28.3 Preoperative Preparation

- The patient should begin using chlorhexidine mouthwash twice daily for oral cleansing 3 days prior to surgery.
- The patient is given prophylactic antibiotics through an IV the day before surgery.

28.4 Steps of the Procedure

1. The use of a mouth opening is optional but may be implemented.
2. To expose the ventrolateral surface of the tongue, a 1-0 suture is introduced through the apex of the tongue or direct traction is performed.
3. The sublingual mucosa, which is behind the lining that separates the dorsum, where the papillae are located, from the rest of the tongue, is where the harvest graft is placed (Fig. 28.2).

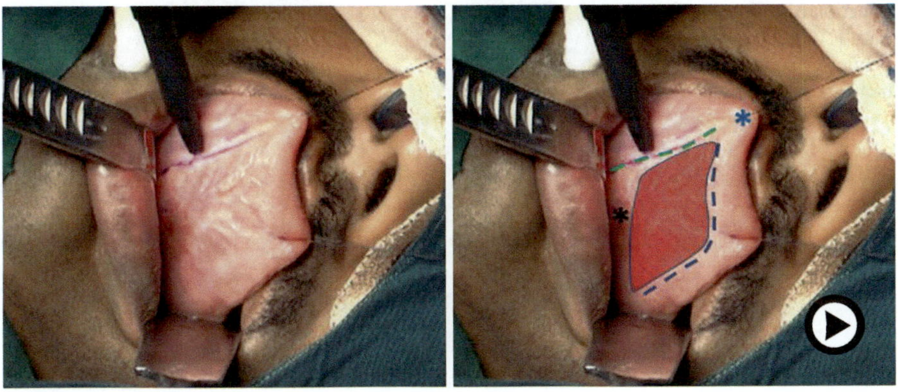

Fig. 28.2 The ventrolateral surface of the tongue, the harvest graft site, is exposed by placing the tip of the tongue (blue asterisk) under traction. The location of where Wharton's duct begins is marked by a black asterisk. The papillary edge (green dot) and the midline frenulum (green dot) define the probable harvest site for the lingual graft mucosa (red region). Buccal (lingual) mucosa graft (https://doi.org/10.1007/000-cnr)

4. Once the Warton's duct hole has been located, the necessary graft is measured and marked with a surgical pen.
5. Along the margins of the graft, a solution containing Lidocaine 1% with 1:100,000 epinephrine is injected to facilitate hemostasis and dissection (Fig. 28.3).
6. Starting at the anterior landmark of the graft, a full-thickness mucosal graft is harvested using sharp instruments. The graft may benefit from being handled with a 4-0 traction stitch (Fig. 28.4).
7. Donor sites are checked for bleeding, and interrupted or continuous polyglactin 3-0 sutures are used to seal them.
8. Graft defatting is done if submucosal tissue is present.
9. When more grafting is required, the operation can be carried out on the contralateral side.

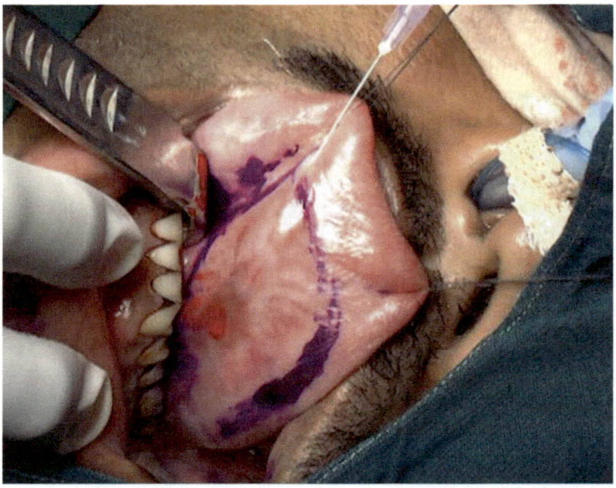

Fig. 28.3 The graft is designed in an elliptical shape and submucosal injection of Lidocaine 1% with 1:100,000 epinephrine is injected to facilitate hemostasis and dissection

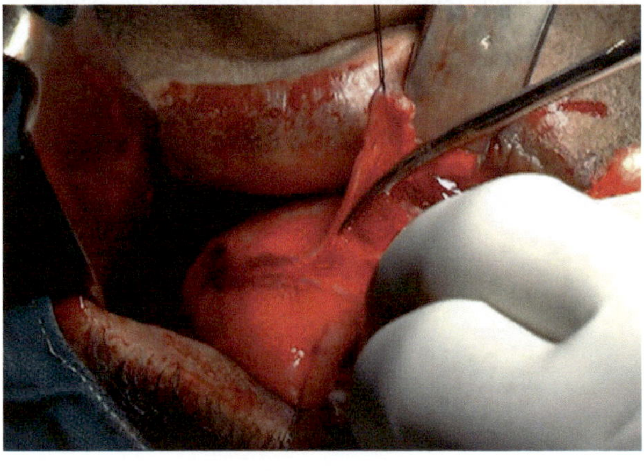

Fig. 28.4 The graft is dissected in the plane between the mucosa and the muscle

28.5 Postoperative Care

- The patient consumes a clear liquid diet on the first postoperative day before progressing to a regular diet the following day.
- The patient continues to use chlorhexidine mouthwash twice daily for 3 days after surgery and is maintained on oral antibiotics until the catheter is removed.

28.6 Tips and Tricks

- A second team operating concurrently with the urethroplasty team could perform LMG harvesting.
- Leave at least 1 cm of mucosa at the tip of the tongue to prevent slurring of speech, and be careful not to include the underlying genioglossus muscle or lingual nerve in the graft, as doing so can lead to contractures, numbness, and increased bleeding, as recommended by Chauhan et al. [10].
- In their study, 65.5% of the LMG was left open, and Lumen et al. [11] recommended close it only if the mucosal borders could be approximated without excessive tension.

28.7 Results and Outcomes

Although the LMG and BMG used in urethroplasty operations have vastly different graft diameters and mucosal and submucosal layer thicknesses, it has been proven that they share the same thickness and blood supply [12]. Since the lateral side of the lingual mucosa serves no functional purpose, approximately half of the tongue can be used as donor tissue (as in tongue cancer) without limiting the tongue's ability to function normally [13]. No significant intraoral problems such as prolonged numbness, salivary alterations, mouth opening difficulty, deviations, or retractions were noted. Tongue graft recipients experienced mild mouth discomfort at the donor location and temporary speech impairment for 1–2 days. Two patients who had grafts taken from the inner cheek experienced temporary (3 months) mouth opening difficulty, neurosensory deficiency, and decreased salivary flow [14]. Cystourethrography did not reveal any major contractures or sacculations in the LMG graft, and urethroscopy described it as being virtually indistinguishable from the patient's own urethra [6]. The imbibition, inosculation, and revascularization characteristics of LMG were also shown to be identical to BMG [14].

References

1. Abbas T, McCarthy L. Foreskin and penile problems in childhood. Surgery (United Kingdom). 2016;34(5):221–5.
2. Abbas TO, editor. Hypospadiology: current challenges and future perspectives. Singapore: Springer; 2023. 190 p.

3. Gopal M, Abbas T, Salle JLP. Management of proximal hypospadias: current challenges and future directions. In: Abbas TO, editor. Hypospadiology [Internet]. Singapore: Springer; 2023. pp. 81–91.
4. Bhargava S, Chapple CR. Buccal mucosal urethroplasty: is it the new gold standard? BJU Int [Internet]. 2004;93(9):1191–3.
5. Wood DN, Allen SE, Andrich DE, Greenwell TJ, Mundy AR. The morbidity of buccal mucosal graft harvest for urethroplasty and the effect of nonclosure of the graft harvest site on postoperative pain. J Urol [Internet]. 2004;172(2):580–3.
6. Simonato A, Gregori A, Lissiani A, Galli S, Ottaviani F, Rossi R, et al. The tongue as an alternative donor site for graft urethroplasty: a pilot study. J Urol [Internet]. 2006;175(2):589–92.
7. Aldaqadossi HA, Shaker H, Youssof H, Kotb Y, Eladawy M. Outcomes of staged lingual mucosal graft urethroplasty for redo hypospadias repair. J Pediatr Urol [Internet]. 2019;15(5):519.e1–7.
8. Abrate A, Gregori A, Simonato A. Lingual mucosal graft urethroplasty 12 years later: systematic review and meta-analysis. Asian J Urol [Internet]. 2019;6(3):230–41.
9. Manoj B, Sanjeev N, Pandurang PN, Jaideep M, Ravi M. Postauricular skin as an alternative to oral mucosa for anterior onlay graft urethroplasty: a preliminary experience in patients with oral mucosa changes. Urology [Internet]. 2009;74(2):345.
10. Chauhan S, Yadav SS, Tomar V. Outcome of buccal mucosa and lingual mucosa graft urethroplasty in the management of urethral strictures: a comparative study. Urol Ann [Internet]. 2016;8(1):36–41.
11. Lumen N, Vierstraete-Verlinde S, Oosterlinck W, Hoebeke P, Palminteri E, Goes C, et al. Buccal versus lingual mucosa graft in anterior urethroplasty: a prospective comparison of surgical outcome and donor site morbidity. J Urol [Internet]. 2016;195(1):112–7.
12. Campos-Juanatey F, Azueta Etxebarria A, Calleja Hermosa P, Marcos Gonzalez S, Alonso Mediavilla E, Correas Gomez MA, et al. Histological comparison of buccal and lingual mucosa grafts for urethroplasty: do they share tissue structures and vascular supply? J Clin Med [Internet]. 2022;11(7):2064.
13. Guerrerosantos J, Dicksheet S, Ruiz-Razura A. Free tongue composite graft for correction of a vermilion defect. Plast Reconstr Surg [Internet]. 1985;76(3):451–4.
14. Simonato A, Gregori A, Ambruosi C, Venzano F, Varca V, Romagnoli A, et al. Lingual mucosal graft urethroplasty for anterior urethral reconstruction. Eur Urol [Internet]. 2008;54(1):79–85.

Cutaneous; Retro-Auricular, Arm Grafts 29

Elias Ramirez-Velazquez, Ricardo A. Arceo-Olaiz, Andres F. Menjívar-Rivera, Marian G. García-Flores, and Andrea Vázquez-Camacho

Abstract

The use of grafts for hypospadias repair was done for the first time in 1897, and it is still a current procedure every pediatric urologist should be familiar with since surgical harvesting technique is highly reproducible and accessible by the appropriate trained hypospadias surgeon. A graft is a lining of skin that has been excised and placed in a new area of the body, in a recipient bed where it

Supplementary Information The online version contains supplementary material available at https://doi.org/10.1007/978-981-99-0795-3_29. The videos can be accessed individually by clicking the DOI link in the accompanying figure caption or by scanning this link with the SN More Media App.

E. Ramirez-Velazquez (✉)
Pediatric Urology Department, Hospital Infantil de México Federico Gómez, Mexico City, Mexico

Hospital Shriners Para Niños A.C, Mexico City, Mexico

Hospital Infantil Privado Starmedica HIP, Mexico City, Mexico

R. A. Arceo-Olaiz
Pediatric Urology Department, Emory University School of Medicine, Atlanta, GA, USA

Children's Healthcare of Atlanta, Atlanta, GA, USA

A. F. Menjívar-Rivera · M. G. García-Flores
Pediatric Urology Department, Hospital Infantil de México Federico Gómez, Mexico City, Mexico

A. Vázquez-Camacho
Adolescent Medicine Department, Hospital Infantil de México Federico Gómez, Mexico City, Mexico

T. O. Abbas (ed.), *Video Atlas of Hypospadias Surgery*,
https://doi.org/10.1007/978-981-99-0795-3_29

needs to develop a new vascular supply. The use of grafts is only indicated in the reconstruction of hypospadias for urethral augmentation, substitution urethroplasty, and/or skin resurfacing. The first graft option should always be the foreskin, when it is not available, there are different options such as mucosa (being buccal the most widely utilized) or skin (retroauricular, upper inner arm, supraclavicular, inner thigh). There are very few reports showing the long-term outcomes of the use of extragenital grafts, the largest series included 93 patients and reported good outcomes, only 8 children (8.6%) had a complication, including keloid formation of the recipient site and revision surgery. The use of upper inner arm skin cannot be routinely recommended due to the lack of long-term outcomes, and should only be considered as a third or fourth graft option.

Keywords

Skin grafting · Extragenital grafts · Full-thickness skin grafts · Retroauricular Wolfe Skin Graft · Inner upper arm skin graft · Redo hypospadias · Cripple hypospadias

29.1 Introduction

Hypospadias repair is one of the most common and technically demanding reconstructive surgeries in pediatric urology. It becomes a passion; however, it also brings challenges, frustration, and failures. As part of our practice, it is not uncommon to treat patients with previous failed surgeries, have significant scarring tissue, or primary proximal hypospadias which do not have the adequate amount and quality of tissue available for reconstruction. Therefore, every hypospadias surgeon must be familiarized with techniques that aid to compensate for ventral tissue deficiency. The use of grafts is a fundamental part of the armamentarium, specifically for complex cases, when flaps are not a viable option [1].

The use of grafts in hypospadias is far from new. Nové-Josserand is credited with the first urethral reconstruction with an inner thigh graft in 1897 [2]. In 1937, Sir Archibald McIndoe reported the use of a split-thickness skin graft from the inner arm to perform the urethroplasty [3]. Since then, they have stayed at the top of the list when it is time to choose a specific strategy. Free skin grafts are linings of skin that have been excised and placed in a different area of the body that serves as, a recipient bed. The goal of this bed is to help develop new vascular supply in order for the donor tissue to survive. On the other hand, a flap has its own primary vascularity from the adjacent tissue, which is mobilized together with the donor tissue, thus avoiding the need of neovascularization. In cases where the surrounding tissue is scarred, fibrotic, or is lacking an adequate blood supply, grafts should be the preferred option [4]. The process by which a graft undergoes neovascularization after excision and transfer to a recipient bed is called "take". It occurs in two phases:

- Initial phase (Plasmatic imbibition). During the first 48 h, the graft temperature is lower than the core body temperature, and the graft survives by taking nutrients from the recipient wound bed.
- Second phase (Inosculation). During next 48 h, the graft temperature rises to core body temperature and a fine vascular network grows from the wound bed that interfaces with the dermis [5].

Then, neovascularization occurs in which new blood vessels invade the graft and establish a permanent vascular supply to provide the nourishment necessary for healing. Certain processes, such as infections or a hematoma, can interfere with the graft taken by damaging the recipient bed [1, 6]. Table 29.1 explains the classification of skin grafts and some of their characteristics.

The ideal extragenital skin donor areas to take grafts and use them in hypospadias reconstruction should be:

- Non-hair-bearing.
- Thin.
- Elastic.
- Accessible/easy to harvest.
- Minimal donor and recipient site morbidity (scarring/retraction).

The extragenital tissues described for use as grafts in urethral plaque reconstruction include:

Table 29.1 Graft classification and characteristics [6, 7].

Classification	General characteristics
Split-thickness skin graft (STSG)	Consist of epidermis and a variable dermal thickness. Harvest method: dermatome with an adjustable depth gauge. Superficial plexus, vascularizes faster than FTSG. Almost does not include lymphatics. Less resistant to trauma. Tendency to be brittle and less durable. Donor site heals by epithelialization, and faster than FTSG.
Full-thickness skin grafts (FTSG)	Include the epidermis and the entire dermis. Harvest method: scissors and/or scalpel. Deeper plexus, vascularizes slowly. Lymphatics are included. Very resistant to trauma. More durable once matured. Less contraction compared to STSG. Superior texture & cosmetic results at donor and recipient sites [8]. Donor site should be closed surgically.

- Mucosa (buccal, bladder, small intestine, rectal). The most popular is buccal mucosa, as it is less invasive and good outcomes have been reported in the literature [9–11].
- Skin (retroauricular/postauricular, inner arm, supraclavicular, and groin, among others) [12–15].

29.1.1 Retroauricular Wolfe Skin Grafts

Retroauricular Wolfe Skin Grafts (RAWG) are a good extragenital graft alternative for patients in whom two-stage repairs are planned, such as revision surgeries, or primary repairs with insufficient foreskin. The RAWG has the advantage of being an affordable full-thickness skin graft, easy to harvest, relatively thin, flexible, and leaves a discrete donor scar. Reports have shown good results when utilized in hypospadias surgery, however it has never been a popular choice. Some disadvantages include fine hair in lumen, creation of a separate surgical site during graft removal, and risk of keloid formation both at the donor and recipient sites [12, 13]. RAWG has also been used in adult patients with urethral stricture disease. Reports have mentioned the possibility of harvesting up to 7–8 cm of full-thickness graft per side, allowing 14–16 cm of graft material if necessary. In pediatric patients with prominent ears, it may be a good option [16].

29.1.2 Inner Upper Arm Skin Grafts

Inner upper arm skin graft is another extragenital alternative for patients in whom it is not possible to harvest a graft with better characteristics. This graft has the advantage of being easy to collect, leaves an inconspicuous scar, and a significant amount can be taken. There are few reports on its use in hypospadias, since other anatomical regions are more popular. Disadvantages include the potential for hair growth in the lumen, thicker skin compared to other sites, creation of a separate surgical site during graft removal, and associated morbidity risk, specifically keloid formation at the donor and recipient sites [15]. Table 29.2 exposes the advantages and disadvantages of the extragenital FTSG exposed in the videos of this chapter.

29.2 Indications

The use of extragenital grafts is only indicated in the reconstruction of hypospadias (for urethral augmentation, substitution urethroplasty, and/or skin resurfacing) when:

(a) **There is no available foreskin, or it is insufficient for surgery,** either because it was used in previous surgeries for correction (cripple hypospadias), previous circumcision, or in newborns with aposthia. **And/or…**

Table 29.2 Advantages and disadvantages of the extragenital FTSG described in the videos of this chapter [1].

Graft type	Advantages	Disadvantages
Retroauricular	Accessible Reasonably thin Inconspicuous donor scar	Two surgical sites Fine hair in lumen Chronic inflammation
Inner upper arm	Accessible Inconspicuous donor scar Significant amount can be taken	Two surgical sites Possible hair growth Chronic inflammation Thick

(b) **There is poor blood supply to local tissues.** This is also related to previous surgeries or deficiency of local skin as in severe cases of hypospadias where a staged approach may be preferred. **And/or…**

(c) **Buccal mucosa is not a viable option.**

29.3 Video Demonstration

29.3.1 Full-Thickness Retroauricular Skin Graft (Fig. 29.1a, b)

- Age at surgery (years): 5
- Gestational age (weeks): 38
- Birth weight (gm): 2750
- Gestational risks (e.g., maternal co-morbidities, IVF, Twin): None
- Family history: None
- Testosterone (if yes, reason, and protocol used): None
- Any features of DSD (e.g., undescended testes): None

29.3.2 Full-Thickness Skin Graft from the Inside of the Upper Arm (Fig. 29.2a, b)

- Age at surgery (years): 12
- Gestational age (weeks): 37
- Birth weight (gm): 2950
- Gestational risks (e.g., maternal co-morbidities, IVF, Twin): None
- Family history: None
- Testosterone (if yes, reason, and protocol used): None
- Any features of DSD (e.g., undescended testes): None

  Video:

  Full-thickness retroauricular skin graft video

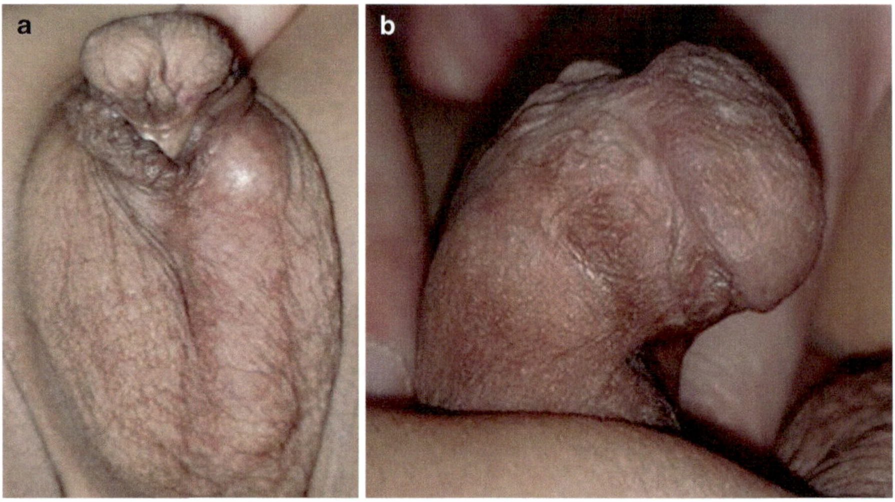

Fig. 29.1 5-year-old male with a history of proximal hypospadias, severe chordee, and multiple failed repairs. He currently has a residual penile chordee with a penoscrotal meatus and fibrotic scar tissue on the glans and shaft. There is no foreskin available for reconstruction. (**a**) Ventral view. (**b**) Lateral view that simulates erection and a severe >30° chordee

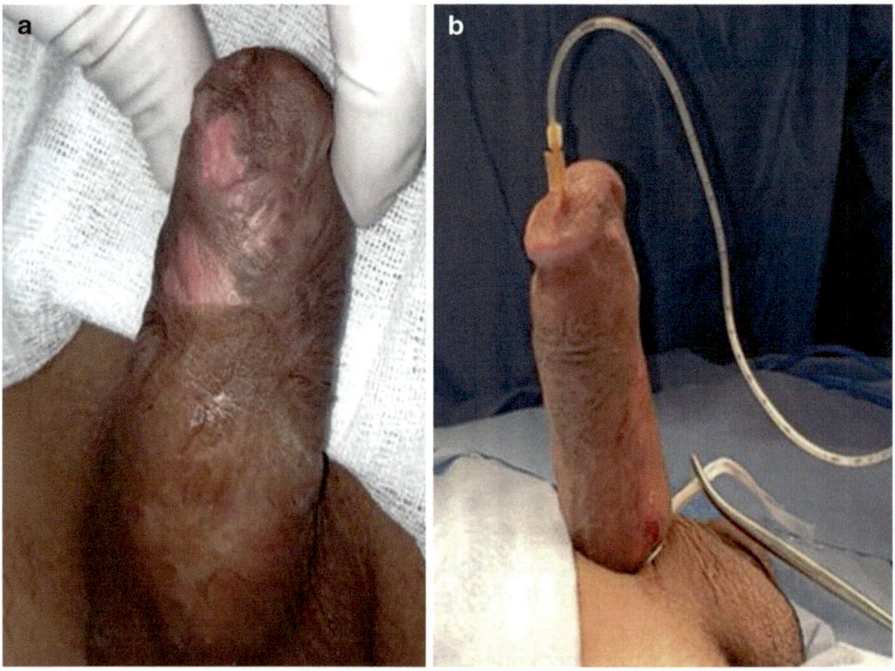

Fig. 29.2 12-year-old male with a history of 4 previous failed surgeries due to proximal hypospadias with severe chordee. He currently has a straight penis, but with a subcoronal meatus, fibrotic scar tissue at the level of the glans and urethral plate. There is no foreskin available for reconstruction. (**a**) Ventral view. (**b**) Lateral view with intraoperative artificial erection demonstrating a straight penis

29.4 Steps of the Procedure

29.4.1 Full-Thickness Retroauricular Skin Graft

29.4.1.1 Traction Sutures

- Two 4-0 silk traction sutures are placed on the lateral aspect of the ear's skin, avoiding puncturing the cartilage (Fig. 29.3a).
  Video:
  Full-thickness skin graft from the inside of the upper arm video

29.4.1.2 Surgical Marking

- Marking on the retroauricular skin is made of the corresponding dimensions, according to the previous measurements of the prepared recipient site. Care must be taken to avoid causing an ear deformity (Fig. 29.3b).

29.4.1.3 Hydrodissection

- Hydrodissection is performed by injecting 2% lidocaine subcutaneously (Fig. 29.3c).

29.4.1.4 Incision

- The skin incision is made with a number 15 blade over the marked area. A fusiform incision is made in order to facilitate a cosmetic wound closure (Fig. 29.3d).

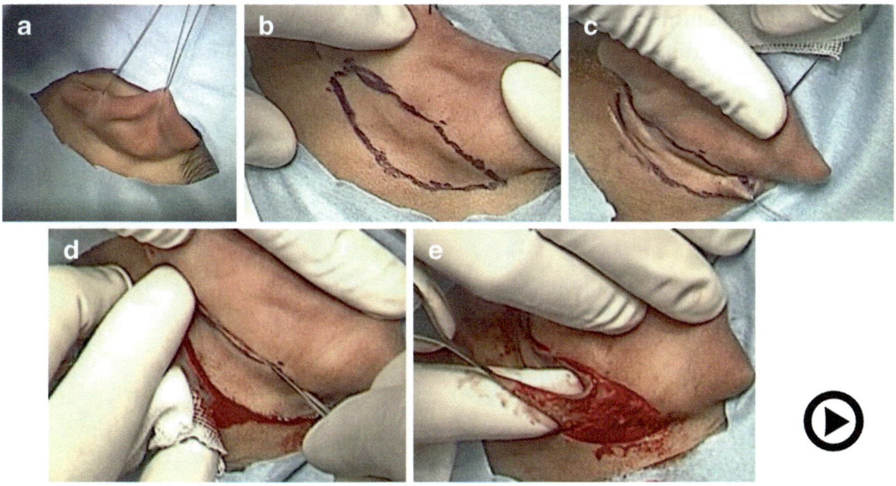

Fig. 29.3 Full-thickness retroauricular skin graft harvest. (**a**) Traction sutures (left ear). (**b**) Surgical marking in fusiform shape. (**c**) Hydrodissection. (**d**) Incision. (**e**) Graft harvest. Cutaneous; retro-auricular grafts. https://doi.org/10.1007/000-cnt

29.4.1.5 Graft Harvest

- The graft is harvested using Iris, Stevens, or Westcott scissors. The dissection plane is at the level of the subcutaneous fat. This step is important, so that very little fat is excised with the graft.
- At the time of skin harvest, use gentle traction with forceps and countertraction with the pad of the ring finger for support to cut down to the dermis (Fig. 29.3e).
- Once the graft is taken, it is placed in saline solution.
- If there is any bleeding, hemostasis is performed with bipolar forceps as needed.

29.4.1.6 Donor Site Wound Closure

If necessary, the defect of donor site can then be closed with deep interrupted sutures either with 4-0 Monocryl or Vicryl. The goal is to reapproximate the skin edges without any tension. In this case, a simple running suture with 5-0 Monocryl is placed into the skin (Fig. 29.4a, b). The wound is covered with a sterile dressing for 24 h (Fig. 29.4c). Antibiotic ointment is placed over the donor site three times per day for a week. As we use absorbable sutures, there is no need to remove any stitches.

29.4.1.7 Contralateral Retroauricular Skin Graft

The same process is performed to obtain a full-thickness contralateral retroauricular skin graft as needed.

29.4.1.8 Graft Preparation

- Once both grafts are taken, the next step is preparing them by defatting with scissors (Fig. 29.5a) and scalpel (Fig. 29.5b) alternatively as needed. It is important to avoid unintentional perforations of the graft.
- The graft should ultimately consist of only dermis and epidermis (Fig. 29.5c).

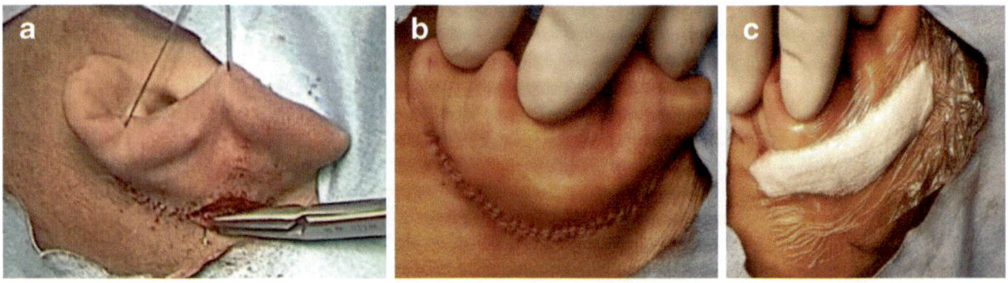

Fig. 29.4 Left retroauricular donor site wound closure. (**a**) Simple running suture in progress at skin with 5-0 absorbable monofilament. (**b**) Wound closure finished. **c** Wound covered with a sterile dressing

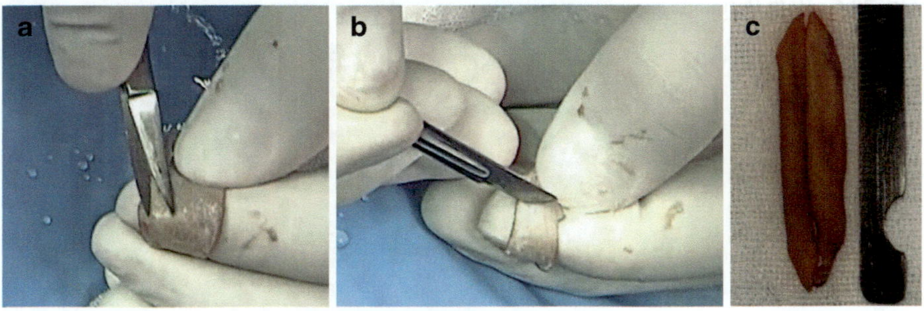

Fig. 29.5 Full-thickness retroauricular skin graft preparation. (**a**) Graft defatting using Iris scissors. (**b**) Graft defatting using scalpel. (**c**) Both appropriate size grafts defatted consisting of only dermis and epidermis

29.4.1.9 Positioning the Graft

The graft is then placed over its recipient bed and sutured with interrupted and running 6-0 or 7-0 fast absorbable suture (Fig. 29.6).

29.4.2 Full-Thickness Skin Graft from the Inside of the Arm

29.4.2.1 Surgical Marking

- A previously measured and marked skin graft of appropriate dimensions is removed from the skin of the upper inner arm. This is a good location for harvesting as the skin is hairless.
- A fusiform shape is preferred to facilitate a more cosmetic wound closure (Fig. 29.7a).

29.4.2.2 Incision

- The skin incision is made with a number 15 blade over the marked area (Fig. 29.7b).

29.4.2.3 Hydrodissection

- Hydro dissection is performed subcutaneously by injecting lidocaine 2%.

29.4.2.4 Graft Harvest

- The graft is then harvested using Iris, Stevens, or Westcott scissors. The dissection plane is at the level of the subcutaneous fat. This step is important, so that very little fat is excised with the graft (Fig. 29.7c).
- At the time of skin harvest, use gentle traction with forceps and countertraction with the pad of the ring finger for support to cut down to the dermis (Fig. 29.7d).
- Once the graft is taken, it is placed in saline solution.

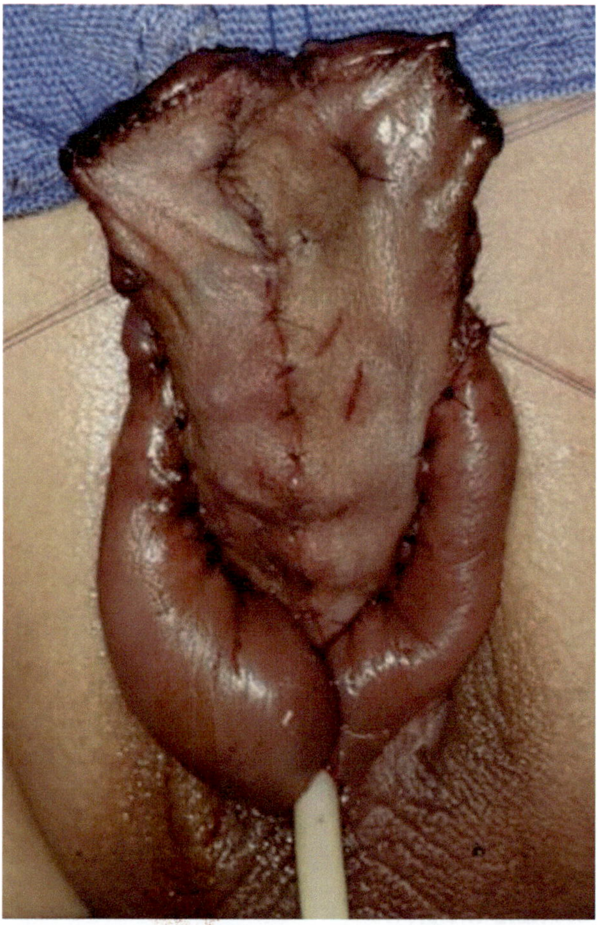

Fig. 29.6 Both (left and right) full-thickness retroauricular skin grafts into position

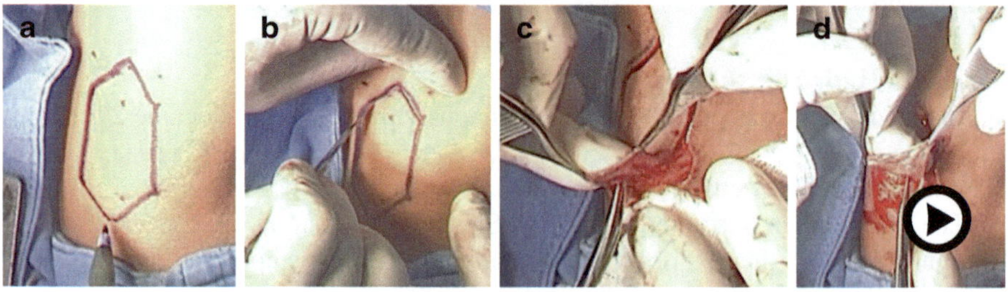

Fig. 29.7 Full-thickness skin graft harvest from the inside of the left arm. (**a**) Surgical marking in fusiform shape. (**b**) Incision. (**c**) Graft harvest using Iris scissors. (**d**) Graft harvest using gentle traction with forceps and countertraction with the pad of the ring finger for support to cut down to the dermis. Cutaneous; arm grafts. https://doi.org/10.1007/000-cns

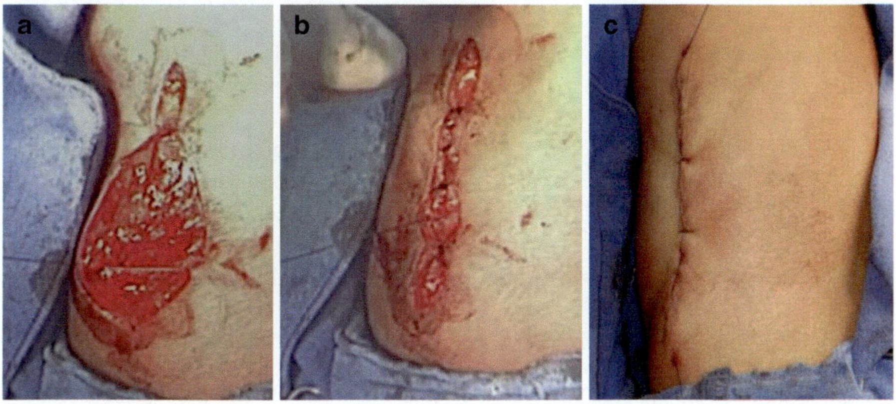

Fig. 29.8 Left inner arm donor site wound closure. **a** and **b** Deep interrupted sutures with 4-0 absorbable monofilament. **c** Skin is closed in a running subcuticular fashion with 5-0 non-absorbable monofilament

29.4.2.5 Hemostasis

- If there is any bleeding, hemostasis is performed with bipolar forceps as needed.

29.4.2.6 Donor Site Wound Closure

- Donor site closure is performed with deep interrupted absorbable sutures, usually 4-0 Monocryl is preferred (Fig. 29.8a, b).
- The skin is closed with a running 5-0 Prolene in a subcuticular fashion (Fig. 29.8c).
- The wound is covered with a sterile dressing for 24 h. Antibiotic ointment is placed over the donor site three times per day for a week.
- Stitches are removed 10 days after the procedure.

29.4.2.7 Graft Preparation

- Once the graft is taken, it is prepared and defatted by using scissors (Fig. 29.9a) and scalpel (Fig. 29.9b) alternatively as needed. It is important to avoid unintentional perforations of the graft.
- The graft should ultimately consist of only dermis and epidermis. It is important to avoid unintentional perforations of the graft.

29.4.2.8 Positioning the Graft

- Graft is then sutured into position with interrupted and running 6-0 or 7-0 fast absorbable suture (Fig. 29.10a).
- Then, an antibiotic ointment is placed over the graft and a roll of sterile Vaseline gauze is pressed over the recipient site secured with absorbable suture (Fig. 29.10b) and covered with a sterile low-compression bandage for 1 week (Fig. 29.10c).

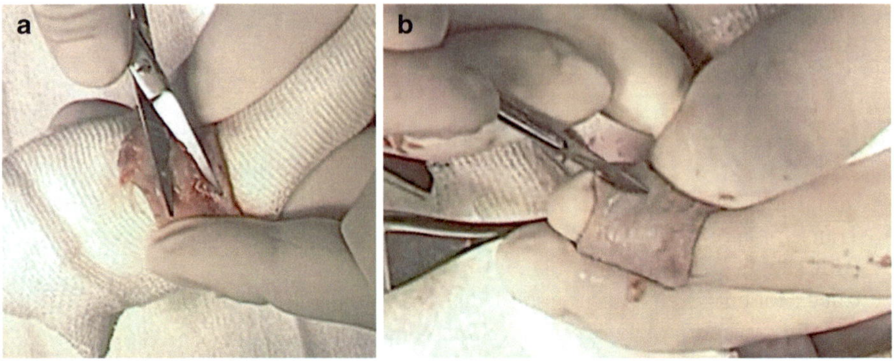

Fig. 29.9 Full-thickness inner arm skin graft preparation. **a** Graft defatting using Iris scissors. **b** Graft defatting using scalpel

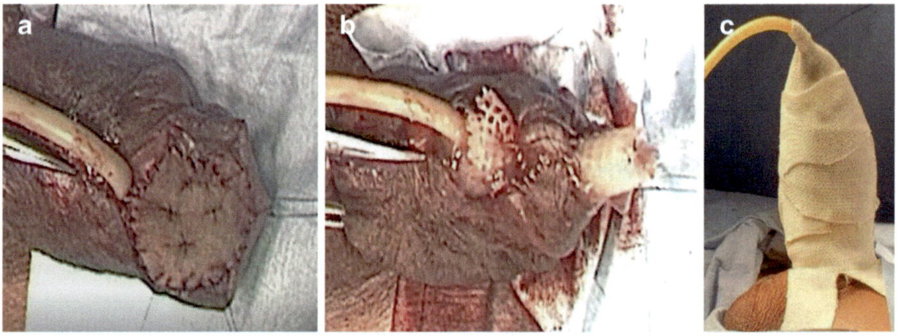

Fig. 29.10 **a** Full-thickness inner arm skin graft into position. **b** Antibiotic ointment over the graft and a roll of sterile Vaseline gauze is pressed and secured over the recipient site. **c** A sterile low-compression bandage in position for 1 week

29.5 Post-operative Care

29.5.1 Full-Thickness Retroauricular Skin Graft

- The donor site wound is covered with a sterile dressing for 24 h.
- After that, the bandage is removed, and the wound is kept uncovered.
- Then, rinsing using soap and water during daily bath is enough.
- Antibiotic ointment is placed on the donor site three times a day for 1 week.
- As we use absorbable sutures, it is not necessary to remove any stitches.
- It is recommended not to expose the wound to the sun, or at least as little as possible for a better cosmetic appearance.
- Analgesics are prescribed, paracetamol 10–15 mg/kg/day is usually sufficient, for 2 or 3 days or as needed.

- In addition, the patient receives antibiotics at the time of the surgical procedure to prevent infection of the graft recipient site. We usually prescribe amoxicillin/clavulanic acid at a dose of 40 mg/kg/day for a week.
- Normal physical activities can be resumed 1 month after surgery.

29.5.2 Full-Thickness Skin Graft from the Inside of the Arm

- The donor site wound is covered with a sterile dressing for 24 h.
- After that, the bandage is removed and the wound is kept uncovered.
- Then, rising using soap and water during daily bath is enough.
- Antibiotic ointment is placed on the donor site three times a day for 1 week.
- The stitches are removed in the office after 10 days.
- It is recommended not to expose the wound to the sun, or at least as little as possible for a better cosmetic appearance.
- Analgesics are prescribed, usually is paracetamol 10–15 mg/kg/day, for 2 or 3 days or as needed.
- In addition, the patient receives antibiotics at the time of the surgical procedure to prevent infection of the graft recipient site. We usually prescribe amoxicillin/clavulanic acid at a dose of 40 mg/kg/day for a week.
- Normal physical activities can be resumed 1 month after surgery.

29.6 Tips and Tricks

- An alternative to measure the receiving site and calculate the size of the donor site, you can use a template of the defect made with a clean drape, and with the marking pen draw the donor site.
- It should be considered that during the healing process, the graft will contract approximately 30%. Thus, harvesting a larger graft compared to the recipient site is preferred.
- Lidocaine hydrodissection is optional, it depends on the preference of the surgeon. In my opinion, it makes it easier to identify the correct dissection plane and gives post-surgical analgesia. Once the surgical area is marked, hydro-dissection can be done before or after incision.
- At the time of skin harvest, use gentle traction with forceps and countertraction with the pad of the ring finger for support to cut down to the dermis.
- During graft preparation, I personally prefer to grab the tissue and stretch it over my index finger, so it has enough tension at the time of defatting. Another option certain surgeon use is to defat it over a silicone bed or plaque, fixing the graft's corners with needles. In case of using curved scissors for defatting, it is recommended to guide the tips up, to avoid cutting or perforating the graft.
- Sometimes, the retroauricular full-thickness skin graft does not provide enough tissue to cover the defect. Consider using a composite graft of RAWG plus buccal mucosa or another extragenital full-thickness skin graft. Try to keep the thin-

ner portion of the graft aligned into the glanular defect, to facilitate the glansplasty during the second stage by avoiding bulky tissue.

– For better cosmetic results, keep the wound site donor area moisturized and avoid sun exposure.

29.7 Results and Conclusion

Whenever there is foreskin available, it should be considered as the first option for correction of complex hypospadias (primary and revision). There are few reports regarding the use and results of extragenital grafts in complicated hypospadias. The largest series reported by Pfistermüller et al. has encouraging results in revision surgeries using retroauricular graft in two staged reconstruction. Of the 93 revision surgeries, 60 were done using retroauricular skin grafts. Good results were reported over the series, eight children (8.6%) required additional procedures. Three cases using RAWG had a complication; one developed a keloid in the graft, and the other two required revision. Two children had dehiscence of the RAWG donor site, which was managed conservatively; and one developed a keloid scar at the donor site [13]. There is insufficient evidence to recommend the routine use of grafts taken from the inner side of the arm for hypospadias reconstruction [15]. It should only be considered as a third or fourth option, once the foreskin, retroauricular skin, and oral mucosa are not available (it is the author's order of preference).

References

1. Herrera O, Gundeti MS. Flaps and grafts in hypospadias repair BT. In: Bhat A, editor. Hypospadiology: principles and practices. Singapore: Springer Singapore; 2022. p. 165–85. Available from: https://doi.org/10.1007/978-981-16-8395-4_12.
2. Hadidi AT. History of hypospadias BT. In: Hadidi AT, editor. Hypospadias surgery: an illustrated textbook. Cham: Springer International Publishing; 2022. p. 3–24. Available from: https://doi.org/10.1007/978-3-030-94248-9_1.
3. McIndoe AH. The treatment of hypospadias. Am J Surg. 1937;38:176–85.
4. Wallis MC, Braga L, Khoury A. The role of flaps and grafts in modern hypospadiology. Indian J Urol. 2008;24(2):200–5.
5. Converse JM, Smahel JB, Donald L, Harper AD. DIRECT connection between the blood vessels of the graft and the host bed as one of the earliest stages in the revascularisation of skin transplants was first described by Bert (1865). He used the term. Br J Plast Surg. 1975;28(1955):274–82.
6. Jordan GH, Rourke KF. Fundamentals and principles of tissue transfer BT. In: Schreiter F, Jordan GH, editors. Urethral reconstructive surgery. Berlin/Heidelberg: Springer Berlin Heidelberg; 2006. p. 19–27. Available from: https://doi.org/10.1007/3-540-29385-X_4.
7. Hadidi AT. Plastic surgery principles BT. In: Hadidi AT, editor. Hypospadias surgery: an illustrated textbook. Cham: Springer International Publishing; 2022. p. 323–33. Available from: https://doi.org/10.1007/978-3-030-94248-9_16.
8. Iwuagwu FC, Wilson D, Bailie F. The use of skin grafts in postburn contracture release: a 10-year review. Plast Reconstr Surg. 1999;103:1198–204.

9. Shebla SE, Akl MM, Abdalrazek M. Buccal versus skin graft for two-stage repair of complex hypospadias: an Egyptian center experience. BMC Urol [Internet]. 2022;22(1):6–10. Available from: https://doi.org/10.1186/s12894-022-01069-6
10. Palmer DA, Marcello PW, Zinman LN, Vanni AJ. Urethral reconstruction with rectal mucosa graft Onlay: a novel, minimally invasive technique. J Urol [Internet]. 2016;196(3):782–6. Available from: https://doi.org/10.1016/j.juro.2016.03.002
11. Memmelaar J. Use of bladder mucosa in a one-stage repair of hypospadias. J Urol [Internet]. 1947;58(1):68–73. Available from: https://www.sciencedirect.com/science/article/pii/S0022534717695181
12. Nitkunan T, Johal N, O'Malley K, Cuckow P. Secondary hypospadias repair in two stages. J Pediatr Urol. 2006;2(6):559–63.
13. Pfistermüller KLM, Manoharan S, Desai D, Cuckow PM. Two-stage hypospadias repair with a free graft for severe primary and revision hypospadias: a single surgeon's experience with long-term follow-up. J Pediatr Urol [Internet]. 2017;13(1):35.e1–7. Available from: https://doi.org/10.1016/j.jpurol.2016.08.014
14. Vanni AJ. New frontiers in urethral reconstruction: Injectables and alternative grafts. Transl Androl Urol. 2015;4(1):84–91.
15. Webster GD, Brown MW, Koefoot RB, Sihelnick S. Suboptimal results in full thickness skin graft urethroplasty using an extrapenile skin donor site. J Urol [Internet]. 1984;131(6):1082–3. Available from: https://doi.org/10.1016/S0022-5347(17)50820-4
16. Manoj B, Sanjeev N, Pandurang PN, Jaideep M, Ravi M. Postauricular skin as an alternative to Oral mucosa for anterior Onlay graft Urethroplasty: a preliminary experience in patients with oral mucosa changes. Urology [Internet]. 2009;74(2):345–8. Available from: https://doi.org/10.1016/j.urology.2009.02.065.

Bladder Mucosa Graft

30

Alaa El-Ghoneimi, Amane-allah Lachkar, Pauline Lopez, Annabel Paye-Jaouen, and Matthieu Peycelon

Abstract

Proximal hypospadias cases often necessitate complex, stepwise reconstruction procedures, with redo surgeries presenting challenges and unpredictable outcomes. The resulting condition, known as hypospadias cripples, is characterized by unhealthy scars, residual curvature, and ineffective urethroplasty. Achieving satisfactory outcomes for these patients remains elusive, particularly due to the lack of healthy penile skin. Early attempts at reconstruction using bladder mucosa tube grafts faced criticism due to complications such as mucosal prolapse and anastomotic strictures. To address skin breakdown issues, the concept of tubularized tunneled bladder mucosa grafts (TBMG) emerged, aiming to provide a pause for tissue revascularization and skin covering.

Keywords

Proximal hypospadias · Redo surgery · Tubularized tunneled bladder mucosa graft (TBMG) · Salvage treatment

Supplementary Information The online version contains supplementary material available at https://doi.org/10.1007/978-981-99-0795-3_30. The videos can be accessed individually by clicking the DOI link in the accompanying figure caption or by scanning this link with the SN More Media App.

A. El-Ghoneimi (✉) · A.-a. Lachkar · P. Lopez · A. Paye-Jaouen · M. Peycelon
Department of Pediatric Surgery and Urology, University Hospital Robert Debré, APHP, University Paris Cité, Paris, France

National Reference Center for Rare Urinary Tract Malformations (MARVU), Paris, France
e-mail: alaa.elghoneimi@aphp.fr; amane-allah.lachkar@aphp.fr; pauline.lopez@chu-limoges.fr; annabel.paye-jaouen@aphp.fr; matthieu.peycelon@aphp.fr

T. O. Abbas (ed.), *Video Atlas of Hypospadias Surgery*,
https://doi.org/10.1007/978-981-99-0795-3_30

30.1 Introduction and Indications

The majority of proximal hypospadias cases would require stepwise reconstruction, and redo surgery is still an intricate procedure with uneven results [1–3]. The unfortunate outcome of numerous unsuccessful reconstruction attempts is hypospadias cripples, characterized by numerous unhealthy scars, residual curvature, and ineffective urethroplasty.

Even after spending a lifelong surgical skill, it's still challenging to classify these patients' care in a way that's satisfactory [4]. It is difficult in these situations because the penile shaft is not covered by healthy skin. Following the second stage, the tubularized flap must be covered by healthy, well-vascularized skin in order for the classical staged free grafts (buccal or bladder mucosa) to be successful.

In 1947, Memmelaar et al. [5] reported the first version of the bladder mucosa tube graft. Mucosal prolapse, proximal anastomosis stricture, and morbidity associated with protracted detrusotomy were among the several problems that led to recurrent criticism of its use [6].

Reducing the pace of skin breakdown following redo surgery was the goal of developing the tunneling strategy of a tubularized free graft [7, 8] The underlying theory was that a pause for tissue revascularization and skin covering would be left following the initial step of repair, which included curvature correction. There is no danger of skin dehiscence or graft necrosis during tunneling since it does not disrupt the vascularization of the neighboring tissues.

For patients who have had numerous unsuccessful reconstructions due to a lack of healthy skin or extensive skin loss, we have now published our findings on the technique of tubularized tunneled bladder mucosa graft (TBMG) and its use as a salvage treatment. is the main procedure for masculinizing genitoplasty or perineal hypospadias long urethroplasty [9].

30.2 Steps of Surgery

30.2.1 First Surgical Procedure

Optimized curvature management using tailored specialized protocols. With a ventral transverse incision made at the point of greatest curvature through the tunica albuginea, extending from 3 to 9 o'clock position, all fibrous tissues were removed and, if necessary, ventral corporoplasty was performed in our hypospadias cases that had severe curvature >45°. The corpora defect was covered with a tunica vaginalis flap. When the tunica vaginalis was not available, a series of fairy cuts were performed for ovotesticular DSD. Until a natural, healthy urethra could be obtained, any urethra that had been repaired or was fibrous was surgically removed from the perineal area (Figs. 30.1 and 30.2).

Redo procedures often involve the use of free skin grafts or local flaps to restore the penile skin. Prior to the TBMG, a minimum of 1 year of delay was observed.

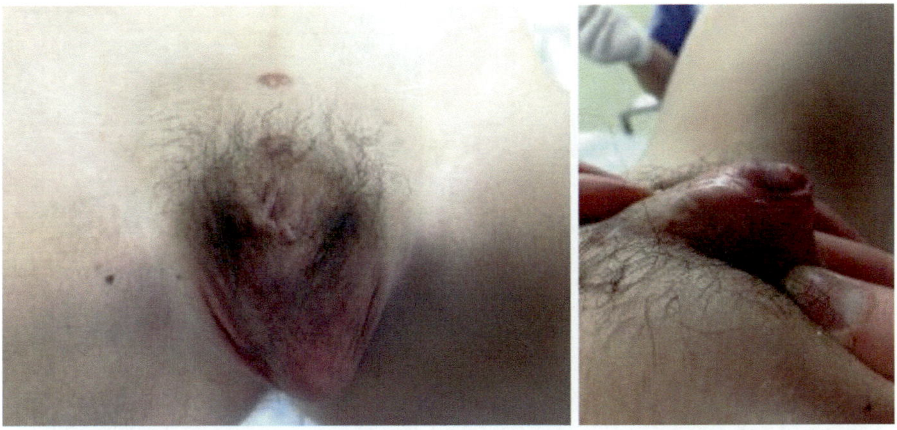

Fig. 30.1 Case 2 is a 12-year-old kid who underwent 12 surgeries to address perineal hypospadias. Sub-total loss of the penile skin. (CC BY 4.0)

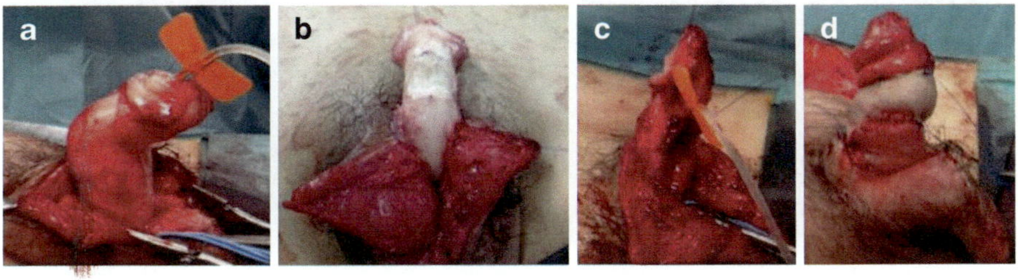

Fig. 30.2 The initial surgical procedure performed: (**a**) Even after undergoing urethroplasty and having all fibrous tissues removed, there is still a significant curvature. The left vaginalis flap covers a large ventral cavernoplasty (**b–c**). (**d**) A total skin-free graft covers the distal portion of the penis, while scrotal flaps cover the base. (CC BY 4.0)

30.2.2 Bladder Mucosa Graft Harvesting by Minimal Detrusotomy

Performing the procedure involves making a small incision across the skin above the pubic region. By making a midline facial incision, the saline-filled bladder can be accessed. Figure 30.3 shows the anterior bladder wall being the site of a brief (2 cm long) transverse detrusotomy. A vertical incision is made in the exposed mucosa, which is then retracted using a 5/0 stitch. To separate a 2-cm-wide section of mucosa, two incisions are made at right angles to each other. The submucosal plane is subjected to blunt and severe dissection, followed by gradual incision along the two parallel lines and slight retraction. The length of these incisions is strictly dictated by the urethra (Video). After inserting a suprapubic catheter, the detrusotomy is closed and a 5/0 absorbable suture is used to seal the mucosal defect.

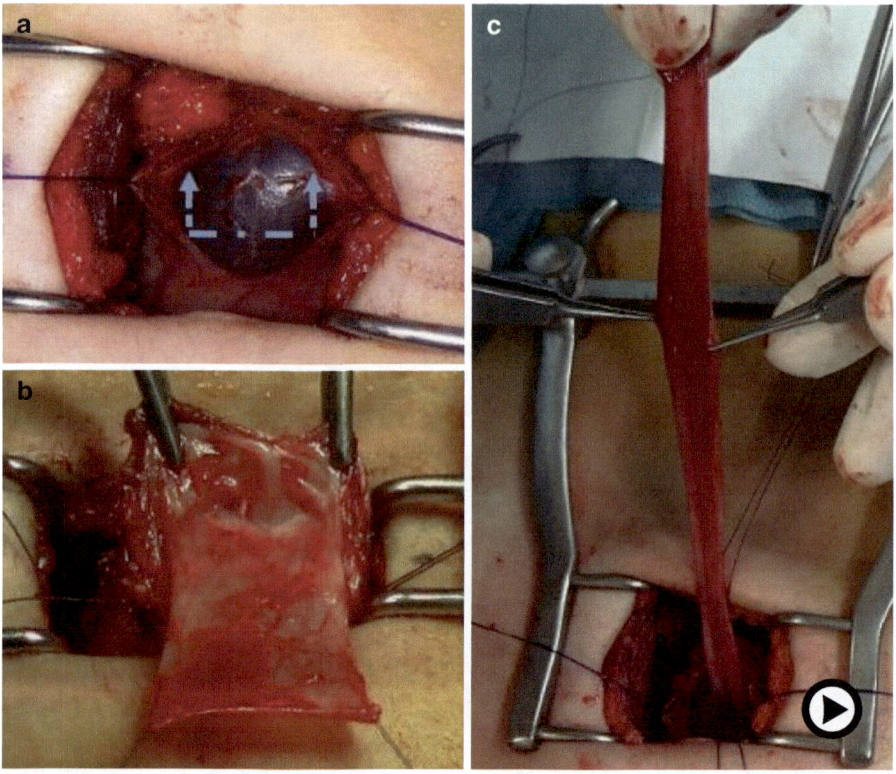

Fig. 30.3 Harvest of lengthy BMG with minimum detrusotomy. After making a 2-cm horizontal incision in the detrusor, the exposed mucosa is incised in two parallel lines and stretched to the necessary length (**a**). Blunt dissection is then used to remove the mucosa from the detrusor (**b**). (**c**) It is possible to extract a 16-centimeter-long section of bladder mucosa. Bladder mucosa graft. (CC BY 4.0) (https://doi.org/10.1007/000-cnv)

30.2.3 Tubularization of the Graft

A 6/0 absorbable PDS round needle is used to tubularize the graft. Depending on the child's age, tubularization is performed around a Foley catheter with a minimum size of 12 CH. Normal saline is continuously irrigated into the graft to keep it hydrated. The graft undergoes tubularization around a catheter size 12 Fr. In order for the graft to fit around the selected catheter, it is necessary to eliminate any extra width (Fig. 30.4).

30.2.4 Tunneling of the Graft (Fig. 30.5)

The perineal urethrotomy is dissected to remove any fibrous tissue and is significantly spatulated. The dissection is performed at the albuginea on the ventral surface of the corpus cavernosum. The identical dissection is performed at the base of

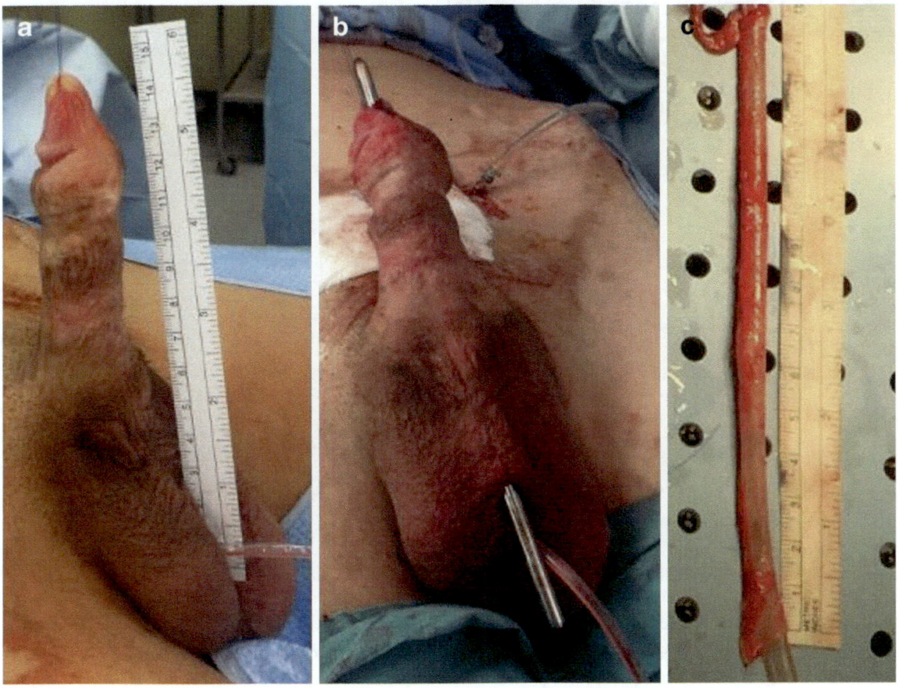

Fig. 30.4 Second stage: tunneling of tubularized bladder mucosa-free graft (CC BY 4.0). (**a**) There was no residual curvature seen during the erection test, a 16 cm urethroplasty was required. The albuginea of the corpus cavernosa is exposed during perineal dissection, which is step **b** in creating the tunnel. The anticipated location of the meatus is the target of a midline incision. To facilitate bougie passage equal to Chap. 18, progressive dilatation with metallic bougie is performed. (**c**) The free graft is tubularized around a Foley catheter Chap. 16

the glans. When the glans is already formed, a precise midline incision is made to separate a line of connection with the inner layer of the glans. Efforts are made to avoid immediately connecting the graft with the skin or fibrous glans margins. Gradual tunneling is performed with a metal bougie of increasing diameter to achieve a caliber greater than that of the urethral catheter (e.g., Bougie 18 Fr for 16 CH catheter). The perineal urethrotomy is dissected free of any fibrous tissue and largely spatulated. Dissection is done close to the albuginea of the ventral surface of the corpus cavernosum. The same dissection is done distally at the base of the glans. If the glans is already constructed, a sharp midline incision is done to isolate a line of anastomosis with the deep mucosa of the glans. Efforts are done not to anastomose directly the graft with skin or fibrous glans edges. Tunneling is then done progressively with increasing diameter of metal bougie to obtain a caliber higher than the urethral catheter (example: Bougie 18 Fr for 16 CH catheter).

A long forceps is introduced from proximal to distal, then the graft, attached to the catheter is pulled smoothly from distal to proximal. If resistance is encountered, perform another dilation.

Two running 6/0 PDS sutures are used to perform the proximal anastomosis with the spatulated urethra. The perineal anastomosis is protected by several layers of

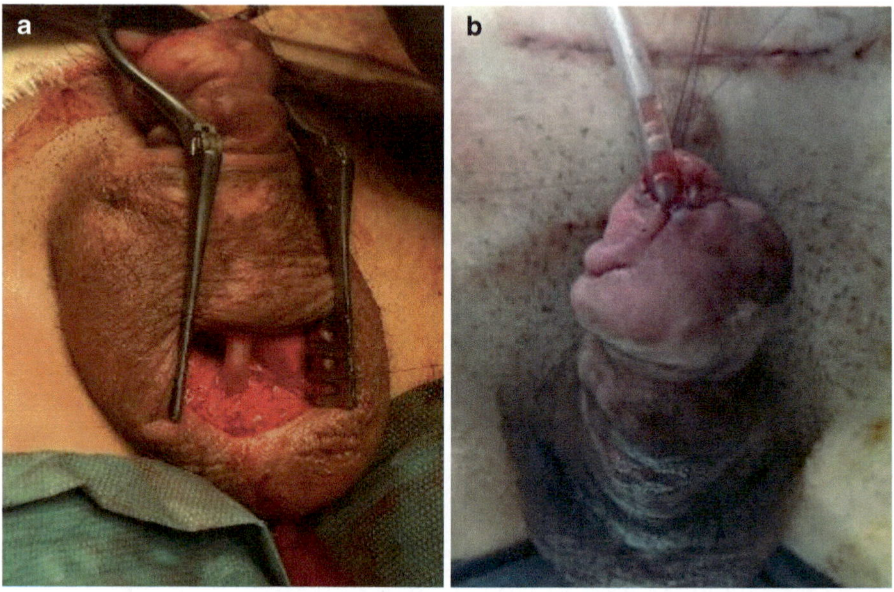

Fig. 30.5 The tubularized graft is tunneled from distal to proximal. The suture line of the graft is positioned carefully opposed to the corpus cavernosum. (**a**) A large anastomosis is performed between the graft and the spatulated perineal healthy urethra. (**b**) The distal anastomosis is performed on the most healthy section of the glans. (CC BY 4.0)

corpus spongiosum and deep fascia. The distal anastomosis is performed using the inner section of the glans, using interrupted 6/0 PDS sutures. A compressive dressing is used for 5 days and then taken off at the outpatient clinic. Anticholinergic therapy is commonly employed. We do not administer antibiotic prophylaxis save for a single dose at the start of operation.

The urethral catheter is withdrawn after a 21-day period, and the suprapubic catheter is then closed. If successful urination is achieved for 48 h, the suprapubic catheter is taken out. If there are symptoms like painful urination, swelling in the perineal area, or severe inflammation, a suprapubic catheter is inserted. An antegrade urethrogram is performed to guide the insertion of a new urethral catheter under general anesthesia until recovery is complete.

The child will have a follow-up appointment 1 month following surgery, followed by appointments every 3 months for a year, and then annually. After each flowmeter procedure, a cystoscopy is performed under general anesthesia when necessary.

30.3 Results

At 105 months of age (range 20–195), the graft operation was performed. The minimal detrusotomy technique was used to effectively extract the graft for urethroplasty procedures with varying lengths, with a median length of 10.5 cm and a range

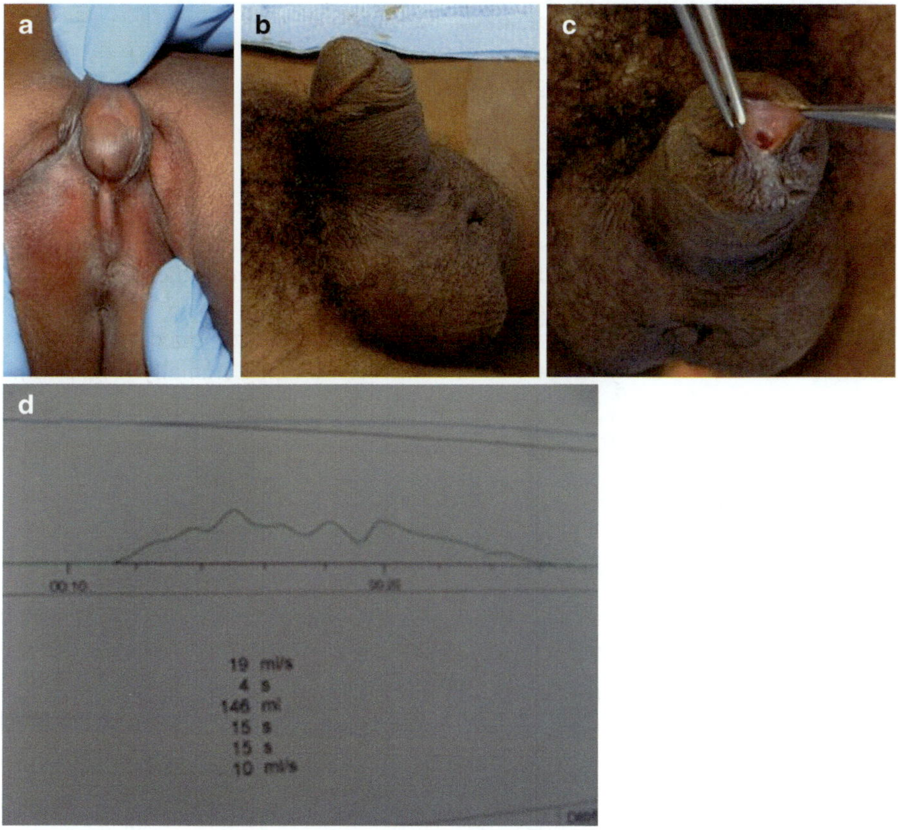

Fig. 30.6 Results of BMG tunneling (CC BY 4.0). (**a**) A 12-year-old boy with ovotesticular 46XX disorder and a perineal urethra. (**b**) Three years post-staged urethroplasty with tunneled buccal mucosa graft, followed by bilateral testicular prosthesis placement. (**c**) The glandular meatus displays a profound connection between a healthy glandular mucosa and the BMG. (**d**) The flowmeter indicates below-normal flow without any postvoid residual

of 8–16 cm. Between 18 and 160 months, the median duration of follow-up was 61.7 months. Five out of ten cases (50%) did not require a redo after TBMG (Fig. 30.6).

One case (case 2, Table 30.1) required self-dilatation with progressive caliber introduced for 3 cm due to stenosis of the distal anastomosis, which cripples redo hypospadias. Normal voiding stream intervals were used to determine the frequency. For the past 3 years, this 15-year-old has opted to maintain the self-dilatation. Additionally, after laser fragmentation, he experienced graft polyps within the artificial urethra and stones that were removed.

Surgical treatment with an onlay buccal mucosal graft has successively alleviated a localized stenosis of the proximal anastomosis in one case of perineal hypospadias.

Table 30.1 Patients' data and results

Case	Indication	Number of previous surgeries	Age (yrs.)	Length of urethroplasty (cm)	Fu (months)	Complications	Treatment of complications
1	Multiple operated perineal hypospadias	7	11.3	12	97	None	
2		12	12.9	15	62	Meatal stenosis, stone	Stone laser fragmentation, Self-dilatation 3 years, no recurrence
3	Ovotesticular 46XX DSD	1	12.5	14	61	Proximal fistula	Fistula closure, no further surgery
4		1	10.5	12	106	Proximal fistula	Fistula closure, no further surgery
5	Perineal hypospadias staged repair	0	1.7	8	160	Proximal stenosis	Onlay buccal mucosal graft, no further surgery
6		0	7.1	9	41	None	
7		0	2	7	30	Stricture	Total redo, staged buccal mucosal graft complicated by proximal fistula needed closure without recurrence
8		0	6.6	8	6	Loss of FU (after 6 months free of complications)	
9	Urethral duplication	2	1.7	8	71	None	
10	Circumcision complication	2	16.3	16	18	None	Preventive self-dilatation 12 months

An extensive penile graft stricture necessitated a complete redo using a phased approach with buccal mucosal graft in one case of perineal hypospadias.

Two instances had a small amount of mucosal prolapse, but there was no dysuria and no additional surgery was necessary.

Case 10 in Table 30.1 shows that an adolescent who had severe penile ischemia following circumcision had to self-dilate the meatus for a whole year to ensure a steady urine flow.

30.4 Discussion

When it comes to lengthy urethroplasty in patients with limited skin, we have found that tunneled BMG to be a dependable option for reconstruction. Additionally, we found the minimum detrusotomy approach to be an appealing option for reducing the morbidity associated with protracted graft retrieval.

After several unsuccessful attempts at hypospadias reconstruction, numerous alternatives exist for urethral reconstruction [10]. Customized reconstruction is the best option for every case because there is no universal procedure that can be utilized today [4].

Repairing salvage hypospadias is difficult because of scarring, obliterated tissue planes, reduced local tissue, and impaired blood flow. In addition, urethral tissue augmentation or replacement may be necessary for patients with long strictures or urethral breakdown to achieve successful surgical outcomes. Barbagli et al. [11] examined information from 1176 individuals following hypospadias failure in their comprehensive multicenter series. According to their findings, in order to get satisfactory outcomes in the end, it usually takes 5 more treatments.

Long segment urethroplasty and skin covering are the two primary obstacles in these instances.

It might be challenging for patients to have additional reconstruction after undergoing several hypospadias procedures since they often have inadequate or weak skin. Although there are several methods for increasing skin coverage, such as using Z-plasties and rotational flaps to augment the skin around the penile shaft, these patients frequently do not have access to redundant skin. There is a lot of hair-bearing skin that will show up after puberty when doing direct scrotal skin transfer, or there is a lot of scarring from these methods, so the cosmetic outcome isn't great. Revisions and updates to established methods, such as the Cecil Culp methodology, were documented by Weis et al. [12] A final complications rate of 21%, including skin disintegration, persisted in their 39-patient series with a Cecil Culp modified approach (3 steps).

In situations when there is a lack of skin and scarring covering tissues, tunneling a tubularized graft seems like a promising alternative to prevent the major complication of skin breakdown.

So far, we haven't had a single patient report skin breakdown.

We also found that tunneling helped avoid urethral fistula. Local closure was used to repair fistulas in two patients in our experience. In contrast to penile fistulas, which can be difficult to close, this one was located deep in the perineum, at the proximal anastomosis, which allowed for numerous well-vascularized accessible layers, making the closure both easy and efficient. There is likely no fistula in the penile shaft since the tubularization suture line is positioned against the corpus cavernosum in a tunneled-in area.

Fine et al. documented the results of a TBMG in 34 kids, 75% of whom had primary proximal hypospadias. A mean of 5.3 cm (ranging from 3.0 to 8.10) was the length of the urethral stent. Over the course of more than a year of follow-up, 32% of patients experienced problems. Of these, 5% had fistulas, 4% had proximal strictures, and 2% had meatal stenosis. The skin of no one was broken. Short FU in comparison to other series may lead to an underestimation of the rate of stricture.

In their study, Zhao et al. [7] detailed the results of TBMG in 57 people who had previously had hypospadias repaired unsuccessfully. The procedure involved tunneling the graft as an initial stage and then anastomosing it 6–12 months later.

In 48 cases where hypospadias surgery failed, Kim et al. [8] recently detailed their experience with TBMG. Every single patient who had difficulties needed a second operation, and just 14.7% of those patients were complication-free. The average length of the graft in their experience was just 3.7 cm, which is relatively short. Despite the fact that no patients experienced skin disintegration, just 22.9% were still free of strictures after 6 years.

The vast lengths required in our instances (median 10.5 cm, maximum 16 cm) surpass the maximal lengths employed in the previous cases, which is why we believe that the use of tubularized tunneled buccal mucosal graft has its limitations in urethral restoration. Buccal mucosal graft harvesting also has a non-negligible morbidity. Among the few data on buccal graft harvesting morbidity, Wood et al. found that 83% of patients experienced severe discomfort post-operatively, with persistent perioral numbness being the predominant long-term consequence at 26% [13].

In 1947, Memmelaar et al. [5] reported the first version of the bladder mucosa tube graft.

It was more or less successful to modify the original approach in order to decrease the problems. In order to decrease the occurrence of distal prolapses, Ransley et al. [6] utilized preputial skin grafts that fused bladder mucosa.

Primary hypospadias [14] and lengthy posterior urethral stricture [15] are two rare cases where TBMG has been reported in the literature. In a recent study, Lanciotti et al. [16] documented the results of a phased bladder mucosal graft procedure in 50 infants with severe hypospadias. The second stage of the procedure involved tunneling the graft. With a range of 35–85 mm, the mean graft length was 5.7 cm. There were 46% of total problems requiring a second surgery at the 5-year follow-up mark. Thirty percent of patients required more than one surgical procedure due to proximal anastomosis tightness.

Out of the four cases where TBMG was used to treat severe primary hypospadias, one patient experienced lengthy stricture, a serious complication that necessitated a two-stage redo operation. No indication of technique superiority has been found in the literature, and this group of hypospadias continues to be hard even as a primary case [17]. When there is enough skin to reconstruct the urethra and adequate vascularization, we now perform one-stage repairs using double-face preputial flaps [18] Although we have only seen skin scarcity on a rare occasion, we do retain the option of a free graft just in case.

Ovotesticular 46XX DSD masculinizing genitoplasty patients make up the second group of patients in our series. These individuals underwent hypospadias reconstructive surgery at an older age than is often recommended. There wasn't enough foreskin to go around, and the penile corpora required cavernotomy to correct their severe curvature. Reconstruction of lengthy urethral segments (12 and 14 cm.) with apical meatus was made possible by the TBGM. Due to a perineal fistula that developed shortly after surgery and was successfully repaired a year later by local anesthesia, neither patient experienced a recurrence. In one instance, mucosal prolapses happened; however, the patient exhibited no symptoms throughout the most recent 9-year follow-up, therefore no surgical intervention was necessary to address the minor prolapse.

Both of our hypospadias cripple patients underwent extensive surgical procedures, which unfortunately left them with unsightly scarring and unhealthy skin. Patients were left with a perineal urethrostomy at the level of their initial normal urethra after the first stage, which involved removing all fibrosed rebuilt urethra and treating substantial residual curvature. There was no skin breakdown and the TBMG proved a dependable salvaging option. After 3 years of self-dilatation to cure distal stenosis, one patient who had been initially covered with a full-thickness free skin transplant gradually stopped. After several surgeries, the glans becomes badly vascularized, which leads to this stenosis. In the second patient, who had seven previous unsuccessful procedures, the TBMG went off without a hitch, and dilatation was unnecessary.

Since the graft stays entirely in the deep tissues and the vascularized local flaps cover the distal and proximal anastomosis, TBMG seemed like a good option in rare cases like urethral duplication; Mouttalib et al. [15] reported a similar experience while successfully reconstructing a long congenital urethral stenosis in two children.

An adolescent who had a serious problem with circumcision at the age of 15 has already undergone this procedure. The skin of the penile shaft, urethra, corpus cavernosum, and glans were all affected by ischemia sloughing. A total skin transplant covering the penis was performed on him elsewhere, with the meatus left 16 cm distant from the penis's tip. One viable approach for salvaging a 16 cm urethra without rupturing the penile skin was TBMG. There was no distal stenosis found after opting to perform prophylactic self-dilatation of the meatus for a year in this case.

The bladder mucosa graft had a few drawbacks, one of which being a morbidity associated with retrieving bladder mucosa. It stands to reason that the lengthy detrusotomy would lead to malfunction, blood in urine, and pain in the bladder after surgery [19]. Through the use of a novel technique, we were able to extract the bladder mucosa graft with a minimal length of detrusotomy (2 cm) and achieve a graft length of 16 cm in our series. Graft retrieval-related morbidity could be lessened using this method.

It should be noted that there are potential difficulties associated with the use of bladder mucosal grafts that are particular to the mucosa of the bladder. These complications can worsen if factors such as urine stagnation in the repaired urethra are present. An article by Weingärtner K et al. [20] detailed six instances of nephrogenic adenoma following urethral reconstruction with bladder mucosa graft.

The incidence of problems may differ according to the particular indications and duration of follow-up, and we must acknowledge that the patient group is diverse and modest in size. Actually, the success rate would be 44% instead of 50% if we consider 1 year to be the lowest follow-up to determine success; removing case number 8 from the study would reduce the valid cohort to 9 patients. We have opted to provide all follow-up periods and treatment outcomes for problems in Table 30.1 so that everyone may see the full picture of our cohort. The ultimate advantage of utilizing our approach in each individual patient will be determined by the surgeon. We fully understand the importance of documenting these complicated situations with extensive follow-up, preferably beyond a year, since difficulties can still arise up to a decade later (post-pubescence and sexual activity).

However, when compared to previously published series, ours had a considerably longer urethral defect, less healthy skin coverage, and a generally similar indication, notwithstanding the heterogeneity of our group.

In conclusion, patients lacking sufficient healthy skin can benefit from a tunneled bladder mucosa tube transplant approach as an alternative to a lengthy urethroplasty. There is hope that the minimum detrusotomy method can lessen the morbidity associated with graft harvesting.

References

1. Verla W, Van Nieuwenhuyse F, Hoebeke P, Oosterlinck W, Sinatti C, Spinoit A-F, et al. Urethroplasty for failed hypospadias repair related strictures in adults: a retrospective analysis with long-term follow-up. Urology. 2020;143:248–54.
2. Badawy H, Soliman A, Moussa A, Youssef M, Fahmy A, Dawood W, et al. Staged repair of redo and crippled hypospadias: analysis of outcomes and complications. J Pediatr Urol. 2019;15(2):151.e1–151.e10.
3. Turkyilmaz Z, Karabulut R, Atan A, Sonmez K. Redo hypospadias repair: comparison of three different methods. Urol Int. 2020;104(5–6):391–5.
4. Mundy AR. Failed hypospadias repair presenting in adults. Eur Urol. 2006;49(5):774–6.
5. Memmelaar J. Use of bladder mucosa in a one-stage repair of hypospadias. J Urol. 1947;58(1):68–73.
6. Ransley PG, Duffy PG, Oesch IL, Van Oyen P, Hoover D. The use of bladder mucosa and combined bladder mucosa/preputial skin grafts for urethral reconstruction. J Urol. 1987;138(4 Pt 2):1096–8.
7. Zhao M, Li Y, Tang Y, Chen W, Yang Z, Li Q, et al. Two-stage repair with buccal mucosa for severe and complicated hypospadias in adults. Int J Urol Off J Jpn Urol Assoc. 2011;18(2):155–61.
8. Kim SW, Lee YS, Han SW. Buccal mucosa tube graft for failed hypospadias repair: worth it or not? Urology. 2020;146:196–200.

9. El-Ghoneimi A, Lachkar AA, Lopez P, Paye-Jaouen A, Peycelon M. Tunneled tubularized bladder mucosalgraft for long urethral reconstruction: is it a reliable option in selected complex cases in children and adolescents? Plast Aesthet Res. 2022;9:39. https://doi.org/10.20517/2347-9264.2021.101.
10. Djordjevic ML, Kojovic V, Bizic M, Majstorovic M, Vukadinovic V, Korac G. "Hanging" of the buccal mucosal graft for urethral stricture repair after failed hypospadias. J Urol. 2011;185(6 Suppl):2479–82. https://doi.org/10.1016/j.juro201101036. Epub 2011 Apr 27.
11. Barbagli G, Perovic S, Djinovic R, Sansalone S, Lazzeri M. Retrospective descriptive analysis of 1,176 patients with failed hypospadias repair. J Urol. 2010;183(1):207–11.
12. Weiss DA, Long CJ, Frazier JR, Shukla AR, Srinivasan AK, Kolon TF, et al. Back to the future: the Cecil-Culp technique for salvage penile reconstructive procedures. J Pediatr Urol. 2018;14(4):328.e1–7.
13. Wood DN, Allen SE, Andrich DE, Greenwell TJ, Mundy AR. The morbidity of buccal mucosal graft harvest for urethroplasty and the effect of nonclosure of the graft harvest site on postoperative pain. J Urol. 2004;172(2):580–3.
14. Valla JS, Takvorian P, Dodat H, Galifer RB, Chavrier Y, Aubert D, et al. Single-stage correction of posterior hypospadias (178 cases). Comparison of three techniques: free skin graft, free bladder mucosal graft, transverse pedicle preputial graft. Eur J Pediatr Surg Off J Austrian Assoc Pediatr Surg Al Z Kinderchir. 1991;1(5):287–90.
15. Mouttalib S, Bouali O, Abbo O, Moscovici J, Galinier P. Free tubularised vesical mucosa graft for congenital stenosis of the urethra in children. Progres En Urol J Assoc Francaise Urol Soc Francaise Urol. 2015;25(2):109–14.
16. Lanciotti M, Betti M, Elia A, Landi L, Taverna M, Cini C, et al. Proximal hypospadias repair with bladder mucosal graft: our 10 years experience. J Pediatr Urol. 2017;13(3):294.e1–6.
17. Castagnetti M, El-Ghoneimi A. Surgical management of primary severe hypospadias in children: systematic 20-year review. J Urol. 2010;184(4):1469–75.
18. Blanc T, Peycelon M, Siddiqui M, Muller C, Paye-Jaouen A, El-Ghoneimi A. Double-face preputial Island flap revisited: is it a reliable one-stage repair for severe hypospadias? World J Urol. 2020;39:1613.
19. Duckett JW, Coplen D, Ewalt D, Baskin LS. Buccal mucosal urethral replacement. J Urol. 1995;153(5):1660–3.
20. Weingärtner K, Kozakewich HP, Hendren WH. Nephrogenic adenoma after urethral reconstruction using bladder mucosa: report of 6 cases and review of the literature. J Urol. 1997;158(3 Pt 2):1175–7.

Part VII

Management of Post Hypospadias Repair Common Complications

31 Repair of Subcoronal Fistula in Cases of Well-Healed Glans without Compromising the Glans

Anil K. Takvani

Abstract

The most typical complication of hypospadias surgery is urethrocutaneous (UC) fistula. In patients with distal hypospadias repairs, coronal and subcoronal fistulas are the most common (Bhat and Mandal, Indian J Urol 24(2):241–248, 2008). It is frequently accompanied by glans dehiscence and necessitates redo distal hypospadias surgery, but occasionally the glans is attractive and the urethral opening is well-positioned and slit. In these instances, we wish to repair the fistula without causing damage to the glans or distal urethral tube. In this video chapter, we describe our subcoronal fistula repair technique with glans and distal urethra preservation.

Keywords

Urethrocutaneous fistula · Hypospadias · Dartos · Cutaneous flap

31.1 Introduction

UC fistula is the most prevalent complication of hypospadias surgery, with a reported incidence of 4–25% [1]. There are numerous techniques for fistula closure, including the simple approximation of the fistula's edges after separating it from the

Supplementary Information The online version contains supplementary material available at https://doi.org/10.1007/978-981-99-0795-3_31. The videos can be accessed individually by clicking the DOI link in the accompanying figure caption or by scanning this link with the SN More Media App.

A. K. Takvani (✉)
Takvani Kidney Hospital, Junagadh, India

T. O. Abbas (ed.), *Video Atlas of Hypospadias Surgery*,
https://doi.org/10.1007/978-981-99-0795-3_31

surrounding tissue; this is technically straightforward but carries a risk of recurrence [2]. The application of the impermeable layer significantly reduces the fistula recurrence rate [3].

For fistula restoration to be successful, a healthy layer of tissue must be interposed above the fistula's subepithelial closure [3]. The local or encircling skin and dartos can be examined to determine their suitability as a waterproof layer. The incision is designed so that the dartos can be mobilized and sutured over the fistula closure with a comfortable skin covering at the conclusion of the operation. This is to be accomplished by averting suture line overlap.

Subcoronal fistulas with comparatively well-healed glans and urethral openings placed at the tip of the glans as vertical slits are encountered by all. The objective is to close the fistula without damaging the glans or the most distal portion of the urethra, which is well-open at the point of the glans. In the past 5 years, we have operated on 40 patients using this technique with 100% success.

31.2 Video Demonstration

Video 1

Factors	Findings
Age at the surgery	3 years
Gestational age	Full term
Birth weight (gm)	2600
Family history	None
Testosterone	Before the first surgery
Age at first hypospadias surgery	18 months

Video 1

Factors	Findings
Age at the surgery	4 years
Gestational age	Full term
Birth weight (gm)	2700
Family history	None
Testosterone	No history
Age at first hypospadias surgery	24 months

Video Links
Video 1: https://1drv.ms/v/s!AnIDekwwlAN-gsY-wvGUGR6MFm1LOQ?e=hLrbUt
Video 2: https://1drv.ms/v/s!AnIDekwwlAN-gsY_wUpyTWQPF8SpNg?e=4yClmm

31.3 Steps of the Procedure

The goal is to repair subcoronal fistula extending beneath the well-healed glans by interpositioning healthy dartos and without disturbing the glans.

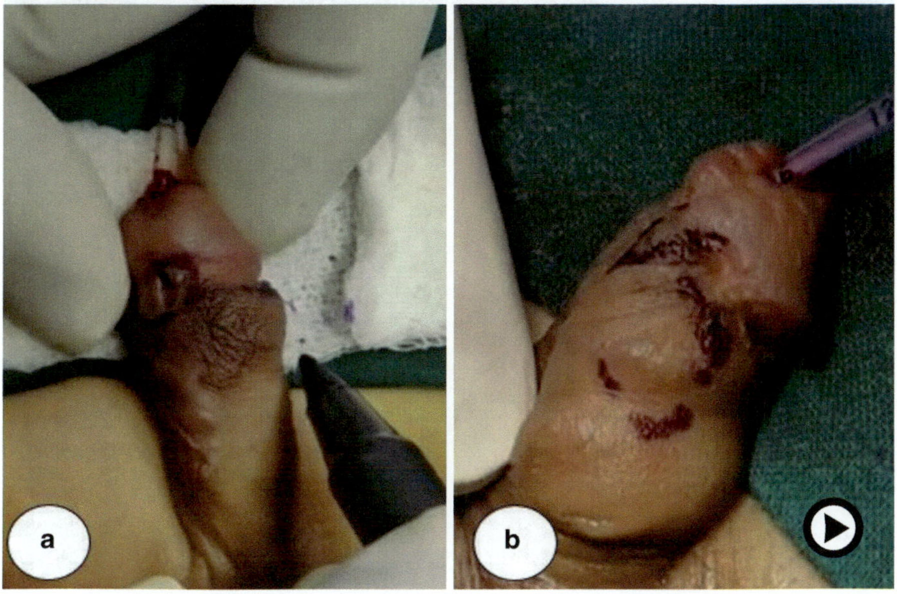

Fig. 31.1 U-shaped marking of fistula and marking of adjacent dartos-skin flap. (**a**) Long fistula extending underneath glans. (**b**) A small fistula with multiple tracts. Management of urethrocutaneous fistula (https://doi.org/10.1007/000-cnx)

31.3.1 Marking of Fistula and Adjacent Dartos-Skin Flap

- A glans penis stay suture is placed.
- A U-shaped marking is made around the fistula (Fig. 31.1).
- Excess skin and underlying dartos were identified and marked on the left side of the penile shaft, adjacent to the lower extremity of the fistula.

31.3.2 Superficial Dissection of Fistula

Care is taken not to damage the urethra proximal to the fistula when performing the superficial dissection of the fistula from the surrounding epidermis (Fig. 31.2).

31.3.3 Preparation of Adjacent Dartos-Cutaneous Flap

- In this case as we marked (Fig. 31.1b) on the left side of the fistula we can see excess skin and underlying dartos. The incision extended on the left side keeping 2–3 mm of skin adjacent to glans as a collar.
- First anterior dissection of dartos flap done from overlying skin for adequate mobilization of dartos flap (Fig. 31.3).

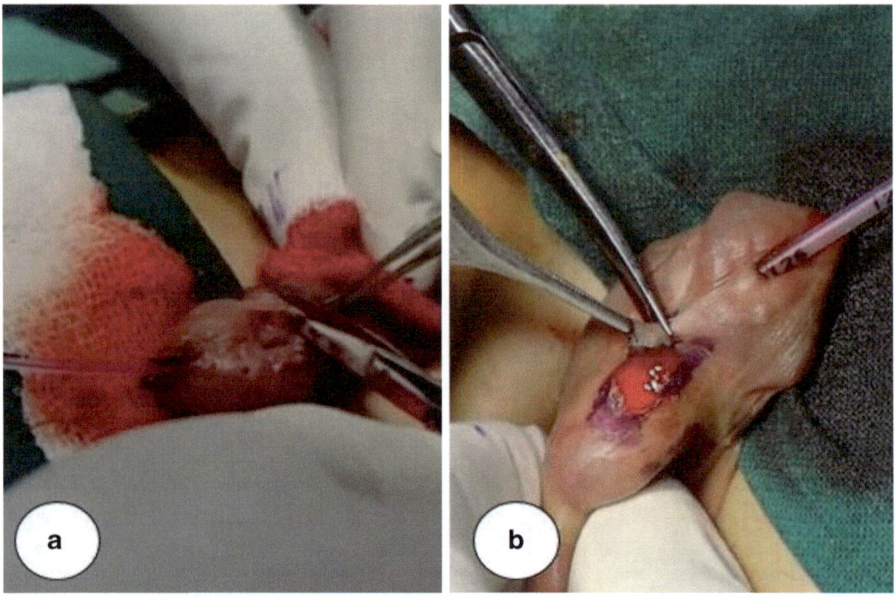

Fig. 31.2 (**a**, **b**) superficial dissection of fistula from the surrounding skin, taking care of not to damage urethra and underneath dartos tissue

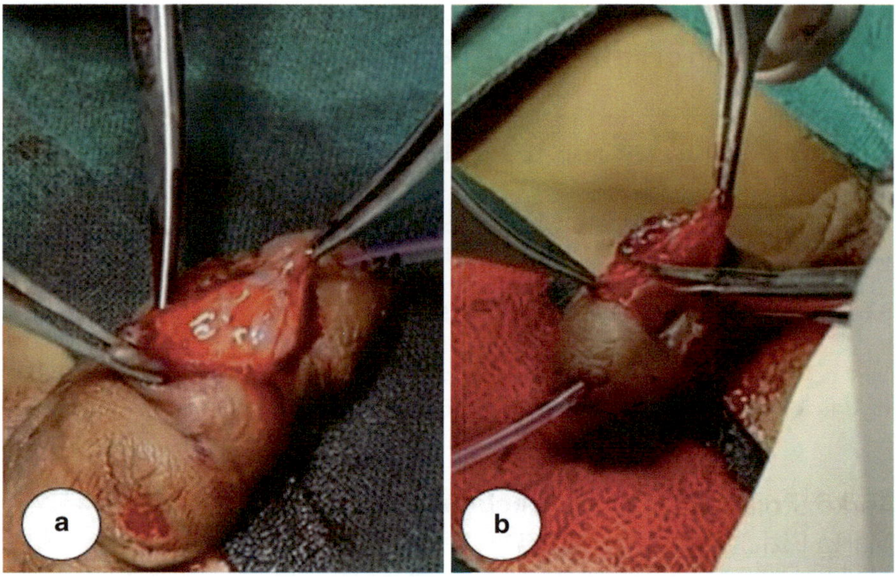

Fig. 31.3 Anteriorly dartos flap dissection (**a**) from the skin (Video 2) and posterior dissection from Buck's fascia (**b**) (Video 1)

- Following that the dartos flap mobilized posteriorly from the underlying buck's fascia. We have to keep the base of the dartos flap broad and the flap should be mobilized adequately so it can be sutured beyond the apex of the fistula without tension.

31.3.4 Deep Freeing of the Fistula

- On either side of the fistula, additional incision and dissection are performed beneath the glans epidermis while taking care not to harm the glans tissue.
- For retraction, stay sutures are placed on both of the glans' wing tips. This step facilitates the dissection and closure of the fistula from the apex and beyond.
- Underneath the healthy glans tissues, adequate fistula mobilization is performed at the fistula's specific upper extremity (Fig. 31.4).

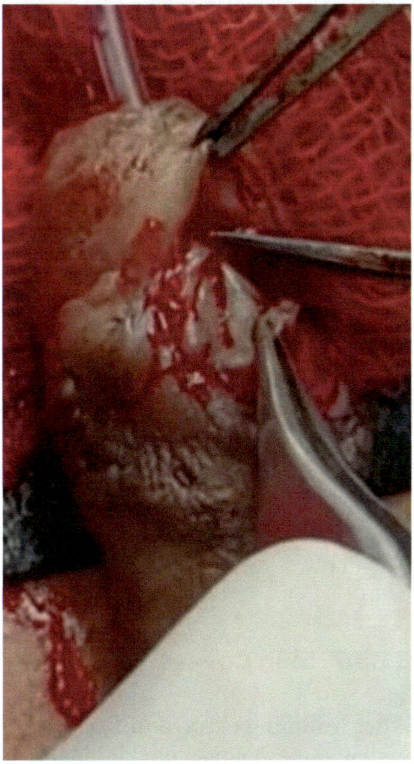

Fig. 31.4 Deep dissection of fistula on upper end from glans tissue (video 1). Freeing of fistula under the glans after upward retraction

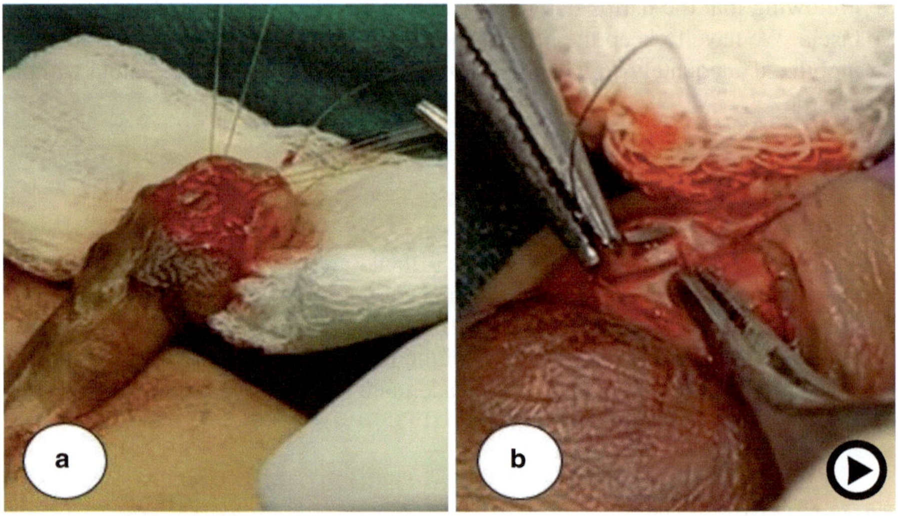

Fig. 31.5 First layer intermittent subepithelial suturing (**a**) and second layer burying continuous suturing (**b**) (https://doi.org/10.1007/000-cnw)

31.3.5 Fistula Closure

- The fistula closed in two layers.
- First layer intermittent, subcuticular sutures from the fistula's upper to lower extremity.
- We must prevent epidermis margins from becoming inverted. The second layer consists of continuous sutures to reinforce the closure of the first layer.
- 6'O Vicryl is utilized for both fistula closure layers (Fig. 31.5).

31.3.6 Inter-positioning of Vascular Flap

Under the glans skin, the mobilized vascular dartos flap is sutured to glans tissue. The flap was secured with 5–6 sutures without tension (Fig. 31.6).

31.3.7 Skin Cover

After trimming extra skin from the outer margins of the flap, the skin was sutured with glans and adjacent skin maintaining cosmesis (the Firtlit collar) (Fig. 31.7).

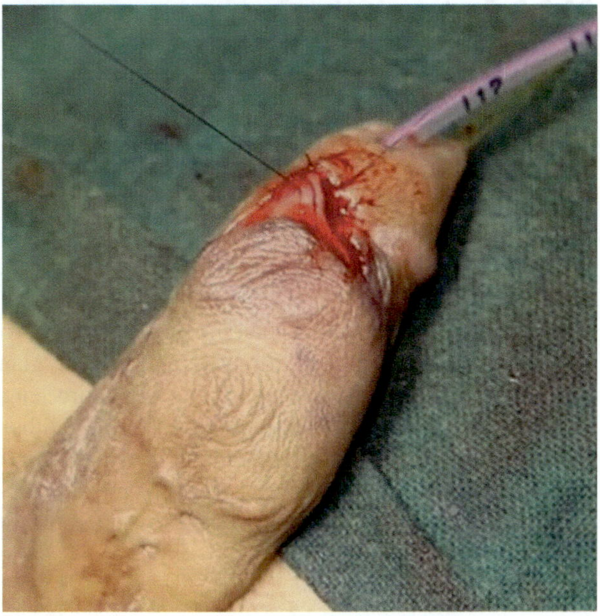

Fig. 31.6 Stitches to fix the dartos flap with underlying glans tissues

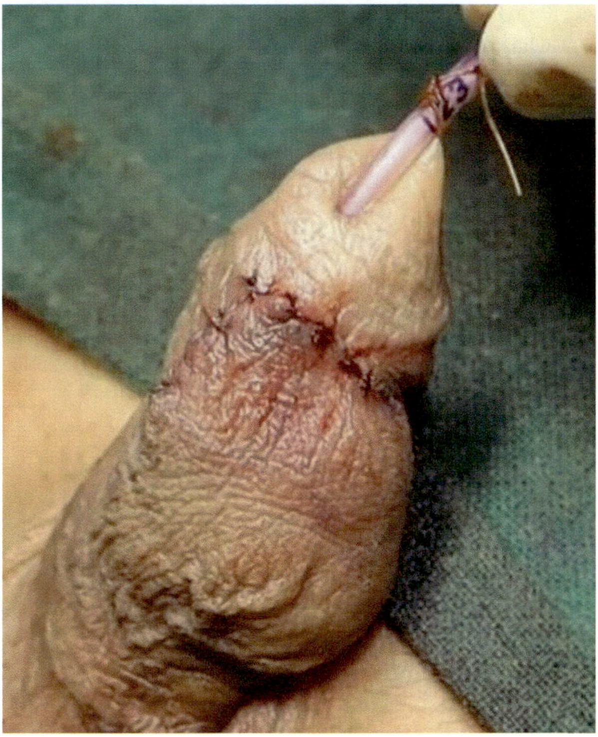

Fig. 31.7 A well-vascularized skin cover with firlit collar

31.3.8 Post-operative Care

- Five days of a light compression dressing were administered.
- 7 F infant feeding tube kept in the bladder for drainage of urine.
- The feeding tube was removed on the sixth day and a voiding trial was administered; the patient voids well with no leakage from the fistula repair site.

31.4 Results and Conclusion

Over the past 5 years, more than 40 similar varieties of fistula have been operated on with the preservation of attractive and healthy glans, with 100% success. This surgical technique involves mobilizing the entire length of the fistula specifically under the healthy glans. The retraction stitch on either side of the glans facilitates the dep dissection of the fistula without causing harm to the glans tissues and under direct vision. The second crucial stage for the success of fistula closure is tension-free interpositioning of adjacent, well-dissected dartos. This procedure is simple, effective, and simple to replicate.

References

1. Belman AB. The de-epithelialized flap and its influence on hypospadias repair. J Urol. 1994;152:2332–4.
2. Walker RD. Outpatient repair of urethral fistula. Urol Clin North Am. 1981;8:573.
3. Shankar KR, Losty PD, Hopper M, Wong L, Rickwood AM. The outcome of hypospadias fistula repair. BJU Int. 2002;89:103–5.

Management of Post-Hypospadias Repair Urethrocutaneous Fistula

32

Pankaj M. Joshi, Tariq O. Abbas, and Sanjay B. Kulkarni

Abstract

The incidence of post-hypospadias urethrocutanoeus fistula varies between 4% and 10% (Kulkarni, Res RepUrol 10:117–126, 2018). The location of fistula varies and is variable and the most usual location is at the corona level. There are numerous surgical treatment options for fistula. We present our algorithm for urethrocutaneous fistula management.

Keywords

Hypospadias · Fistula · Corona · Stricture · Penile urethra

32.1 Introduction

Post-operative urethrocutaneous fistula is a possible complication of hypospadias correction [2]. They are found in the area where ischemia has taken place [3]. Fistulas can develop for a number of different reasons in the different types of hypospadias phenotypes [4] post-surgery. It is important to take a thorough history and perform a

Supplementary Information The online version contains supplementary material available at https://doi.org/10.1007/978-981-99-0795-3_32. The videos can be accessed individually by clicking the DOI link in the accompanying figure caption or by scanning this link with the SN More Media App.

P. M. Joshi (✉) · S. B. Kulkarni
UROKUL, Pune, India

T. O. Abbas
Urology Division, Surgery Department, Doha, Qatar

T. O. Abbas (ed.), *Video Atlas of Hypospadias Surgery*,
https://doi.org/10.1007/978-981-99-0795-3_32

physical examination on a child who develops with fistula. Fistulae are typically fixed at least 3 months following the initial procedure [5]. Several fundamental concepts are required for the proper healing of this injury. Although technically simple, a simple closure carries the danger of visible suture lines and higher recurrence rates. Several methods have been explored to repair larger or multiple fistulas, but this is only possible if the skin neighboring the fistula is vascularized and flexible. An interposition waterproofing layer significantly decreases the recurrence incidence of bigger or recurrent fistulas with compromised local vascularity. We have standardized the management of fistula depending on the size and location [1].

Urethrocutaneous fistula can be classified according to several factors as follows:

A. *Size:* less than 5 mm, more than 5 mm.
B. *Location:* Proximal penile, distal penile.
C. *Associated factors:* distal stricture, stricture at site of fistula.

32.2 Video Demonstration

Factors	Findings
Age at surgery (months)	26
Gestational age (weeks)	Full term
Birth weight (gm)	2800
Gestational risks (e.g., maternal co-morbidities, IVF, Twin)	None
Family history	None
Testosterone (if yes, reason, and protocol used)	None
Any features of DSD (e.g., undescended testes)	None

32.3 Steps of Procedure

32.3.1 Depending on Size of Fistula

- Place a traction suture on glans.
- Inject methylene blue in the urethra (Fig. 32.1).
- Assess the size of fistula using a scale.

32.3.1.1 For Fistula Larger than 5 mm

- Make a circumferential incision.
- Dissect the fistula till its base to the urethra.
- Excise the fistula tract.
- Take everting sutures with 5-0 polydioxanone.
- Close the fistula employing continuous sutures.
- Second layer closure with dartos that is prepared and covers the fistula closure site.

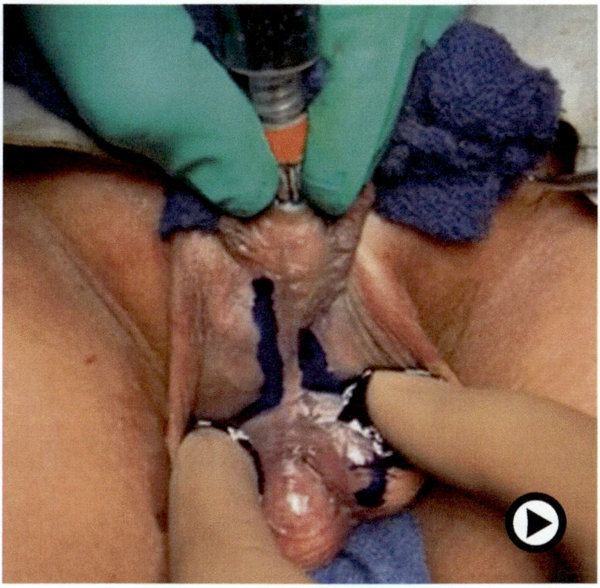

Fig. 32.1 Injection of methylene blue in urethra in a retrograde manner to determine the locations and numbers of the urethrocutaneous fistulas. Fistula Repair-adult perspectives (https://doi.org/10.1007/000-cny)

32.3.1.2 For Small Fistulas Less than 5 mm Width (Inversion Technique)

- Pass a mosquito forceps from meatus into the fistula (Fig. 32.2).
- Take everting stich so that fistula gets everted in the urethral lumen.
- Close the dartos.
- Catheter can be removed next day.

32.3.2 Depending on the Presence and Location Stricture

32.3.2.1 If There Is Distal Glanular or Meatal Stenosis

- Incise the urethra across meatus ventrally.
- Put a graft as dorsal inlay [6] (Fig. 32.3).
- Close urethra over a catheter/stent

32.3.2.2 If the Stricture Is Only Focal at Site of Fistula

- Enlarge the fistula
- Insert a graft as dorsal inlay (Fig. 32.4)
- Close urethra [7].

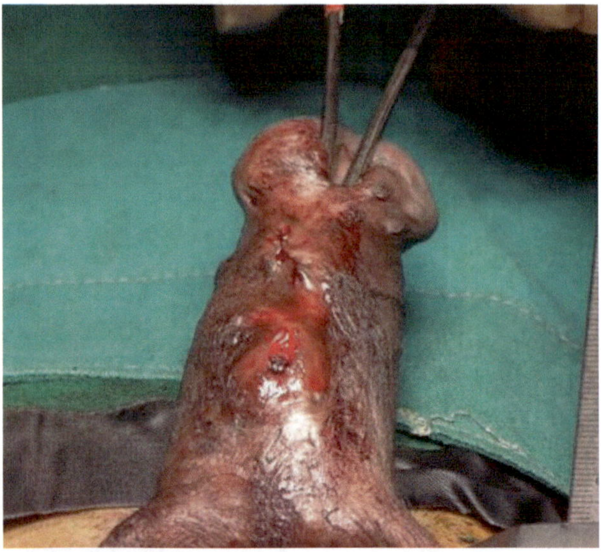

Fig. 32.2 Inversion technique for the repair of the small urethrocutaneous fistulas. A mosquito forceps is inserted from meatus into the fistula

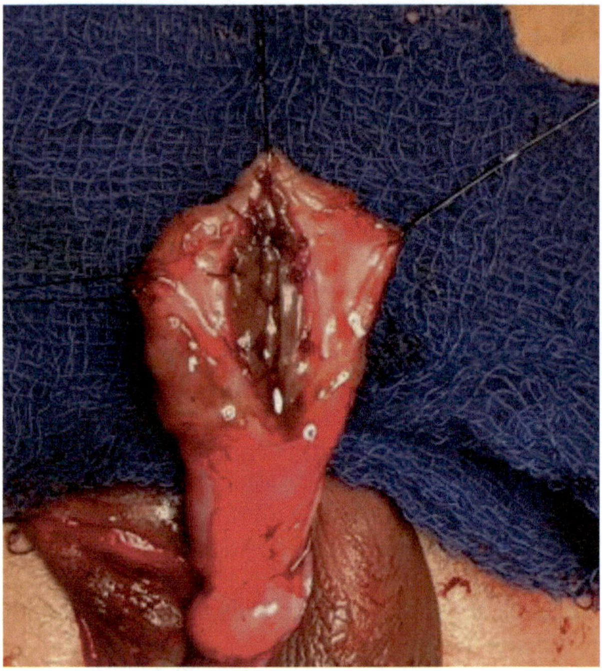

Fig. 32.3 Dorsal inlay graft for meatal stenosis with complete repair of urethra

Fig. 32.4 Dorsal inlay graft at site of stricture

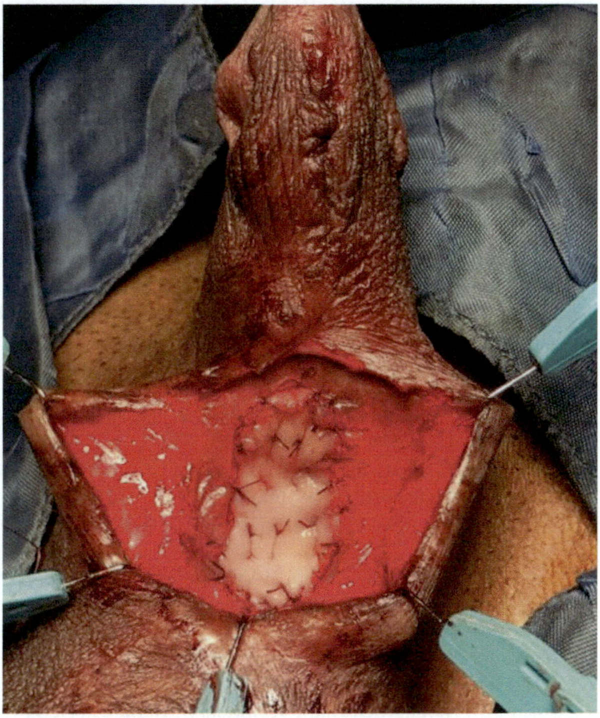

32.3.3 Multiple Fistula

- Lay open the urethra ventrally across all fistulae.
- Johansson stage I urethroplasty [8]
- 6 months later, perform a dorsal inlay BMG and close the urethra [9]
- Refrain of inserting grafts in the first stage, as grafts can contract.

32.4 Results and Conclusion

It is not clear why some fistulas persist in recurrence [10]. There is no definitive answer beyond possible flaws in surgical technique or postoperative treatment; nevertheless, decreased local vascularity due to scarred surrounding skin may provide a reasonable explanation. The findings demonstrate that the first success rates for both simple and multilayer fistula closure are poor [11].

When only a simple closure was tried, success rates for the second and third attempts were significantly lower, ranging from 50% to 80%, but no recurrence was detected when a waterproofing layer was also used [12]. In addition to the fistulas being small, easily controllable, and reducing the psychological trauma [13, 14] of the patient suffering recurrent surgeries, the application of tunica vaginalis or scrotal dartos tissue in a scarred area as a waterproofing cover at the earliest reintervention minimizes the recurrence risk [12].

References

1. Kulkarni SB, Joglekar O, Alkandari MH, Joshi PM. Redo hypospadias surgery: current and novel techniques. Res Rep Urol [Internet]. 2018;10:117–26.
2. Abbas T, McCarthy L. Foreskin and penile problems in childhood. Surg (United Kingdom). 2016;34(5):221.
3. Abbas TO, editor. HYPOSPADIOLOGY : current challenges and future perspectives. 2023. 190 p.
4. Abbas TO. An objective hypospadias classification system. J Pediatr Urol [Internet]. 2022;18(4):481.e1–8.
5. Baaklini GT, Abbas T, Hofer MD. Urethral anatomy, physiology, and regeneration. In: Abbas TO, editor. Hypospadiology [Internet]. 2023. p. 25–35.
6. Abbas TO, Pippi Salle JL. Dorsal inlay TIP (DTIP). In: Hypospadias Surgery [Internet]. 2022. p. 451–60.
7. Shaw NM, Mallahan C, Joshi P, Venkatesan K, Kulkarni S. Novel use of Asopa technique for penile urethrocutaneous fistula repair. Int Urol Nephrol [Internet]. 2021;53(6):1127–33.
8. Al-Ali M, Al-Hajaj R. Johanson's staged urethroplasty revisited in the salvage treatment of 68 complex urethral stricture patients: presentation of total urethroplasty. Eur Urol [Internet]. 2001;39(3):268–71.
9. Joshi PM, Barbagli G, Batra V, Surana S, Hamouda A, Sansalone S, et al. A novel composite two-stage urethroplasty for complex penile strictures: a multicenter experience. Indian J Urol [Internet]. 2017;33(2):155–8.
10. Abbas T, Vallasciani S. Toward an ecosystem model of hypospadiology. In: Abbas TO, editor. Hypospadiology [Internet]. 2023. p. 1–23.
11. Cimador M, Castagnetti M, De Grazia E. Urethrocutaneous fistula repair after hypospadias surgery. BJU Int [Internet]. 2003;92(6):621–3.
12. Srivastava RK, Tandale MS, Panse N, Gupta A, Sahane P. Management of urethrocutaneous fistula after hypospadias surgery—an experience of thirty-five cases. Indian J Plast Surg [Internet]. 2011;44(1):98–103.
13. Bethell GS, Chhabra S, Shalaby MS, Corbett H, Kenny SE, BAPS NOAH Contributors. Parental decisional satisfaction after hypospadias repair in the United Kingdom. J Pediatr Urol [Internet]. 2020;16(2):164.e1–7.
14. Spinoit A-F, Waterschoot M, Sinatti C, Abbas T, Callens N, Cools M, et al. Fertility and sexuality issues in congenital lifelong urology patients: male aspects. World J Urol [Internet]. 2020; 39:1013.

33 Approach to Redo Surgery for Failed TIP Urethroplasty

Pedro López Pereira, M. J. Martinez Urrutia, and Susana Rivas Vila

Abstract

Urethroplasty reinterventions are complicated procedures that should only be performed by surgeons with extensive experience in this type of surgery. The success of these surgeries depends not only on the surgeon's experience but also on many other factors. A meticulous evaluation of the skin and its vascularization as well as the quality of the urethral plate after failed attempts for urethral repair are very important factors that we must consider when considering the type of urethroplasty we should perform. When the urethral plate is narrowed and scarred and there is redundant skin on the penile shaft after the original repair, a vascularized flap may be a good option for urethroplasty. If the urethral plate is unavailable, a buccal mucosa graft and a two-stage urethroplasty would be the best choice.

Keywords

Hypospadias · Fistula · Re-urethroplasty · Urethral plate · Unfavorable urethral plate · Flap · Graft · Failed TIP

Supplementary Information The online version contains supplementary material available at https://doi.org/10.1007/978-981-99-0795-3_33. The videos can be accessed individually by clicking the DOI link in the accompanying figure caption or by scanning this link with the SN More Media App.

M.J.M. Urrutia
S.R. Vila

P. L. Pereira (✉)
Pediatric Urology Department, University Hospital La Paz, Madrid, Spain

T. O. Abbas (ed.), *Video Atlas of Hypospadias Surgery*, https://doi.org/10.1007/978-981-99-0795-3_33

33.1 Introduction

Despite continuous modifications and technical advances, successful hypospadias repair remains a major challenge. A combination of factors threatens to compromise even the most meticulous repair.

A meta-analysis by Pfistermuller et al. [1] examined 49 studies that included 4675 children who had undergone tubularized incised urethroplasty (TIP) repair. They identified an overall complication rate of 10.6%, with fistulas (5.7%) being the most frequent complication, followed by meatal stricture (3.6%) [1]. Fistula correction following failed hypospadias repair should not be lightly dismissed and, in some series, there has been a 20% recurrence rate [2].

Large fistulas or those occurring at the corona with only a thin bridge of skin connecting the gland wings distally represent a failure of the original urethroplasty. Surgery that is limited to fistula closure in these cases is generally doomed to failure, and in these circumstances a repeat urethroplasty is invariably required. Depending upon the initial approach to hypospadias repair; techniques like Mathieu, Thiersch Duplay, and redo TIP have been described in instances with a reasonable degree of success [3, 4]. Alternatively, placement of an inlay graft after incision of the urethral plate can improve outcomes in reoperated hypospadias. However, surgeons still must use caution when using tissue that has already failed closure in the past and now has a more variable blood supply [5–7].

Before considering a new urethroplasty in a failed hypospadias repair, we must have information about the type of surgery done previously. We must keep in mind that the quality of the tissue and its vascularity decreases with each procedure performed on the penis; the options for using that tissue in reconstruction are reduced, which will result in increased complications. It is therefore important to carefully evaluate the skin and tissues for their potential use and to plan the surgery to be performed [6, 8].

The urethroplasty technique used will depend on the characteristics of the urethral plate after previous surgeries and the surgeon's preferences. When the urethral plate is narrow and scarred and there is redundant skin of the penile shaft after the original repair, a combined meatal-based flap may be a good choice for urethroplasty. If preputial mucosa is present, another option could be to place of an inner preputial graft (dorsal inlay graft) or buccal mucosa graft inlay if preputial mucosa is not available [6, 8].

Due to the variable nature of non-virgin tissue and its possible diminished vascularity, we must add additional layers of covering (tunica vaginalis or dartos) to increase the likelihood for tissue survival [9–11].

33.2 Steps of the Procedure

33.2.1 Scenario 1

- When the boy has a narrow and scarred urethral plate and there is redundant skin on the penile shaft and preputial mucosa after the original repair and penile curvature <30° we recommend using a *flap of preputial mucosa rather than an inner preputial graft* (Figs. 33.1, 33.2, 33.3 and 33.4).

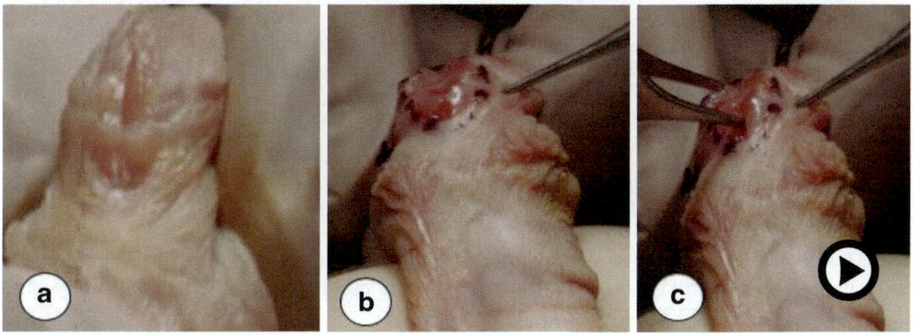

Fig. 33.1 (**a**) Subcoronal fistula and glans dehiscence. (**b**) Landmarks that delineate the urethral plate. (**c**) Preparation of the urethral plate with mucosal bridge sectioning. Redo after TIP Repair. https://doi.org/10.1007/000-cnz

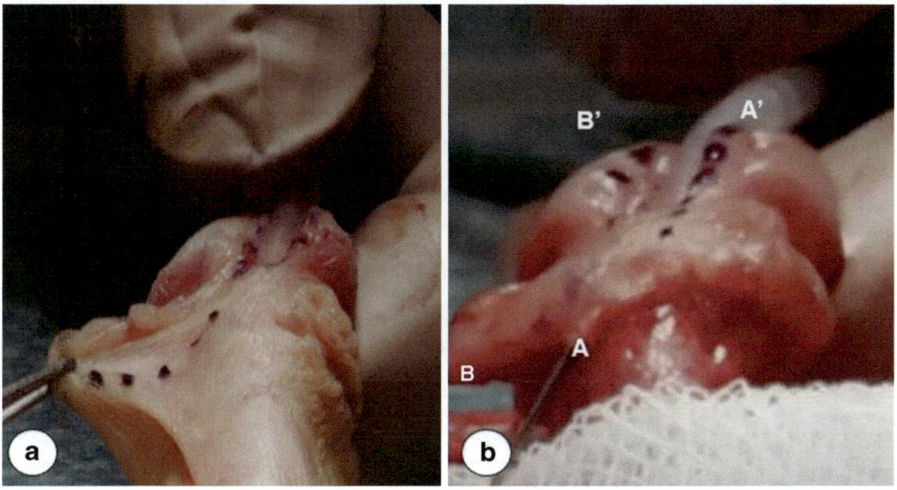

Fig. 33.2 (**a**) Landmarks to create the mucosa collar flap for the neo-urethroplasty. (**b**) Exposition for periurethral plate incision. A: edge of the distal mucosa of the collar flap, to be suture in the gland at A′ and B: edge of the distal mucosa of the collar flap, to be suture in the gland at B′

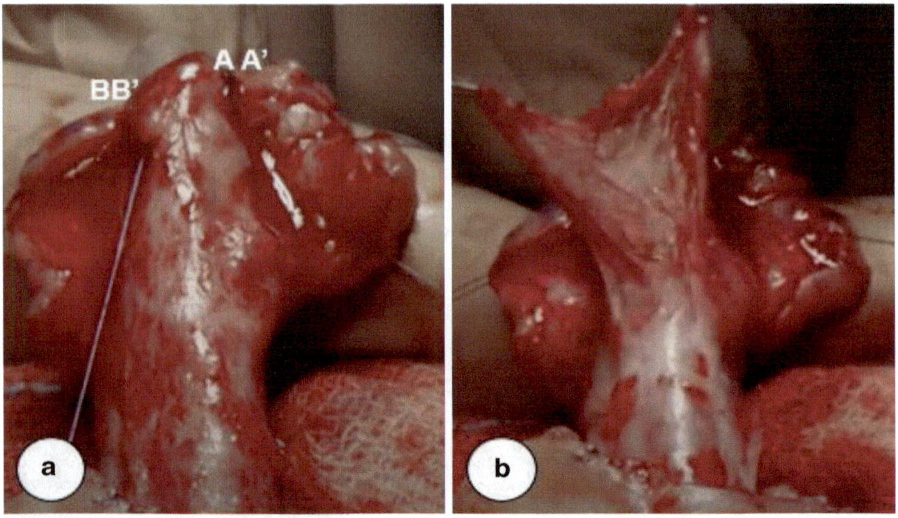

Fig. 33.3 (**a**) Finished neo-urethroplasty. A: edge of the distal mucosa of the collar flap sutured in the gland at A′. B: edge of the distal mucosa of the collar flap sutured in the gland at B′. (**b**) Ventral dartos flaps

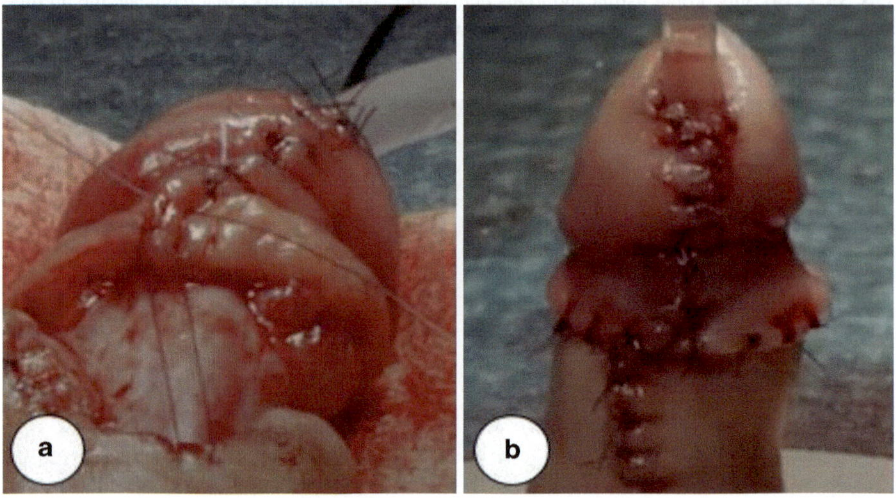

Fig. 33.4 (**a**) Glanuloplasty. (**b**) Skin closure

33.2.2 Scenario 2

– In those cases where we have neither enough skin nor preputial mucosa and the urethral plate is scarred and fibrotic or unavailable, and penile curvature <30° we would advise a buccal mucosa graft and two-stage urethroplasty (Fig. 33.5).

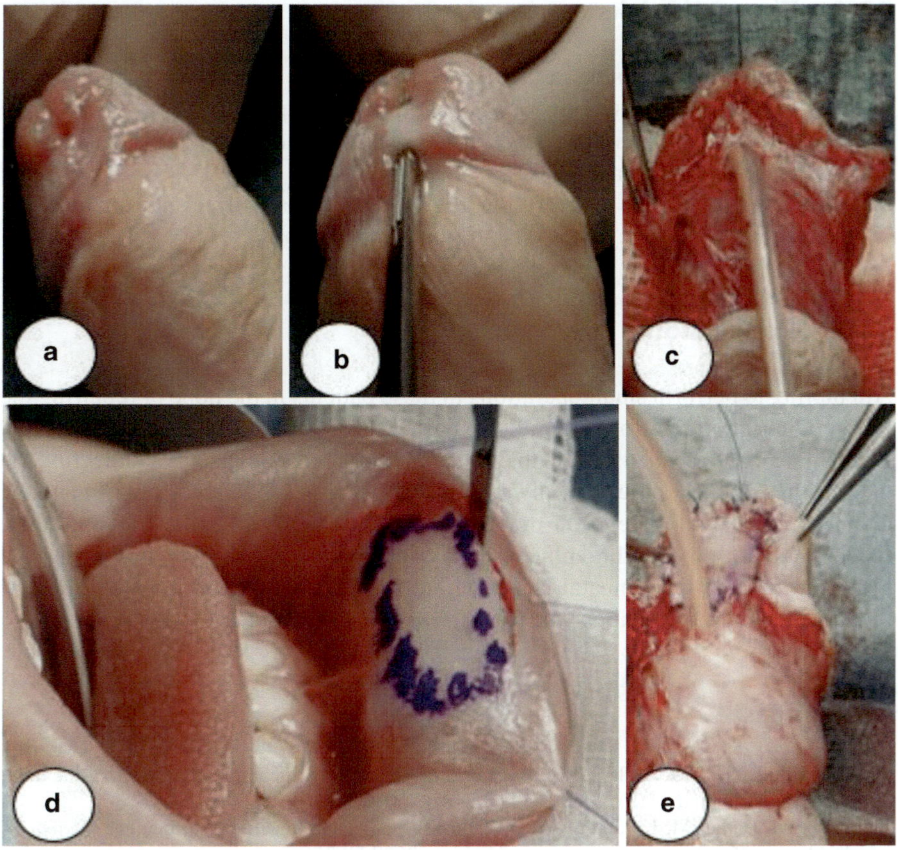

Fig. 33.5 (**a**, **b**) 3-year-old boy underwent 2 previous TIP operations; he has a fistula at the corona with only a thin bridge of skin connecting the gland wings. (**c**) Urethral plate unavailable. (**d**, **e**) Buccal mucosa graft

33.3 Video Demonstration

https://drive.google.com/file/d/1xW9-hbhTqz7-5xLGgjvqI38R_7kLu4ah/view?usp=sharing

Patient	Findings
Age at first surgery	14 months
Age at second surgery	24 months
Family history	None
Testoterone	None
	None

33.4 Tips and Tricks

- Before making a decision, a careful examination of the penis is mandatory in order to take into account all the possible treatment options.
- Adequate immobilization during surgery allows the suture to be performed without the need for a tourniquet.
- Wide dissection of the wings of the glands allows tension-free suturing and protects the urethroplasty.

33.5 Conclusions

Attempting to perform small operations in these patients in the hope of repairing the failure with minimal effort generally makes matters worse. We should not attempt to repair a large coronal fistula with only a thin bridge of skin distally connecting the gland wings. In these cases, it is always necessary to repeat the urethroplasty and the technique used will depend on the anatomy of the penis after the failed urethral reconstruction. If the urethral plate is thick, rigid, and less stretching, it is preferable to perform a combined meatal-based flap to augment the urethroplasty, if there is redundant skin of the penile shaft from the original repair [12, 13].

References

1. Pfistermuller KL, McArdle AJ, Cuckow PM. Meta-analysis of complication rates of the tubularized incised plate (TIP) repair. J Pediatr Urol. 2015;11:54–9.
2. Sunay M, Dadali M, Karabulut A, et al. Our 23-year experience in urethrocutaneous fistulas developing after hypospadias surgery. Urology. 2007;69:366–8.
3. Bar-Yosef Y, Binyamini J, Matzkin H, et al. Salvage Mathieu urethroplasty: reuse of local tissue in failed in failed hypospadias repair. Urology. 2005;65:1212–5.
4. Nozohoor Ekmark A, Svensson H, Arnbjornsson E, et al. Failed hypospadias repair: an algorithm for secondary reconstruction using remaining local tissue. J Plast Reconstr Aesthet Surg. 2015;68:1600–9.
5. Kolon TF, Gonzales ET. The dorsal inlay graft for hypospadias repair. J Urol. 2000;163:1941–3.
6. Snodgrass WT, Bush N, Cost N. Algorithm for comprehensive approach to hypospadias reoperation using 3 techniques. J Urol. 2009;182:2885–91.
7. White CM, Hanna MK. Salvaging the dehisced glans penis. J Pediatr Urol. 2018;14:422.e1–5. https://doi.org/10.1016/j.jpurol.2018.04.028.
8. Snodgrass W, Bush NC. Re-operative urethroplasty after failed hypospadias repair: how prior surgery impacts risk for additional complications. J Pediatr Urol. 2017;13:289.e281–6.
9. Gapany C, Grasset N, Stéphane Tercier S, Ramseyer P, Frey P, Meyrat BJ. A lower fistula rate in hypospadias surgery. J Pediatr Urol. 2007;3:395–7.
10. Fahmy O, Khairul-Asri MG, Schwentner C, et al. Algorithm for optimal urethral coverage in hypospadias and fistula repair: a systematic review. Eur Urol. 2016;70:293–8.

11. Savanelli A, Esposito C, Settimi A. A prospective randomized comparative study on the use of ventral subcutaneous flap to prevent fistulas in the Snodgrass repair for distal hypospadias. World J Urol. 2007;25:641–5.
12. Abbas TO, Salle JLP. When to graft the incised plate during TIP repair? A suggested algorithm that may help in the decision-making process. Front Pediatr. 2018;6:326. https://doi.org/10.3389/fped.2018.00326.
13. Khalil M, Gharib T, El-shaer W, Sebaey A, Elmohamady B, Elgamal K. Mathieu technique with incision of the urethral plate versus standard tubularised incised-plate urethroplasty in primary repair of distal hypospadias: a prospective randomized study. Arab J Urol. 2017;15:242. https://doi.org/10.1016/j.aju.2017.03.007.

Management of Penile Stricture After Hypospadias Repair

34

Pankaj M. Joshi, Tariq O. Abbas, and Sanjay B. Kulkarni

Abstract

Typically, a two-stage urethroplasty is used to treat complex penile strictures, such as post-hypospadias repair. The initial placement of a buccal mucosal graft (BMG) may result in a substantial contraction rate, necessitating revision surgery. We describe our experience and approach to the care of penile strictures associated with hypospadias.

Keywords

Hypospadias · Dorsal inlay · Buccal graft · Urethroplasty

34.1 Introduction

Hypospadias is one of the commonest congenital diseases and occurs in 1:150 boys born world over [1]. Many surgical procedures have been described as to repair hypospadias [2]. The overall success rate is approximately 85%. The reported incidence of urethral stricture after hypospadias surgery in the pediatric population is

Supplementary Information The online version contains supplementary material available at https://doi.org/10.1007/978-981-99-0795-3_34. The videos can be accessed individually by clicking the DOI link in the accompanying figure caption or by scanning this link with the SN More Media App.

P. M. Joshi (✉) · S. B. Kulkarni
UROKUL, Pune, India

T. O. Abbas
Urology Division, Surgery Department, Sidra Medicine, Doha, Qatar

T. O. Abbas (ed.), *Video Atlas of Hypospadias Surgery*,
https://doi.org/10.1007/978-981-99-0795-3_34

6.5% with short follow-up [3]. Independent of the original site of urethral reconstruction, more than 25% of all strictures found in adult patients treated for hypospadias as children are located in the bulbar region [4]. The patient then presents with poor urine flow and recurrent urinary tract infections. With hypospadias repair, urethral dilatation cannot address all urethral strictures; hence, recurrent dilatation is not indicated. If first dilatation fails, urethroscopy and imaging of the urinary system should be performed as soon as feasible to determine the severity of the stricture. Depending on the length of the stricture, both direct vision internal urethrotomy and urethral augment with buccal mucosa inlay are viable treatments [5]. We present our systematic approach to the management of penile stricture associated with hypospadias [6–8].

34.2 Indications

- Stricture seen on retrograde urethrogram.
- Associated hypospadias fistula or multiple fistulae (Fig. 34.1a).

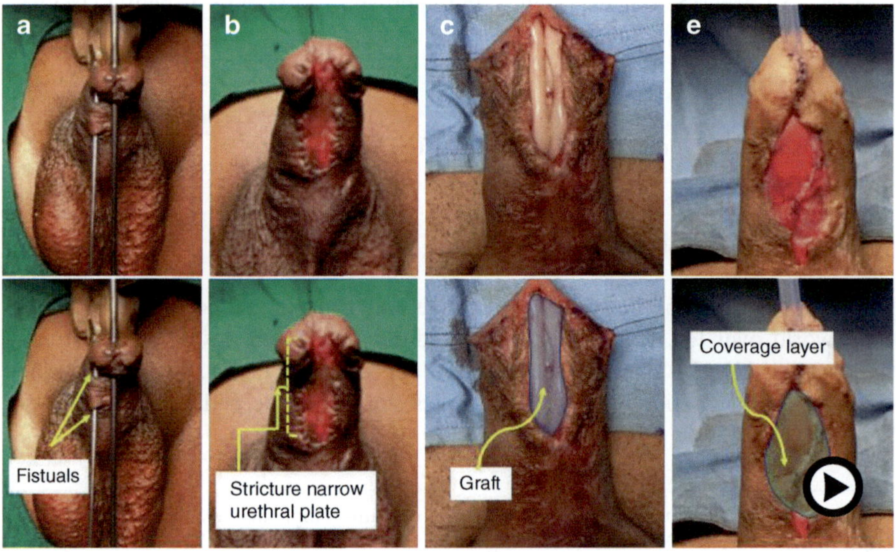

Fig. 34.1 Multiple urethrocutaneous fistulas (**a**) associated with urethral stricture. Stage I Johansons surgery performed (**b**) followed by dorsal inlay after 6 months (**c**) that is applied and a robust coverage layer is used (**d**). Management of penile stricture after hypospadias repair (https://doi.org/10.1007/000-cp0)

34.3 Video Demonstration

Factors	Findings
Age at surgery (months)	26
Gestational age (weeks)	Full term
Birth weight (gm)	2800
Gestational risks (e.g., maternal co-morbidities, IVF, Twin)	None
Family history	None
Testosterone (if yes, reason, and protocol used)	None
Any features of DSD (e.g., undescended testes)	None

34.4 Steps of the Procedure

We present three approaches to the management of penile urethral stricture after hypospadias repair. The decision is based on the size of the urethra as measured by urethrogram.

34.4.1 Approach 1 (Ventral Urethrotomy)

- Stay stich is taken on the glans.
- Urethra is incised ventrally across the stricture (Fig. 34.1b).
- The urethrotomy is performed till good 1 cm proximal urethra is seen.
- Measure the caliber of the native urethral plate.
- *If caliber is less than 8 mm,* then staged procedure is performed.
- The spongiosa is underrun with absorbable vicryl sutures.
- The urethral mucosa is sutured to the native skin.
- Silicone catheter is inserted.
- The catheter is removed after 48 h.
- The patient is assessed at 3 and 6 months.
- After 6 months, a midline incision is made in urethral plate, buccal graft is inserted as dorsal inlay and urethra tubularized (Fig. 34.1c). The advantage of using graft is second stage is it avoids graft contracture.

34.4.2 Approach 2 (Dorsal Inlay BMG Urethroplasty)

If urethral plate is >8 mm wide:

- An incision is made in urethral plate in midline.
- Dorsal inlay BMG urethroplasty is performed.

- Urethra is tubularized over a Silicone catheter.
- Skin is closed.
- Catheter is removed after 21 days.

34.4.3 Approach 3

This is a novel approach which is cosmetic and reduces the risk of fistula formation after urethroplasty.

- A semicircular incision is made at corona between 3 and 9 o'clock (Fig. 34.2).
- The skin is dissected below the dartos tissue on the ventral aspect of penis.
- The skin flap is then retracted down to expose the urethra.
- The urethra is incised ventrally, and width of urethral plate assessed.
- A dorsal inlay BMG urethroplasty is performed [9].
- The urethra is closed.
- The skip flap is sutured at original location.
- As there are no overlapping sutures, the risk of fistula formation is very minimal.

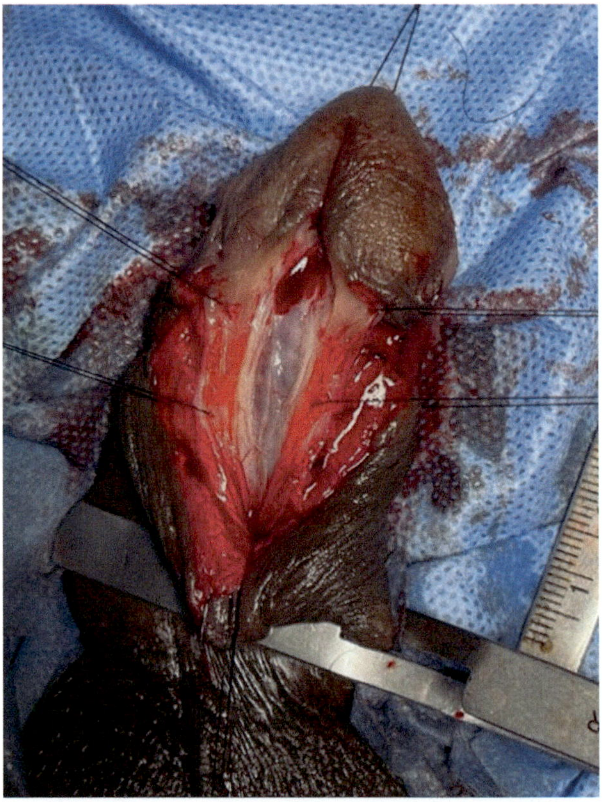

Fig. 34.2 Semicircular incision, skin flap reflected down. Urethra exposed and dorsal inlay BMG Urethroplasty is performed

34.5 Post-operative Care

- To keep the Coban dressing for 24 h.
- Antibiotic prophylaxis while the urethral catheter/stent in place.

34.6 Tips and Tricks

- In staged surgery spongiosa needs to be closed separately.
- Do not insert graft in first stage.

34.7 Results and Conclusion

In a group of 34 patients with urethral stricture following hypospadias treatment, the overall success rate was 75% (83% for one-stage repairs and 68% for multistage repairs). Those who required multistage repair plans were obviously at a greater risk of failure because of the severity of their strictures and the poor quality of their native tissue, compared to those on whom surgeons would risk a single-stage repair [10]. In patients with distal strictures, urethroplasty was considerably more successful than less invasive techniques (52% versus 12%, P = 0.02), although the success rates did not differ in patients with midshaft or proximal strictures [11].

References

1. Abbas T, McCarthy L. Foreskin and penile problems in childhood. Surg [Internet]. 2016;34(5):221–5.
2. Abbas TO, editor. Hypospadiology: current challenges and future perspectives. 2023. 190 p.
3. Duel BP, Barthold JS, Gonzalez R. Management of urethral strictures after hypospadias repair.—PubMed—NCBI. J Urol [Internet]. 1998;1(160):170–1.
4. Faraj S, Loubersac T, Bouchot O, Heloury Y, Leclair M-D. Adults with previous hypospadias surgery during childhood: beware of bulbar strictures. J Pediatr Urol [Internet]. 2022;18(1):4.e1–8.
5. Ye W, Ye M, Jiang X. How to treat urethral stricture after hypospadias repair. J Pediatr Urol [Internet]. 2020;16:S58.
6. Kulkarni SB, Joglekar O, Alkandari MH, Joshi PM. Redo hypospadias surgery: current and novel techniques. Res reports Urol [Internet]. 2018;10:117–26.
7. Shaw NM, Mallahan C, Joshi P, Venkatesan K, Kulkarni S. Novel use of Asopa technique for penile urethrocutaneous fistula repair. Int Urol Nephrol [Internet]. 2021;53(6):1127–33.
8. Joshi PM, Barbagli G, Batra V, Surana S, Hamouda A, Sansalone S, et al. A novel composite two-stage urethroplasty for complex penile strictures: a multicenter experience. Indian J Urol [Internet]. 2017;33(2):155–8.
9. Abbas TO, Pippi Salle JL. Dorsal Inlay TIP (DTIP). In: Hypospadias surgery [Internet]. 2022. p. 451–60.
10. Barbagli G, De Angelis M, Palminteri E, Lazzeri M. Failed hypospadias repair presenting in adults. Eur Urol [Internet] 2006;49(5):887–95.
11. Gargollo PC, Cai AW, Borer JG, Retik AB. Management of recurrent urethral strictures after hypospadias repair: is there a role for repeat dilation or endoscopic incision? J Pediatr Urol [Internet]. 2011;7(1):34–8.

Cecil Culp Procedure

35

Karl Godlewski and Christopher Long

Abstract

Every hypospadias surgery presents unique challenges to surgeons striving for a successful repair. As no two surgeries are completely alike there are numerous technical variations surgeons utilize to optimize outcomes. Paucity of skin and lack of vascularized tissue can be significant barriers for healing in re-operative but also primary hypospadias repairs. Wounds closed under tension can lead to poor capillary vascular flow resulting in skin breakdown and potentially breakdown of the entire repair. In this chapter, we discuss the Cecil Culp technique first described in the 1950s for proximal hypospadias cases (Cecil, J Urol 56(2):237–242, 1946). As with most procedures, the technique has evolved over time but remains a fairly simple solution for complex reconstruction in patients with a lack of ventral skin during closure. With time, indications for this technique have expanded beyond hypospadias surgery, within our institution we utilize it in select cases of chordee correction, circumcision injuries as well as degloving genital trauma cases (Weiss et al., Urology 106:196–199, 2017). The Cecil Culp technique is an excellent option to provide skin and soft tissue coverage in select cases of hypospadias and beyond.

Supplementary Information The online version contains supplementary material available at https://doi.org/10.1007/978-981-99-0795-3_35. The videos can be accessed individually by clicking the DOI link in the accompanying figure caption or by scanning this link with the SN More Media App.

K. Godlewski (✉) · C. Long
Children's Hospital of Philadelphia, Philadelphia, PA, USA
e-mail: godlewskk1@chop.edu; longc3@chop.edu

T. O. Abbas (ed.), *Video Atlas of Hypospadias Surgery*,
https://doi.org/10.1007/978-981-99-0795-3_35

Keywords

Hypospadias · Re-operative hypospadias · Ventral skin deficiency · Vascular coverage

35.1 Introduction

Cecil first described the repair in 1946 to provide skin coverage in hypospadias cases that were left with insufficient ventral shaft skin after constructing the neourethra [1]. He did this by making a scrotal incision that "mirrored" the area of deficient ventral penile skin and burying the penis into the open wound in the scrotum. In this first stage, he also created a perineal urethrostomy for urinary diversion. A second stage procedure would then follow approximately 6 weeks later, releasing the penis from the scrotum and leaving a strip of scrotal skin on the ventral shaft to relieve tension during shaft skin closure. Culp modified the technique from a two- to a three-stage hypospadias repair [2, 3]. The first stage involved chordee correction without urethroplasty, the second a urethroplasty and Cecil repair using a catheter for urinary diversion, and the third release of the penis from the scrotum. Currently, our practice is to wait at least 12 months before a release is performed to allow for optimal shaft skin expansion for a tension-free ventral shaft skin closure. Although the Cecil Culp repair can be used in the primary hypospadias setting, in more modern times at least and at our institution, its use has primarily been in redo or salvage hypospadias cases where skin is limited and adjacent tissue vascularity is in question. In this setting, multiple prior failed repairs and poor tissue quality, despite utilizing a Cecil procedure, complications such as fistulae, diverticulum, urethroplasty dehiscence, and stricture can occur; however, the rehabilitated ventral shaft tissue allows for great success in addressing these complications at the time of Cecil release [4].

35.2 Indications

35.2.1 Redo Hypospadias Repair

In patients with a history of multiple failed hypospadias repairs the quality of skin is often of poor, frequently requiring grafting prior to urethral reconstruction [5, 6]. Once urethroplasty has been completed, coverage over the repair can be challenging due to poorly vascularized or absent dartos tissue and less elastic skin, making robust coverage (waterproofing) layers and a tension-free closure problematic [7]. As mentioned previously, poor vascularization and tension put the entire repair at risk [8]. The Cecil-Culp procedure lessens these concerns in reoperative hypospadias repairs by transferring the well-vascularized bed of scrotal dartos to the penile shaft and utilizing the tension of the scrotal skin to increase the elasticity of the penile shaft skin to complete the closure [9]. Alternatively, in patients with multiple prior repairs and a relative lack of penile shaft skin, a Cecil at the time of the first stage repair can improve the vascularity of the ventral penile shaft and stretch the deficient penile shaft skin for closure at subsequent stages (Fig. 35.1).

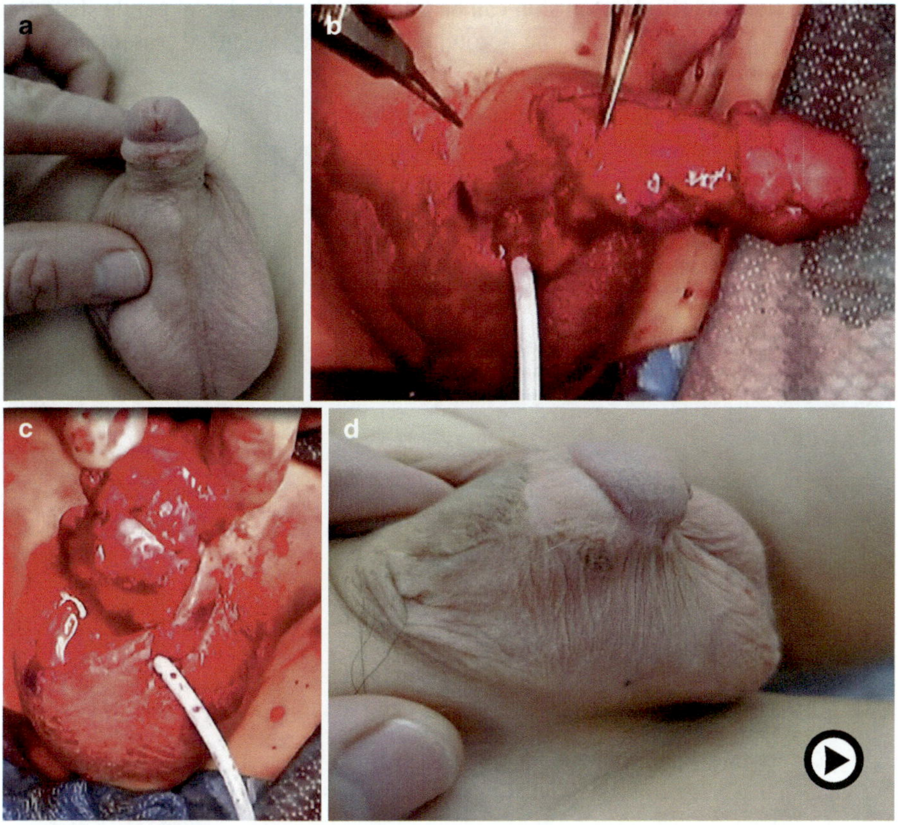

Fig. 35.1 9-year-old male with a history of a midshaft hypospadias corrected initially with a single-stage repair. He later developed recurrent chordee and a fistula requiring buccal mucosal grafting and dorsal plication. He began to develop urinary tract infections with flattening of his uroflow curve and elevated post-void residuals. Cystoscopy revealed a urethral stricture and he was found to have persistent chordee. He underwent a first-stage hypospadias repair (dermal patch corporal graft) with cut back of his neourethra to the penoscrotal junction and Cecil-Culp procedure. In this case the Cecil-culp procedure was utilized at the time of the first stage repair given the paucity of skin after chordee correction. (**a**) Initial appearance prior to first stage hypospadias repair with dermal patch graft—note the lack of any excess shaft skin. (**b**) Post chordee correction illustrating lack of ventral shaft skin available for coverage. (**c**) Urethral meatus matured to the penoscrotal junction and a lateral scrotal incision was made mimicking the defect on the penile shaft to bury the penis in the scrotum (**d**) 1 year post Cecil-Culp procedure with well-healed lateral suture line. Cecil Culp Procedure (https://doi.org/10.1007/000-cp1)

35.2.2 Non-Hypospadias Repair (Trauma)

The Cecil-Culp procedure can also be utilized in clinical scenarios other than hypospadias repair. It can be considered in any setting where there is deficiency of ventral shaft skin such as chordee secondary to hypoplastic ventral skin during circumcision, after resection of ventral scarring as in the case of lichen sclerosis or following trauma [10]. Ventral skin can be transferred to the dorsal penile shaft and the penis sutured down into the scrotum to provide enhanced vascularity and increase pliability of the shaft skin (Fig. 35.2).

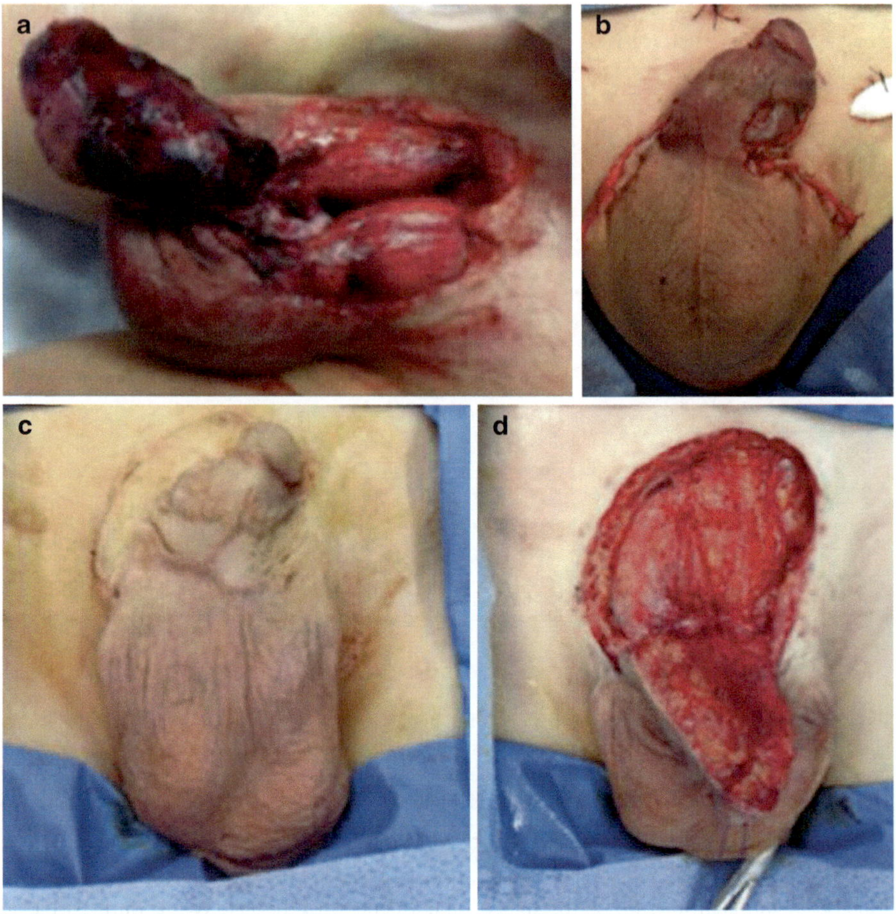

Fig. 35.2 This is a 12-year-old boy who sustained a close-range shotgun wound to the penis resulting in severe injuries to the dorsum of the penis. He was taken emergently to the operating room for exploration. He was found to be missing the proximal corporal bodies bilaterally to the level of the crus and thrombosed distal corpora. The decision was made to embed the dorsal shaft into the suprapubic area in a modified Cecil-Culp procedure to allow for sufficent tissue to reconstruct the penis in a delayed fashion. (**a**) Initial photo with intact ventral shaft skin and absent proximal corporal bodies. (**b**) The dorsum of the penis is embedded into the suprapubic fat. (**c**) Postoperative photo 8 months after initial surgery. (**d**) Release of the penis from the suprapubic fat. (**e**).Tubularized penile shaft. (**f**) Postoperative photo taken 5 years after release

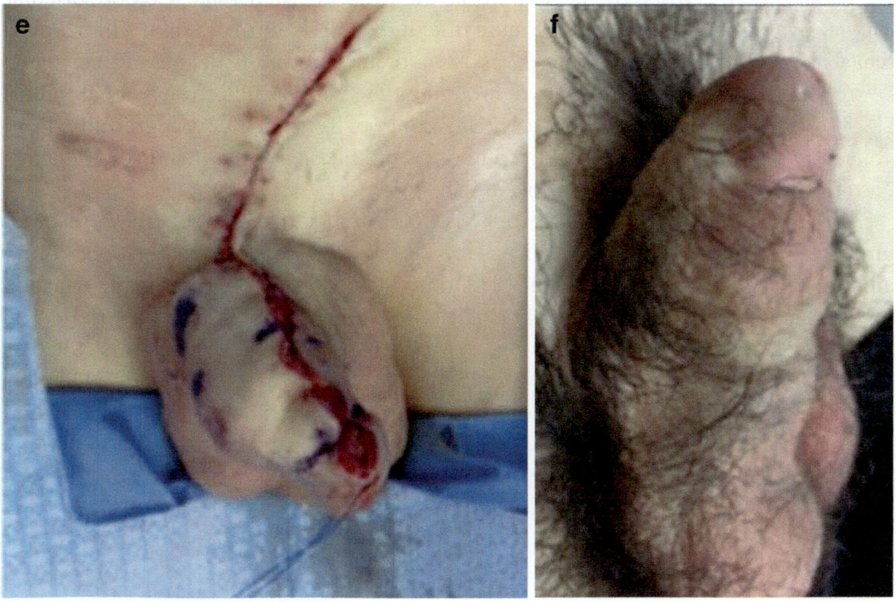

Fig. 35.2 (continued)

35.3 Video Presentation

35.4 Steps of the Procedure

35.4.1 Penile and Urethroplasty Reconstruction

- Complete the urethral reconstruction with available ventral skin, graft as needed to augment urethra.
  - Urinary diversion with urethral catheter
  - Consider suprapubic catheter placement
- Begin shaft skin reconstruction dorsally suturing the shaft skin to the preputial collar in a simple interrupted fashion using 5-0 Monocryl
  - If insufficient skin to cover dorsally make relaxing incisions at the level of the penoscrotal junction of ventral shaft skin to gain mobility
- If ventral shaft skin can be approximated either proximally or distally without tension close in two layers (4-0 or 5-0 Monocryl based on age)
- If possible approximate the ventral preputial collar distally with simple interrupted 5-0 Monocryl (Fig. 35.3)

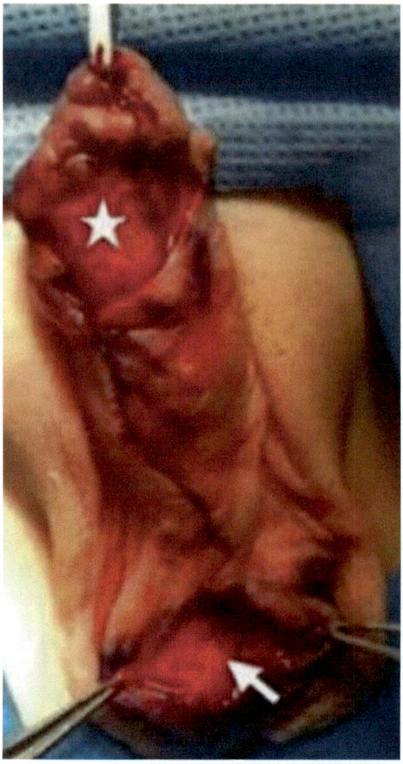

Fig. 35.3 Ventral shaft defect marked with star, scrotal incision marked with white arrow. Note proximal ventral shaft skin has been partially closed.

35.4.2 Scrotal Incision

- Measure distance between penoscrotal junction and proximal aspect of ventral skin defect if applicable
- Mark this measurement on the scrotum measuring from the penoscrotal junction
- Measure the length of the ventral shaft defect and again mark on scrotum
- Make a vertical incision between these two marks deepening the incision such that the scrotal defect width is similar to the shaft skin defect

35.4.3 Embedding Penis into Scrotum

- Begin proximally (if hinge point is present proximally) and suture the proximal aspect of ventral shaft defect to superior edge of scrotal incision
  - Interrupted 5-0 Monocryl or 4-0 Monocryl for older children
  - Ideally done in two layers—dartos and skin for added reinforcement to prevent separation with erections. Particular attention should be placed on the distal aspect of the closure, where the maximal amount of pressure tends to occur, especially with erections. This is an area that has a higher risk of dehiscence

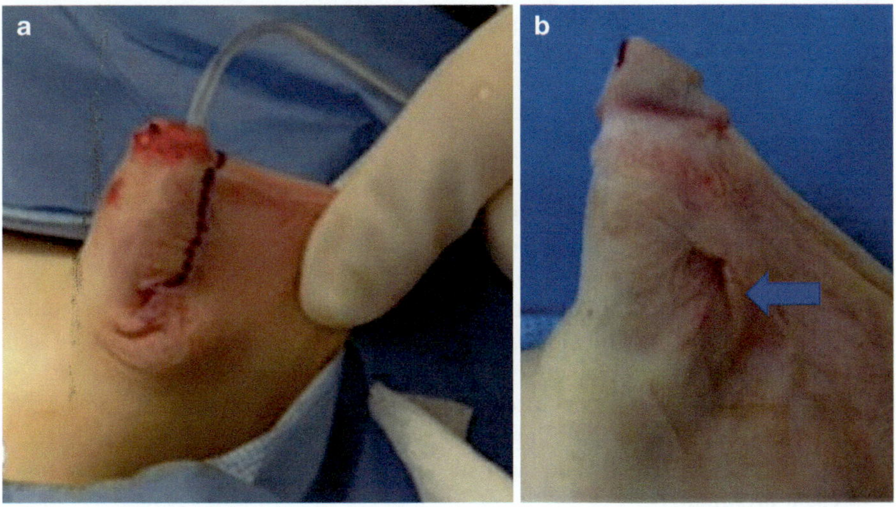

Fig. 35.4 (**a**) Marking indicating suture line of shaft skin to scrotum– pinch skin edges to ensure lateral shaft skin can be closed without tension prior to incision. (**b**) Hinge point (blue arrow) that should be identified and re-established at the time of penile release

  - If proximal shaft skin is closed and penis is hinged over this, leave ¼ inch penrose at this hinge point for 5–7 days postoperatively (Fig. 35.4)
- Complete closure circumferentially
- *Leave penis embedded for 1 year to allow for maximal dorsal shaft skin expansion and to prevent transfer of hair bearing scrotal skin to the penile shaft*

35.4.4 Release of Penis

- Mark suture line of scrotum and shaft skin
- Pinch to ensure ventral skin will approximate tension free before incision
- If penis was hinged at penoscrotal junction attempt to clearly identify hinge point and place vessel loop through this to facilitate retraction and visibility
- Place a urethral catheter during dissection to prevent harm to urethra
- Incise skin and separate scrotal dartos from penile shaft
  - Err towards undermining scrotal skin leaving more dartos on penile shaft
- Close scrotal and shaft defects in two layers
  - Interrupted horizontal mattress 5-0 Monocryl on shaft skin

35.5 Postoperative Care

- Apply Vaseline to suture lines for 3 weeks with each diaper change or 4–5× daily if potty trained

- Penrose removal 5–7 days postoperatively
- Urethral catheter removed in 10–14 days

35.6 Tips and Tricks

- Close proximal ventral shaft skin or distal preputial collar, if possible, to create a gap between urethral closure and scrotal anastomosis
  - Leave ¼ inch penrose drain if hinge point is created (Fig. 35.4)
- Measure the ventral shaft defect and create a mirrored incision in the scrotum
  - Typically in the midline but can be off center if asymmetric dorsal shaft skin or as in Fig. 35.2 where urethral meatus needs to be matured.
- Ideally perform a two-layer closure (dartos and skin) of lateral shaft skin to scrotum to prevent separation during erections
- Begin closure proximally and move distally for better visualization if hinge point present proximally
- Consider placing suprapubic catheter for additional urinary drainage
- **Keep penis embedded in scrotum for at least 1 year**
- During release pinch lateral shaft skin in midline to ensure closure without tension is possible before making incision
- Err toward undermining scrotal skin when releasing penile shaft

35.7 Conclusion

Z-plasties, rotational flaps, tissue expanders, transferred dorsal island flaps and grafts can all be utilized to overcome shaft skin deficiency during hypospadias repair [11–15]. At our institution the Cecil Culp procedure is a proven, effective, and reproducible means of dealing with paucity of skin during redo hypospadias repair, primary hypospadias repair, and in the trauma setting. In 2017 we published our series of 39 failed hypospadias repairs of which 23 underwent a Cecil Culp repair. Seven of these patients developed complications despite the Cecil, however most were successfully addressed at the time of penile release from the scrotum likely a direct effect of the robust vascularized tissue present for coverage. As surgery evolves this long-standing technique has endured the test of time and remains an invaluable technique for select reconstructive cases.

References

1. Cecil AB. Repair of hypospadias and urethral fistula. J Urol. 1946;56(2):237–42. https://doi.org/10.1016/S0022-5347(17)69802-1.
2. Culp OS. Early correction of congenital chordee and hypospadias. J Urol. 1951;65(2):264–78. https://doi.org/10.1016/S0022-5347(17)68481-7.
3. Culp OS. Struggles and triumphs with hypospadias and associated anomalies: review of 400 cases. J Urol. 1966;96(3):339–51. https://doi.org/10.1016/S0022-5347(17)63266-X.

4. Weiss DA, Long CJ, Frazier JR, Shukla AR, Srinivasan AK, Kolon TF, DiCarlo H, Gearhart JP, Canning DA. Back to the future: the Cecil-Culp technique for salvage penile reconstructive procedures. J Pediatr Urol. 2018;14(4):328.e1–7. https://doi.org/10.1016/j.jpurol.2018.04.026. Epub 2018 May 30.
5. Duckett JW, Coplen D, Ewalt D, Baskin LS. Buccal mucosal urethral replacement. J Urol. 1995;153(5):1660–3.
6. Metro MJ, Wu HY, Snyder HM, Zderic SA, Canning DA. Buccal mucosal grafts: lessons learned from an 8-year experience. J Urol. 2001;166(4):1459–61.
7. Choudhury P, Saroya KK, Jain V, Yadav DK, Dhua AK, Anand S, Mawar S, Verma V, Kapahtia S, Acharya SK, Shah R, Bajpai M, Goel P. 'Waterproofing layers' for urethrocutaneous fistula repair after hypospadias surgery: evidence synthesis with systematic review and meta-analysis. Pediatr Surg Int. 2023;39(1):165. https://doi.org/10.1007/s00383-023-05405-1.
8. Amukele SA, Stock JA, Hanna MK. Management and outcome of complex hypospadias repairs. J Urol. 2005;174:1540.
9. Ehle JJ, Cooper CS, Peche WJ, Hawtrey CE. Application of the Cecil-Culp repair for treatment of urethrocutaneous fistulas after hypospadias surgery. Urology. 2001;57(2):347–50. https://doi.org/10.1016/s0090-4295(00)00997-3.
10. Weiss DA, Smith ZL, Taylor JA, Canning DA. Old tools, old problems, new solution: the use of a modified Cecil-Culp concept in the trauma setting. Urology. 2017;106:196–9. https://doi.org/10.1016/j.urology.2017.04.023. Epub 2017 Apr 25. PMID: 28454986.
11. Fam MM, Hanna MK. Resurfacing the penis of complex hypospadias repair ("hypospadias cripples"). J Urol. 2017;197(3 Pt 2):859–64. https://doi.org/10.1016/j.juro.2016.09.075. Epub 2017 Jan 26.
12. Mendez-Fernandez MA, Hollan C, Frank DH, Fisher JC. The scrotal myocutaneous flap. Plast Reconstr Surg. 1986;78(5):676–8. https://doi.org/10.1097/00006534-198611000-00020.
13. Castañares S, Belt E. Surgical reconstruction of the penis in skin losses, using scrotum skin. Br J Plast Surg. 1968;21(3):253–7. https://doi.org/10.1016/s0007-1226(68)80032-3.
14. Zöllner AM, Buganza Tepole A, Gosain AK, Kuhl E. Growing skin: tissue expansion in pediatric forehead reconstruction. Biomech Model Mechanobiol. 2012;11(6):855–67. https://doi.org/10.1007/s10237-011-0357-4. Epub 2011 Nov 4. PMID: 22052000; PMCID: PMC3425448.
15. Zhuo Q, Li S, Wu J, Wang Z, Yang D, Tao L. Clinical application of scrotal flap on penis lengthening. Saudi Med J. 2009;30(3):418–21.

Part VIII

Miscellaneous Procedures

Foreskin Reconstruction in Hypospadias Cases

36

Fernando Jose Gonzalez Ledon, Omar Sanchez Alvarez, and Byron Pacheco

Abstract

Hypospadias correction aims to enhance psychosocial and psychosexual adaptation in affected children, emphasizing the importance of achieving a natural penile appearance. Righini's pioneering work on foreskin reconstruction and preservation (FRP) in hypospadias surgery underscores the multifaceted role of the foreskin beyond cosmetic concerns, acknowledging its potential sexual and immunological functions. While circumcision carries risks, FRP has been successfully employed in hypospadias repair, with studies reporting favorable outcomes and minimal complications. Despite inherent risks such as postoperative phimosis, FRP presents a viable option supported by various authors for its reproducibility and satisfactory results.

Supplementary Information The online version contains supplementary material available at https://doi.org/10.1007/978-981-99-0795-3_36. The videos can be accessed individually by clicking the DOI link in the accompanying figure caption or by scanning this link with the SN More Media App.

F. J. G. Ledon (✉)
Children's Hospital of Mexico "Federico Gomez", Mexico City, Mexico

Pediatric Urology, Universidad Autonoma de Mexico, Mexico City, Mexico
e-mail: doctorfer@uroped.com

O. S. Alvarez
Pediatric Urologist Hospital Civil de Guadalajara "Fray Antonio Alcalde", Guadalajara, Jalisco, Mexico

B. Pacheco
Hospital de Especialidades Portoviejo-Ecuador, Portoviejo, Ecuador

Universidad de Guayaquil-Ecuador, Guayaquil, Ecuador

T. O. Abbas (ed.), *Video Atlas of Hypospadias Surgery*,
https://doi.org/10.1007/978-981-99-0795-3_36

Keywords

Hypospadias correction · Foreskin preservation · Psychosocial adaptation Surgical outcomes

Key Points

- It should be used in hypospadias with adequate foreskin in size and symmetry.
- The reconstructed foreskin should be fully retracted postoperatively.
- Foreskin preservation (FRP) is possible in glanular, subcoronal, and some distal penile hypospadias cases, although having adequate skin, it could be done in other more complex cases.
- Foreskin preservation in hypospadias is an extra intervention within the correction, it is important to discuss the risk of complications with the child's parents.

36.1 Introduction

The main objective in hypospadias correction is to improve the future psychosocial and psychosexual adaptation of surgically treated children. This involves getting an as natural as possible penile appearance; with this principle, Righini [1] described the reconstruction and preservation of the foreskin (FRP) in hypospadias surgery [1]. It is important to consider that the FRP is not just a matter of cosmetic results. Whether or not we agree with the functions of the foreskin, there is no doubt that mammals have had a foreskin for over sixty million years, so it does not appear to be just excess skin left over during hypospadias correction, but rather, the aim is to maintain the previously reported natural functions of the foreskin, such as sexual and immunological ones [2, 3].

Circumcision is not free of complications. For example, Fink et al. [4], in a descriptive cross-sectional study of 123 circumcisions, reported worsening of erectile function ($p = 0.01$) [4]. FRP has been described in patients with phimosis, traumatic injuries, and penile cancer, as Haseebuddin et al. have reported [5]. In hypospadias, Leclair et al. [6], and Castagnetti et al. [7], among others, have reported prepuce preservation without major complications [6, 7].

Pradyumna et al. [8] carried out a prospective cohort of 80 patients in distal hypospadias and some penile hypospadias, comparing preservation of the foreskin against circumcision, where the main outcome was complications (they did not measure post-preservation phimosis), without finding significant differences in both groups in complications such as fistulas, strictures or dehiscences ($p > 0.05$) [8]. Snodgrass et al. [9], in a prospective cohort, comparing circumcision (343 patients) against preputioplasty (85 patients), where complications were the main outcome; found no statistically significant differences in more than 5 years of follow-up ($p = 1$) [9].

In another context, the functional and cosmetic results of FRP have been evaluated in hypospadias [10]. Fasching et al. [11] conducted an analytical cross-sectional study of 64 children, 33 of whom underwent foreskin preservation. They were assessed with The Hypospadias Objective Scoring Evaluation (HOSE), Pediatric Penile Perception Score (PPPS), and uroflowmetry, without finding statistical significance in both groups ($p = 0.012$) [11].

Just like any other surgery, the reconstruction and preservation of the foreskin (FRP) presents complications inherent to the prepuce, such as dehiscences and post-operative phimosis, the latter being the most frequent [6, 12]. Leclair et al. [6] reported 316 foreskin reconstructions in which 18 children (6%) presented partial or total dehiscence. In this same study, 40 cases (12%) of phimosis were reported after foreskin reconstruction and preservation, of which 30 received 0.1% betamethasone, which resolved the phimosis in 26 cases [6].

Our goal is not to try to convince whether or not to preserve the foreskin in hypospadias repair, but rather to consider it as an option in hypospadias correction as various authors have described such as Klijn et al. [13], Rampersad et al. [14], and Özer et al. [15], among others; since it is a reproducible procedure, with adequate cosmetic results and with minimal complications [6–15].

36.2 Indications

- Distal hypospadias.
- Penile hypospadias that can be corrected in a single step.
- The hypospadias correction technique should not influence the foreskin preservation unless a technique that requires extra foreskin for correction is used, such as Matthiew.

36.3 Steps of the Procedure

- Delimit cut sites, with Firlit's principle [16], measure that the circumferential distance of the closed foreskin is wide enough to slide the foreskin over the glans (Fig. 36.1).
- Infiltration with epinephrine 1:100,000
- Incision of delimited sites, with cold cutting (scissors or scalpel) of the lateral edges that will be the midline (Fig. 36.2)
- Exposure of the entire wound to assess closure of the preserved foreskin and penile midline over the shaft of the penis (Fig. 36.3)
- Foreskin midline suture separating the internal (Fig. 36.4) and external face
- One or two internal skin planes closure, with 6–0 or 7–0 polydiaxonone. We prefer to make subcuticular stitches so that we don't lose length in the circumferential closure, one plane per face.
- Midline suture in the outer face of the foreskin, one plane, with simple or continuous 6–0 or 7–0 polydiaxonone.
- Check that the foreskin is completely retracted after its reconstruction (Fig. 36.5).

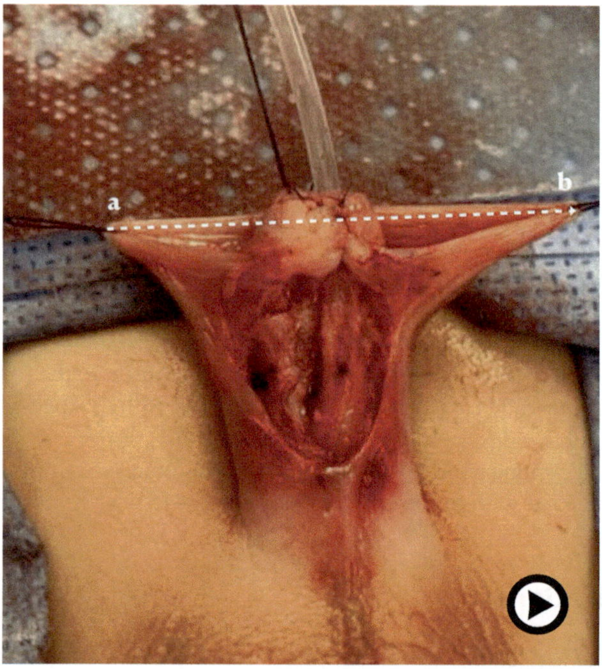

Fig. 36.1 It is important to evaluate the total length of the skin to be closed; the distance from point a to point b must be of a sufficient circumference to allow the foreskin to slide over the glans. Foreskin reconstruction in hypospadias cases (https://doi.org/10.1007/000-cp2)

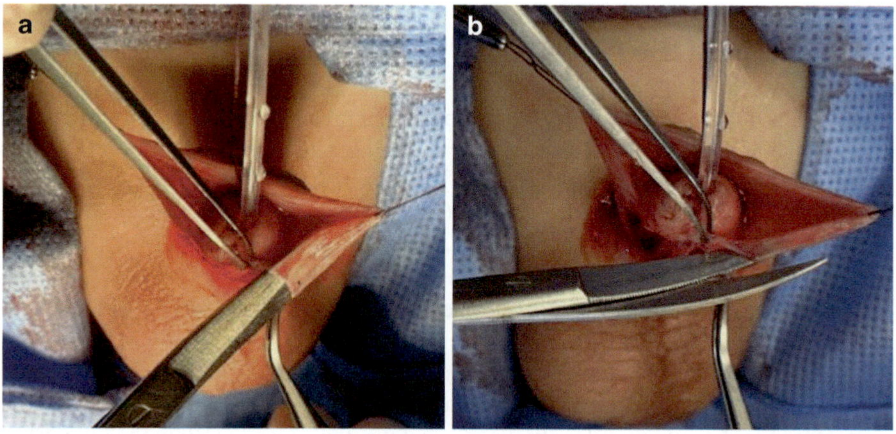

Fig. 36.2 Foreskin lateral edge cut, (**a**) blunt separation between the internal and external skin planes, (**b**) longitudinal cut between the lateral traction point that will be the midline separating internal and external skin

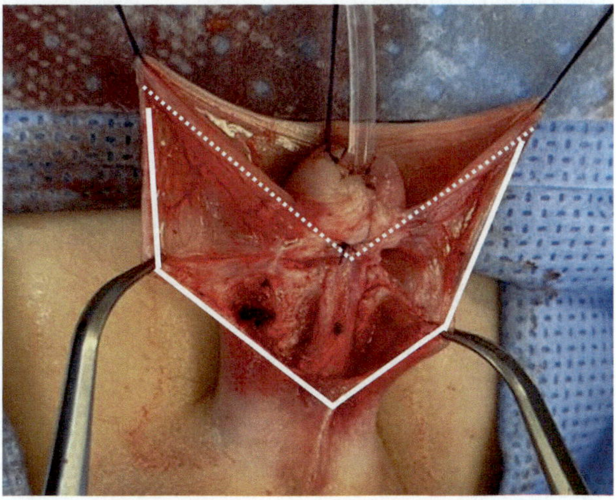

Fig. 36.3 Foreskin in its maximum extension prior to midline closure, dotted line is the edge of the inner face, continuous line outer skin prepuce distal segment and midline of the shaft of the penis proximal segment

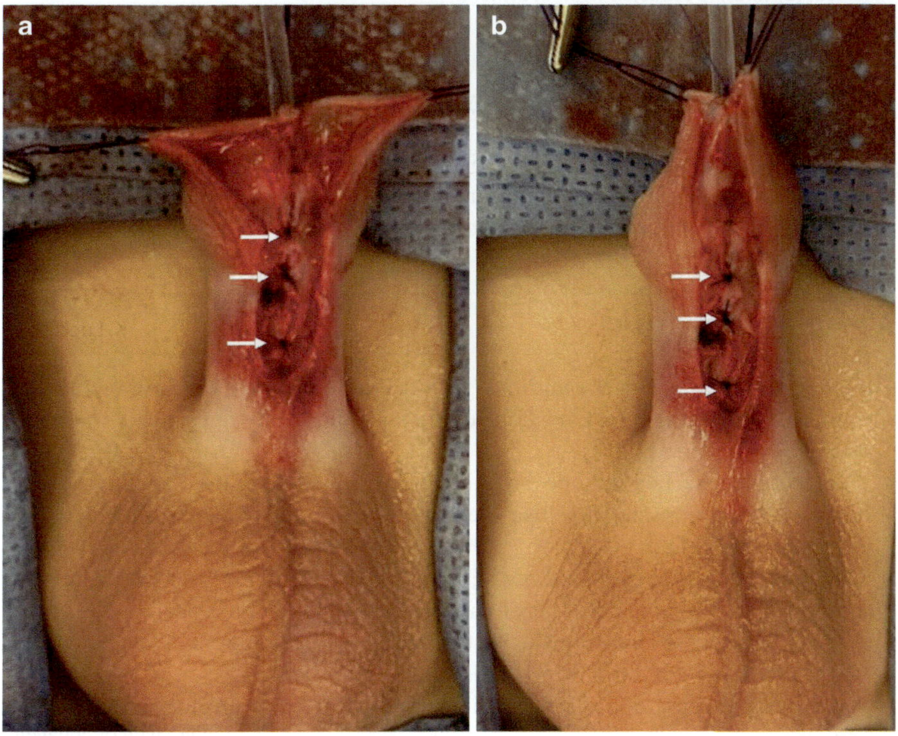

Fig. 36.4 (**a**) Partial proximal closure of the internal face of the prepuce, (**b**) close-up continuous complete closure with 6–0 subcuticular suture, arrows reinforcement points with 6–0 pds of darts on the groove and subcoronal urethra, do not reinforce on the free skin of the foreskin (distal)

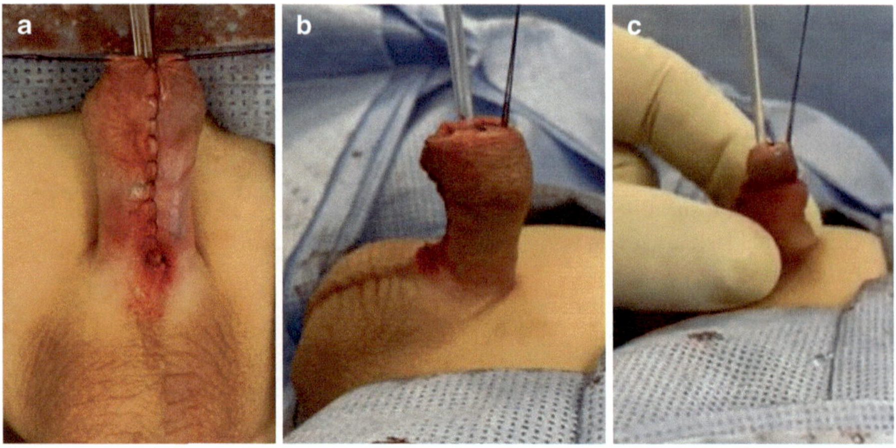

Fig. 36.5 Final view (**a**) complete closure of the ventral face with continuous suture anchored 6–0, (**b**) lateral view where absence of cord and symmetry of the ventral and dorsal skin can be observed, (**c**) foreskin retracted without difficulty

- Sometimes the skin is not completely symmetrical, so the stitches can be distributed to leave a symmetrical closure.
- If the dorsal skin is longer and cannot close the ventral midline, a midline cut can be made with the Byars principle, making sure we leave a symmetrical ventral dorsal cylinder shape (see the case in video).

36.4 Tips and Tricks

- Join foreskin angles in the midline (with dissecting forceps), before reconstruction, to define if the foreskin can be easily and completely retracted at the end of the FRP.
- Polypropylene or polydaxone 5–0 stitches at each angle of the foreskin to facilitate reconstruction and not lose the anatomy and the objective of length and width of the cylinder.
- The inner face stitches should not be very deep and preferably subcuticular so as not to lose skin that is necessary to achieve a wide circumference.
- When placing the dressing, leave the penis with the foreskin extended, not retracted.
- Do not force retraction after dressing removal, usually until 2–3 weeks after surgery.
- In case of having some phimosis, leave a 0.1% mometasone scheme.
- Hypospadias follow-up should not be different from cases without preservation and depends on each surgeon

36.5 Results and Conclusion

In our 5 years experience, we have performed FPR in 41 patients (22 glandular, 11 coronal, and 8 subcoronal). Seven patients (17%) had complications inherent to preservation, 2 total dehiscences, 3 partial dehiscences (fistula), and 2 phimosis. of which a phimosis also had a foreskin fistula. The complications were resolved with 4 representations and 3 with circumcisions (two of them because there was not enough skin to preserve the foreskin and the last one due to the parent's desire to have a circumcision performed).

It is clear to us that the FRP can be offered in duly selected distal hypospadias and penile hypospadias. Complications occur in about 8%. To prevent subsequent surgeries it is imperative that the foreskin retracts completely and easily at the end of the surgery. Making it clear that if the appearance is not as natural as possible, it is better for patients than not having a foreskin in many cases.

References

1. Righini A. Symposium sur l'hypospadias. Ann Chir Infant. 1969;10:314.
2. Nayyar C, Chander R, Gupta P, Sherwal B. Co-infection of human immunodeficiency virus and sexually transmitted infections in circumcised and uncircumcised cases in India. Indian J Sex Transm Dis. 2014;35:114–7.
3. Gebremedhin S. Assessment of the protective effect of male circumcision from HIV infection and sexually transmitted diseases: evidence from 18 demographic and health surveys in Sub-Saharan Africa. East Afr J Public Health. 2010;7:295–9.
4. Fink K, Carson C, DeVellis R. Adult circumcision outcomes study: effect on erectile function, penile sensitivity, sexual activity and satisfaction. J Urol. 2002;167:2113–6. PMID: 11956453.
5. Haseebuddin M, Brandes S. The prepuce: preservation and reconstruction. Curr Opin Urol. 2008;18:575–82. https://doi.org/10.1097/MOU.0b013e32831 1c9c2.
6. Leclair M, Benyoucef N, Héloury Y. La reconstruction du prépuce dans la chirurgie d'hypospade distal: quelle morbidité? Prog Urol. 2008;18:475–9. https://doi.org/10.1016/j.purol.2008.03.019.
7. Castagnetti M, Bagnara V, Rigamonti W, Cimador M, Esposito C. Preputial reconstruction in hypospadias repair. J Pediatr Urol. 2017;13:102–9. https://doi.org/10.1016/j.jpurol.2016.07.018.
8. Pradyumna P. A prospective study comparing modified foreskin reconstruction versus circumcision with tubularized incised plate urethroplasty for distal and mid penile hypospadias. J Pedatr Urol. 2020;16:674.e1–7. https://doi.org/10.1016/j.jpurol.2020.07.040.
9. Snodgrass W, Dajusta D, Villanueva C, Bush N. Foreskin reconstruction does not icrease urethroplasty or skin complications after distal TIP hypospadias repair. J Pediatr Urol. 2013;9:401–6. https://doi.org/10.1016/j.jpurol.2012.06.008.
10. Esposito C, Savanelli A, Escolino M, et al. Preputioplasty associated with urethroplasty for correction of distal hypospadias: a prospective study and proposition of a new objective scoring system for evaluation of esthetic and functional outcome. J Pediatr Urol. 2014;10:294–09. https://doi.org/10.1016/j.jpurol.2013.09.003.
11. Fasching G, Arneitz C, Gritsch-Olipp G. Foreskin reconstruction and preservation of a thin distal urethra: a challenge in tubularized incised plate urethroplasty. Pediatr Surg Int. 2011;27:755–60. https://doi.org/10.1007/s00383-011-2891-7.
12. Shoor G, Sugandhi N, Acharya S, et al. Outcomes of preputioplasty in patients undergoing TIP urethroplasty (tubularization of incised urethral plate) for distal and mid penile hypospadias.

J Pediatr Urol. 2020;16(319):e1–319.e7. https://doi.org/10.1016/j.jpurol.2020.04.014. Epub 2020 Apr 21.
13. Klijn A, Dik P, De Jong T. Results of preputial reconstruction in 77 boys with distal hypospadias. J Urol. 2001;165:1255–7. PMID: 11257696.
14. Rampersad R, Nyo Y, Hutson J, O'Brien M, Heloury Y. Foreskin reconstruction vs circumcision in distal hypospadias. Pediatr Surg Int. 2017;33:1131–7. https://doi.org/10.1007/s00383-017-4151-y.
15. Özer M, Timmermans F. An insight into circumcised men seeking foreskin reconstruction: a prospective cohort study. Int J Impot Res. 2020;32:611–6. https://doi.org/10.1038/s41443-019-0223-y.
16. Firlit C. The mucosal collar in hypospadias surgery. J Urol. 1987;137:80–2. https://doi.org/10.1016/s0022-5347(17)43878-x.

Preputioplasty in Hypospadias Surgery

37

Massimo Garriboli, Azad Mathur, and Hazem Mosa

Abstract

Hypospadias repair seeks to restore normal penile anatomy, yet cultural and religious factors influence perceptions of normality. In regions where circumcision is less prevalent, preputioplasty has become a routine component of primary hypospadias repair, especially when parents prioritize foreskin preservation. This video book chapter illustrates our approach for prepucioplasty in hypospadias cases.

Keywords

Penile anatomy, Circumcision, hypospadias, Foreskin preservation

Key Points

- Preputioplasty is an essential part of a true anatomical penile reconstruction.
- Preputioplasty is technically simple and does not increase operative time.
- Preputioplasty does not increase the risk of urethral/skin complications and reoperation.

Supplementary Information The online version contains supplementary material available at https://doi.org/10.1007/978-981-99-0795-3_37. The videos can be accessed individually by clicking the DOI link in the accompanying figure caption or by scanning this link with the SN More Media App.

M. Garriboli (✉)
Evelina London Children's Hospital, St Thomas' Hospital, London, UK
e-mail: massimo.garriboli@gstt.nhs.uk

A. Mathur · H. Mosa
Addenbrookes Hospital, Cambridge, UK
e-mail: azad.mathur@nnuh.nhs.uk

T. O. Abbas (ed.), *Video Atlas of Hypospadias Surgery*,
https://doi.org/10.1007/978-981-99-0795-3_37

37.1 Introduction

The aim of hypospadias repair is restoration of normal penile anatomy. However, religion and culture play an important role in defining what is normal. In European and Latin countries, most of the population is uncircumcised [1] while in Muslim countries and the United States circumcision of new-borns is widely practiced [2]. Righini first reported preputioplasty at the time of primary hypospadias repair in 1969 [3] and, since then, the technique has been adopted by many surgeons. Preputioplasty is currently offered as routine part of hypospadias repair by many, particularly if parents favour foreskin preservation [4, 5].

37.2 Indications

1. Distal hypospadias: preputioplasty can be routinely offered.

   During the preoperative counselling, parents are asked whether, regardless of the presence of hypospadias, they would have had their son circumcised for any reason (e.g., culture, religion). If the answer is no, a foreskin reconstruction can be offered as a standard part of the procedure of primary single-stage hypospadias repair.
2. Proximal hypospadias: recommended in only selected cases with less than 30 degrees of curvature after ventral degloving.

37.3 Contraindications

1. Monk-hood deformity of the foreskin: reconstructing this type of foreskin results in a suboptimal cosmetic outcome as dorsal bulky whorls of skin persist despite a successful reconstruction [6].
2. Severe curvature (>30 degrees) after ventral degloving: in this cases a preputial skin graft is needed for a 2-stage repair. In rare cases, when parents insist on foreskin preservation, a buccal mucosal graft can be used for the urethral reconstruction to allow the prepuce to be reconstructed.

37.4 Steps of the Procedure

1. A 5–0 Prolene glans is placed as stay suture and ×2 6–0 polydioxanone (PDS) stay sutures are used at the distal end of the hooded foreskin, one on each side.
2. By bringing the edges of the foreskin together using a fine-toothed forceps we can test if the foreskin can be easily retracted to allow the glans to emerge fully through the proposed preputial opening. If this appears too tight, reposition the stays more proximally until a wide enough opening can be achieved (Fig. 37.1). Alternatively, a dorsal preputial release incision (DPRI) can be considered.
3. Make a ventral incision along the visible junction between the inner preputial mucosa and the outer preputial skin starting from the stays and extending below

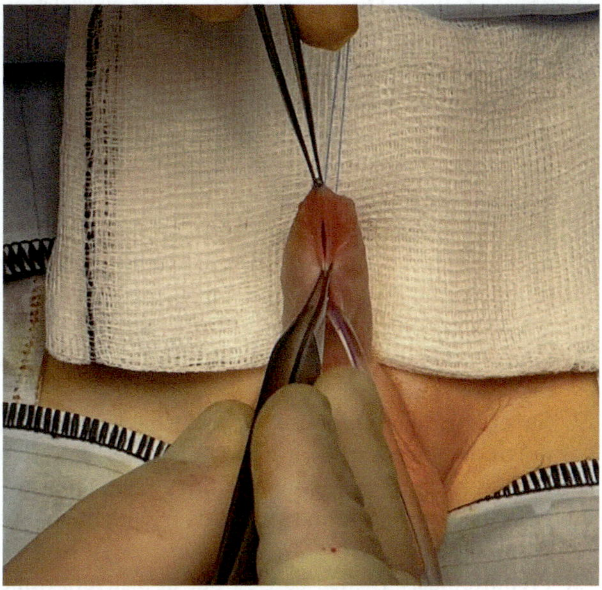

Fig. 37.1 Testing the prepuce retractability to decide the position of stays

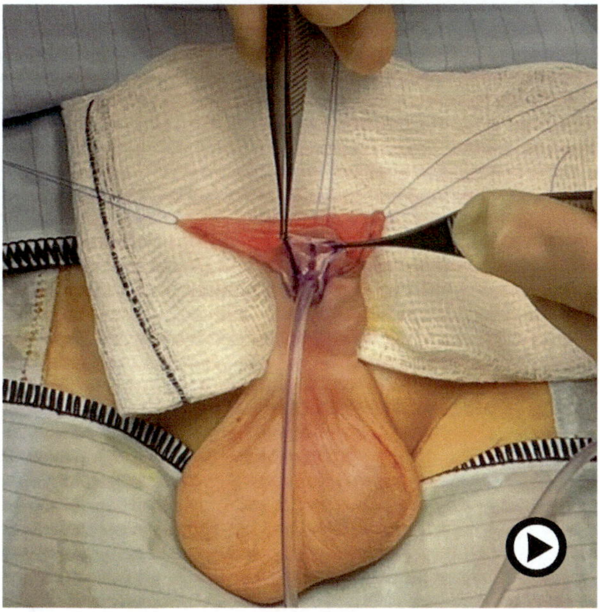

Fig. 37.2 Markings for ventral incisions. Preputioplasty in hypospadias surgery (https://doi.org/10.1007/000-cp3)

the meatus making sure your incision is at least 2 mm away from the glans to allow enough tissue for a tension-free closure of inner preputial mucosa (Fig. 37.2).

4. This is followed by ventral degloving down to the penoscrotal junction.
5. Perform an artificial erection test to confirm straightness of the penis using a 21 G butterfly needle injecting normal saline into the glans with a tourniquet applied at the penoscrotal junction.
6. A small finger goniometer or smartphone app goniometry can be used to assess the angle of curvature. If the penis is straight or <30 degrees of curvature is noted, a single-stage repair can be safely carried out.
7. Dorsal midline plications (Baskin or Yachia) are used to correct curvature <30 degrees. The ventral dissection is extended laterally around the corporal bodies to access the dorsal midline for placement of dorsal midline plication sutures without making an incision in the dorsal prepuce.
8. Glans wings are then developed, and a deep incision of the urethral plate is made down to the corpora.
9. Subepithelial urethroplasty is performed in 1 or 2 layers with a continuous 7–0 polydioxanone for the first layer and interrupted sutures for the second layer.
10. Urethroplasty is then covered with a ventral dartos "waterproof" layer.
11. Glansplasty is performed in 2 layers with subepithelial 6/0 polydioxanone and 5/0 polyglactin.
12. Preputioplasty is then carried out in 3 layers (inner prepuce, dartos and skin) with interrupted 6/0 polydioxanone (Figs. 37.3 and 37.4).

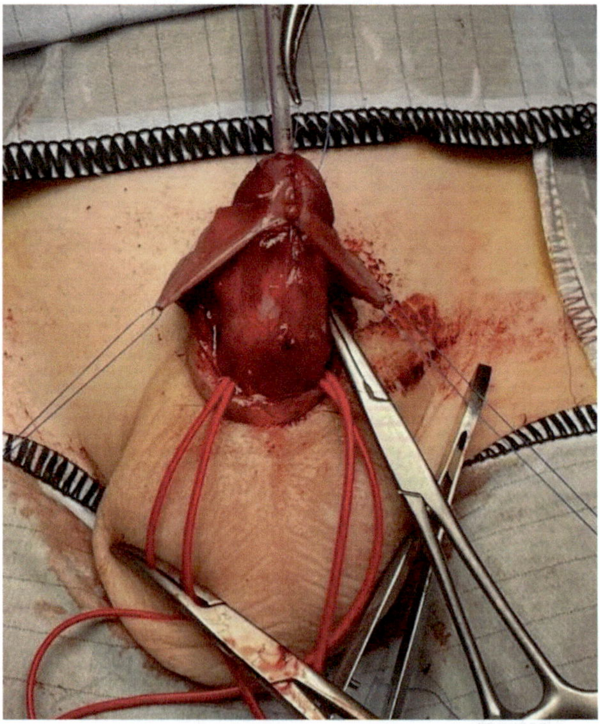

Fig. 37.3 Appearance after ventral degloving, urethroplasty, and glansplasty

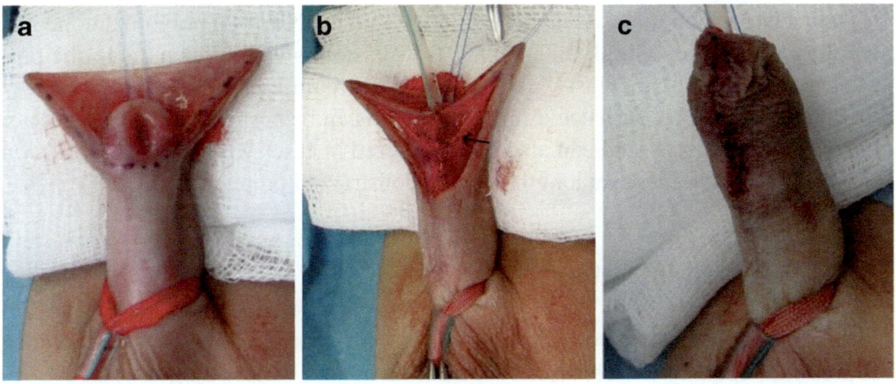

Fig. 37.4: Three layers of prepuce closure: (**a**) inner mucosa, (**b**) dartos, (**c**) outer skin

13. For curvature >30 degrees, we would not recommend performing a preputioplasty. If foreskin preservation is requested by parents, a buccal mucosal graft can be used to reconstruct the urethra.
14. An absorbent and (gently) compressive dressing and a 6 Fr. or 8 Fr. feeding tube catheter are kept for approximately 7 days (this may not be necessary in case preputioplasty is performed without urethroplasty).
15. Parents are instructed to instil antibiotic ointment inside the reconstructed prepuce for 2 weeks after dressing removal in order to prevent recurrence of preputial adhesions between the raw surfaces of the ventral inner prepuce and the healing glans [6]. Parents are also instructed to not retract the foreskin for at least 6–8 weeks after surgery.
16. After the first post-operative review, if the result is satisfactory and partial or complete retraction is possible in clinic, parents can attempt retraction once daily when the child is having their evening bath.

37.5 Tips and Tricks

37.5.1 Retractability at the End of Procedure

It is important to make sure the foreskin can be retracted with ease at the end of the procedure. Kallampallil et al. have shown that retractability at the end of surgery predicts the likelihood of future retractability [7].

37.5.2 Dorsal Preputial Release Incision (DPRI)

If the preputial skin closure is identified to be too tight, we perform a dorsal preputial release incision (DPRI). This is a vertical incision placed dorsally in the midline across the inner and outer prepuce.

The incision is then closed transversely with interrupted 6–0 polydioxanone following in a Heineke- Mikulicz fashion. This incision is well hidden along the preputial opening and increases the preputial circumference and allows easy retractability of the reconstructed foreskin. DPRI can be performed either before or after the preputioplasty and can also be considered in cases with severe ventral skin shortage in order to increase length of the reconstructed prepuce.

37.5.3 Pan's Modification

Pan et al. described closing the last part of the ventral incision transversely to widen the preputial opening and reported no phimosis in their series [8].

37.5.4 Securing the Catheter at the End of Surgery

Make sure when tying the glans to the catheter that the knot stays outside the reconstructed foreskin as it is difficult to completely remove the suture if the knot is too close to the glans.

37.5.5 Defining Postoperative Phimosis

It is important to note that postoperatively, non-complete retraction of the reconstructed foreskin may be observed, and this can still be considered normal before puberty. Balanitis Xerotica Obliterans (BXO) or presence of fibrotic scar should be ruled out on examination and in the absence of urinary symptoms, parents should be reassured.

37.6 Results and Conclusion

Foreskin reconstruction carries excellent functional and cosmetic results with low complication rates [9–11]. It does not increase operative time when associated with hypospadias repair [4]. It does not increase the likelihood of urethroplasty or skin complications or reoperation [4, 11]. Foreskin dehiscence and foreskin fistula are potential complications. Foreskin fistulae should be closed in layers after confirmation that there is no connection to the urethra. Preputioplasty can be attempted again after dehiscence, or a circumcision may be performed based on parental preference. Phimosis is non-retractability of the foreskin beyond puberty and should be treated based on the wishes of these young men and their parents.

Preputioplasty can therefore be offered to almost all children with distal hypospadias undergoing a single-stage repair if parents request it. The monkhood variety of foreskin should not be reconstructed for an optimal aesthetic outcome (Fig. 37.5).

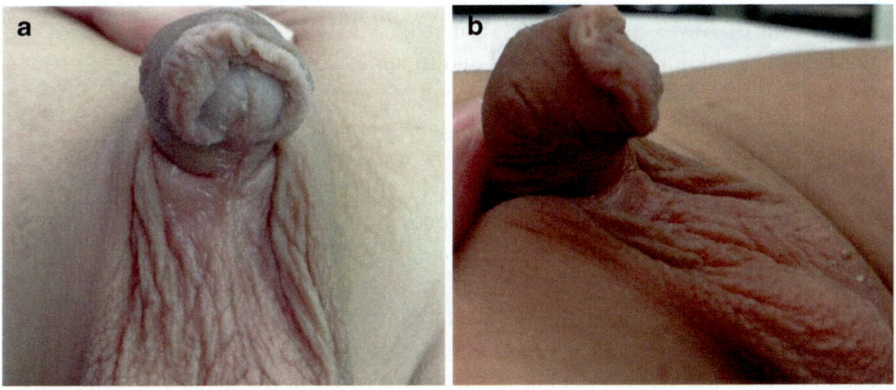

Fig. 37.5 Monkhood deformity of the prepuce

References

1. Dave SS. Male circumcision in Britain: findings from a national probability sample survey. Sex Transm Infect. 2003;79:499–500.
2. Jacobson DL, Balmert LC, Holl JL, Rosoklija I, Davis MM, Johnson EK. Nationwide circumcision trends: 2003 to 2016. J Urol. 2021;205(1):257–63.
3. Righini A. Symposium sur l'hypospadias. Ann Chir Infant. 1969;10:314.
4. Manuele R, Senni C, Patil K, Taghizadeh A, Garriboli M. Foreskin reconstruction at the time of single-stage hypospadias repair: is it a safe procedure? Int Urol Nephrol. 2019;51:187–91.
5. Bethell GS, Chhabra S, Shalaby MS, Corbett H, Kenny SE, Godse A, et al. Parental decisional satisfaction after hypospadias repair in the United Kingdom. J Pediatr Urol. 2020;16(2):164–e1.
6. Shoor G, Sugandhi N, Acharya SK, et al. Outcomes of preputioplasty in patients undergoing TIP urethroplasty (tubularization of incised urethral plate) for distal and mid penile hypospadias. J Pediatr Urol. 2020;16:319.
7. Kallampallil J, Hennayake S. Foreskin retractility following hypospadias repair with preputioplasty—medium term outcomes. J Pediatr Urol. 2013;9:1204–9.
8. Pan P. A prospective study comparing modified foreskin reconstruction versus circumcision with tubularized incised plate urethroplasty for distal and mid penile hypospadias. J Pediatr Urol. 2020;16:674.
9. Mosa H, Olczak B, Paul A, Mishra P, Taghizadeh A, Garriboli M. Are there anatomical limiting factors to foreskin reconstruction at the time of single-stage hypospadias repair? J Pediatr Urol. 2023;19:700.e1.
10. Castagnetti M, Gnech M, Angelini L, et al. Does preputial reconstruction increase complication rate of hypospadias repair? 20-year systematic review and meta-analysis. Front Pediatr. 2016;4:4.
11. Snodgrass W, Dajusta D, Villanueva C, et al. Foreskin reconstruction does not increase urethroplasty or skin complications after distal TIP hypospadias repair. J Pediatr Urol. 2013;9:401–6.

Correction of Penoscrotal Transposition

38

Pankaj M. Joshi, Tariq O. Abbas, and Sanjay B. Kulkarni

Abstract

Penoscrotal transposition (PST) is a rare congenital abnormality. There are various kinds of PST, ranging from an overriding scrotum to a bifid scrotum, and the surgical options are challenging. We describe here an effective surgical procedure for correcting penoscrotal transposition.

Keywords

Penoscrotal transposition · Hypospadias · Scrotoplasty

38.1 Introduction

Penoscrotal transposition is an uncommon condition linked to hypospadias [1–3]. There is minimal literature discussing surgical procedures for PST repair. Several procedures have been documented, although edema and skin necrosis are possible risks. The surgical procedures vary according to the degree of the PST [4]. The aesthetics of the genitalia should be given priority. Diverse surgeons elected to treat

---

Supplementary Information The online version contains supplementary material available at https://doi.org/10.1007/978-981-99-0795-3_38. The videos can be accessed individually by clicking the DOI link in the accompanying figure caption or by scanning this link with the SN More Media App.

P. M. Joshi (✉) · S. B. Kulkarni
UROKUL, Pune, India

T. O. Abbas
Urology Division, Surgery Department, Sidra Medicine, Doha, Qatar

T. O. Abbas (ed.), *Video Atlas of Hypospadias Surgery*,
https://doi.org/10.1007/978-981-99-0795-3_38

hypospadias while delaying the management of PST. Finally, the PST is occasionally left uncorrected. The fundamental pathology is scrotal skin covering the penis. The scrotum appears to be divided, and the penis had a downward orientation. The penis will not return to its normal location if the transposition is simply corrected and it is essential to repair the penile suspensory ligament. This chapter describes the process of transposition repair with reconstruction of genital aesthetics [2].

38.2 Video Demonstration

Factors	Findings
Age at surgery (months)	26
Gestational age (weeks)	Full term
Birth weight (gm)	2800
Gestational risks (e.g., maternal co-morbidities, IVF, Twin)	None
Family history	None
Testosterone (if yes, reason, and protocol used)	None
Any features of DSD (e.g., undescended testes)	None

38.3 Steps of the Procedure

The objective is to position the scrotal fold below the penis and to ensure that the rugosity of the scrotum is transverse and that the scrotal folds on either side are identical.

38.3.1 Preparation of Flap

- A stay suture is taken on the glans penis.
- Marking of the blood supply of scrotal flaps is done.
- The incision should never be circumferential.
- There should be a dorsal region about 1 cm which should be left intact as described by Glenn-Anderson [5] (Fig. 38.1).

38.3.2 Reforming the Suspensory Ligament

- The suspensory ligament lies free, and many times attached to the scrotal skin.
- The suspensory ligament is dissected from the skin.
- Interrupted sutures are taken, and suspensory ligament is reformed.
- The penis which was looking down initially starts looking cranially (Fig. 38.2).

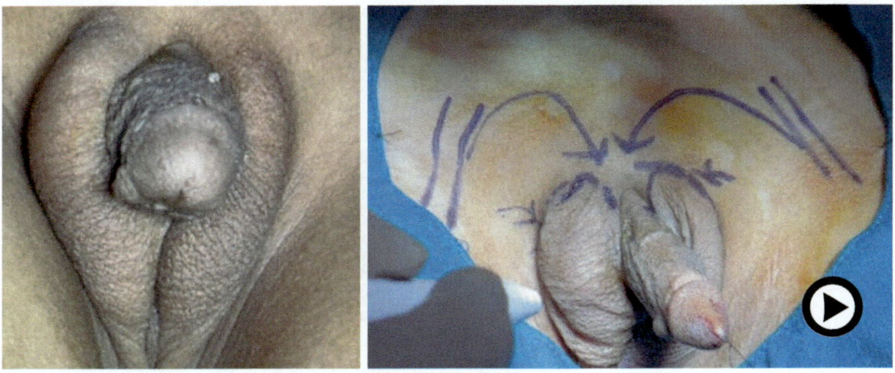

Fig. 38.1 (**a**) Severe penoscrotal transposition. (**b**) Marking of scrotal folds and direction of blood supply to the skin of penis and scrotum. Correction of penoscrotal transposition (https://doi.org/10.1007/000-cp4)

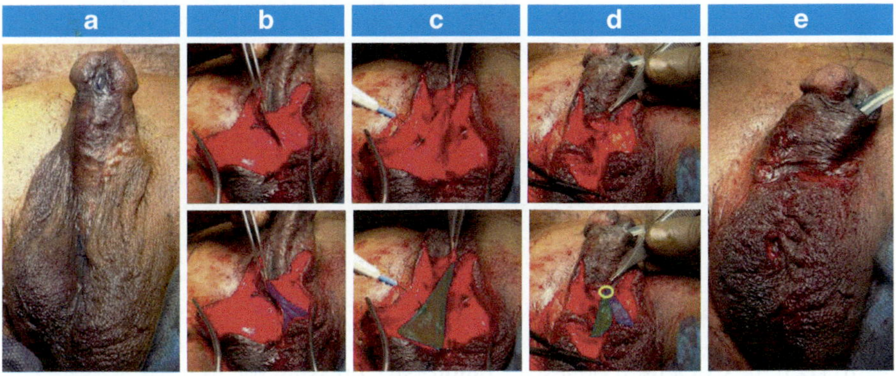

Fig. 38.2 Reforming the suspensory ligament. (**a**) Shows a case of peno-scrotal transposition that was not corrected. Detection of the abnormal attachments of the penile suspensory ligament (PSL) in the right side (**b**) and left (**c**), release of the testes and cord from the incorrectly positioned PSL, isolation of both the PSL and the midline (**d**), and restoration of the ligaments with fixation to the penile shaft (**e**)

38.3.2.1 Scrotoplasty

- The scrotal folds are rotated medially (Fig. 38.3).
- Both sides of scrotum are matched with the rugosity.
- The dartos is sutured in the midline.
- The scrotum is sutured in layers with interrupted sutures.

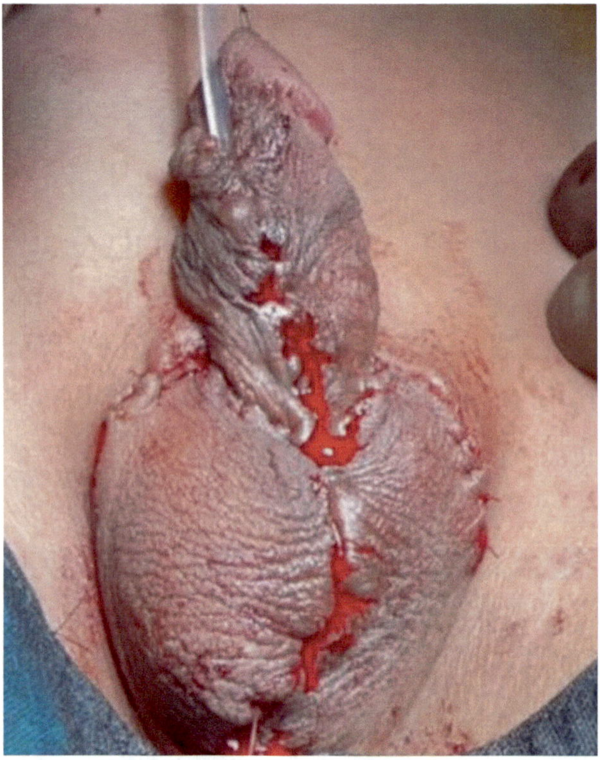

Fig. 38.3 Scrotoplasty is performed by rotating the scrotal folds medially

38.4 Post-operative Care

- To keep the Coban self-adhesive compressive dressing for 24 h.
- The urethral catheter/stent to be removed depending on the type of hypospadias repair.

38.5 Tips and Tricks

- Look at the lines of fusion of scrotal skin with penile skin.
- Mark incisions before making them.
- There should be no circumferential incision at the base of the penis, need to leave a dorsal skin area of 1–2 cm intact.
- Finding and reconstructing the penile suspensory ligament reforms the direction of penis.
- Scrotal skin should be sutured with interrupted sutures.

38.6 Results and Conclusion

Modified Glen Anderson technique if performed properly stand the test of time. It is the anatomical dissection which avoids complication of edema and skin necrosis. It is essential to correct the genital esthetics in patients with hypospadias and penoscrotal transposition. After surgery, complications included urethral and testicular damage, urinary fistula, flap necrosis, and penile edema. Circular incision near the base of the penis impairs lymphatic drainage, which may impede with neourethral healing. Widely used Glenn-Anderson technique demonstrated extensive edema that remained for lengthy durations (6–9 months) and, following resolution, left the penile skin black and pigmented, resembling scrotal skin. Saleh et al. found a 10% complication risk when only the dorsal strip of penile skin was preserved [5].

References

1. Abbas TO. An objective hypospadias classification system. J Pediatr Urol [Internet]. 2022;18(4):481.e1–8.
2. Abbas T, McCarthy L. Foreskin and penile problems in childhood. Surg [Internet]. 2016;34(5):221–5.
3. Abbas TO, editor. Hypospadiology: current challenges and future perspectives. 2023. 190 p.
4. Perović S, Vukadinović V. Penoscrotal transposition with hypospadias: 1-stage repair. J Urol [Internet]. 1992;148(5):1510–3.
5. Saleh A. Correction of incomplete penoscrotal transposition by a modified Glenn-Anderson technique. Afr J Paediatr Surg [Internet]. 2010;7(3):181–4.

Tips and Tricks in Post-hypospadias Repair Dressing

39

Aykut Akinci and Berk Burgu

Abstract

The surgical correction of male genital anomalies has seen progress in recent years, but choosing the right dressing remains challenging. The ideal dressing should provide mechanical protection against contamination and reduce edema caused by surgical trauma, while being easily removable and having minimal adverse reactions. The use of dressings is controversial due to the risk of pain and necrosis if applied too tightly. Different types of dressings have been attempted, but all have the potential to become contaminated and wet. Postoperative dressing is given to all patients who undergo hypospadias surgery in our clinic. In our clinic, a chlorhexidine gauze dressing followed by an elastic compression bandage is applied without tension.

Keywords

Hypospadias · Dressing · Elastic bandage · Bleeding · Edema

Supplementary Information The online version contains supplementary material available at https://doi.org/10.1007/978-981-99-0795-3_39. The videos can be accessed individually by clicking the DOI link in the accompanying figure caption or by scanning this link with the SN More Media App.

A. Akinci
Pediatric Urology, Denizli State Hospital, Denizli, Turkey

B. Burgu (✉)
Department of Pediatric Urology, Ankara University School of Medicine, Ankara, Turkey

T. O. Abbas (ed.), *Video Atlas of Hypospadias Surgery*,
https://doi.org/10.1007/978-981-99-0795-3_39

39.1 Introduction

Over the years, there has been progress in the surgical correction of male genital anomalies in children and adolescents, thanks to the development of new techniques, instruments, and sutures that have improved the outcomes. However, choosing the appropriate dressing remains a difficult task. Different materials have been utilized with varying degrees of success, and there is no agreement regarding their application [1]. The appropriate dressing for clinical use is determined by the tissue's protective function and its ability to serve as a mechanical barrier against contamination and to reduce edema caused by surgical trauma. The structural material should have specific physical properties such as elasticity, flexibility, and resistance, and it must fit tightly on the tissue surface. The dressing should have minimal adverse reactions when in contact with living tissue or organic fluids, and it should be easily removable.

There is a lack of consensus on the use of dressings in the medical literature due to the risk of pain and necrosis if applied too tightly, according to Sanders. Gormley et al. state that the purpose of a dressing is to protect the suture line, reduce swelling (edema), and immobilize the penis for a period of 2–10 days. Sanders further argues that dressings serve the purpose of preventing bleeding, maintaining sterility in the wound, keeping the penis upright to minimize urethral trauma at the penoscrotal angle through stenting, aiding lymph drainage, and allowing early detection of complications through visualization [2, 3].

Various types of dressings have been attempted for hypospadias, such as silastic foam elastic velcro dressings. Despite the kind of dressing used, removing it can cause stress, anxiety, and pain, and requires careful planning, often requiring a bath to soak off the dressing. Although this process can be time-consuming, particularly with uncooperative children, dressings are still commonly used. They are prone to becoming wet from urine, wound exudate, soiling, and sweat. To prevent any contamination of the dressing, it is recommended to apply double nappies [4–6].

All patients who undergo hypospadias surgery are given postoperative dressing. In our clinic, we apply a chlorhexidine gauze dressing to the penis first, followed by an elastic compression bandage (coban, 3M), which is applied without any tension.

39.2 Indications

Various techniques for hypospadias dressing have been described, and there are no strict rules. However, in our clinic, dressing is routinely applied after hypospadias repair surgery to reduce edema, bleeding, and infection. An elastic bandage-supported dressing has been used in our clinic for years. Although some surgeons have concerns about compression related to the elastic bandage, there are no serious side effects observed when it is applied correctly.

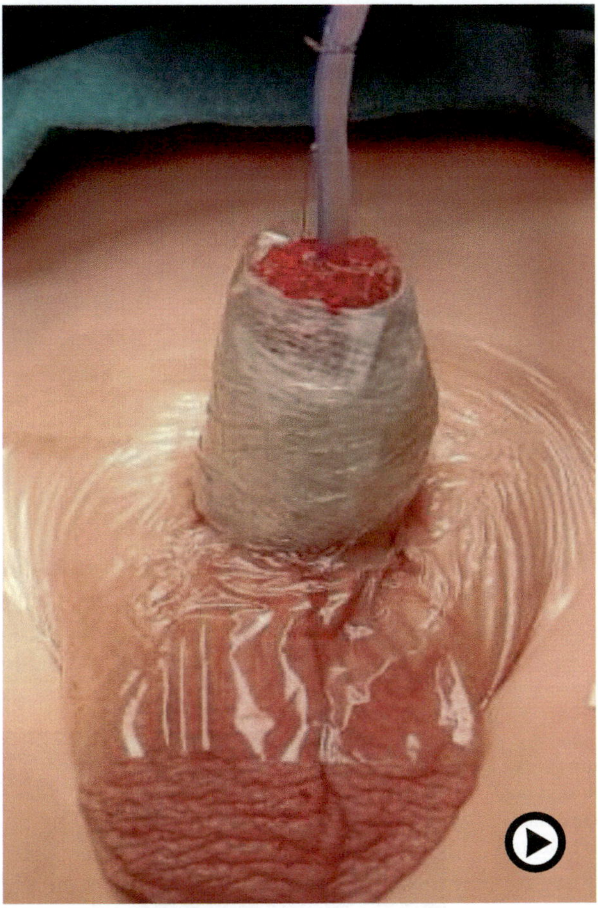

Fig. 39.1 Dressing applied in one-stage hypospadias. Tips and tricks in post hypospadias repair dressing (https://doi.org/10.1007/000-cp5)

In single-stage hypospadias surgery performed in our clinic, a chlorhexidine-soaked gauze is wrapped around the penis, followed by an elastic bandage applied without tension (Fig. 39.1).

In cases where a flap or graft is used in the first stage, a small roll is made from the chlorhexidine-containing gauze. This roll is placed on top of the flap or graft to apply pressure. Then, an elastic bandage is wrapped around the penis (Fig. 39.2).

In cases where the ventral skin is reconstructed and there are many stitches, especially along the ventral line, we also use a technique where the penis is gently pulled and fixed to the abdominal skin using traction (Fig. 39.3).

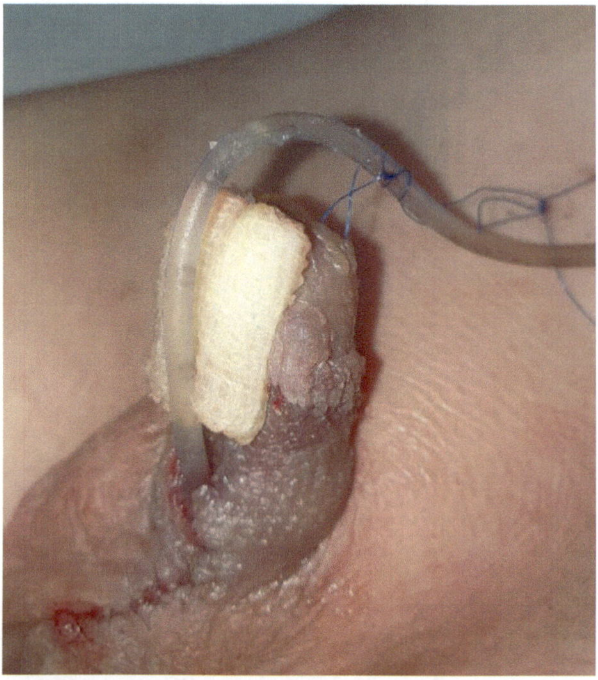

Fig. 39.2 Dressing applied when using graft or flap in two-stage hypospadias

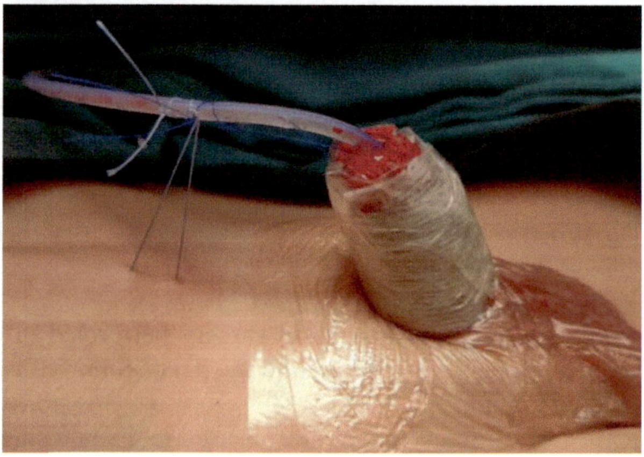

Fig. 39.3 Traction modification of the glans penis to the pubic skin that we apply in hypospadias repairs with serious ventral skin reconstruction

39.3 Video Demonstrations

Video link:
https://we.tl/t-ZIx35XQ9qp

39.4 Steps of the Procedure

- After the completion of the hypospadias repair, the traction suture previously passed through the glans is held with forceps. The surgical area is cleaned, sterilized again with an antiseptic solution, and dried. Afterward, materials to be used for dressing are brought close to the surgical field (Fig. 39.4).
- A ready-made gauze soaked in chlorhexidine is prepared in a suitable size for the penis. It is wrapped around the penis without being too tight. Due to its wetness, it can stay in place for a short time without loosening (Fig. 39.5).
- Afterward, we move on to the application of the previously cut elastic bandage, which is tailored to the length of the penis. The elastic bandage is wrapped around the penis at least 2 times, covering the entire penis and ensuring that the glans penis is not exposed, while allowing for some tension (Fig. 39.6).

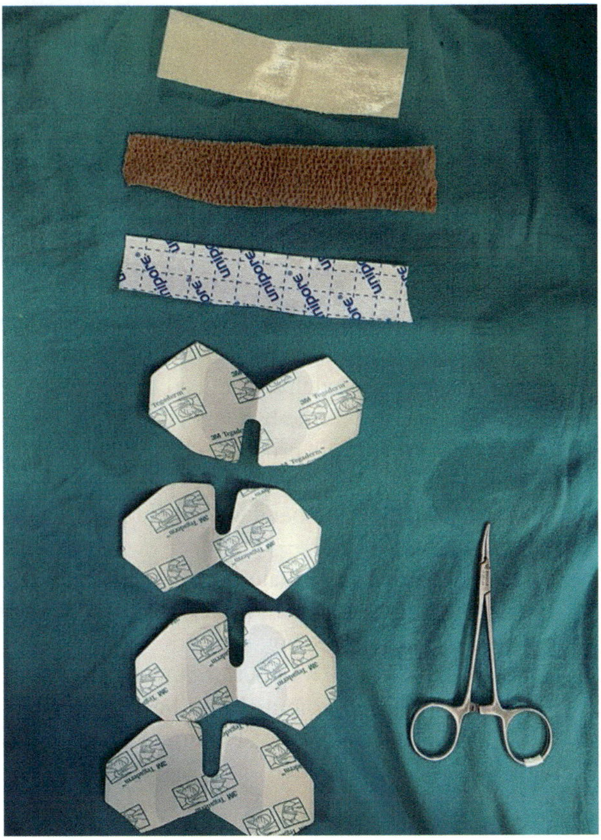

Fig. 39.4 Materials to be used for dressing

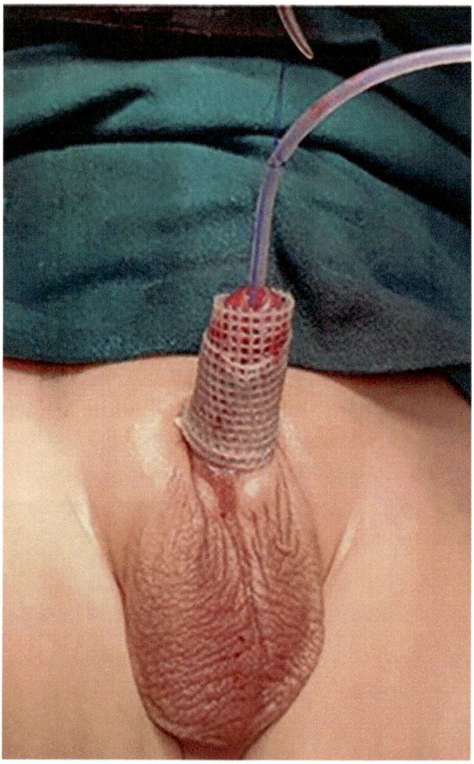

Fig. 39.5 Wrapping the penis with gauze soaked in chlorhexidine

- If the elastic bandage is not tight enough or too tight, it should be removed and reapplied. It is important to ensure that the bandage is not too tight, as this can cause complications such as reduced blood flow to the penis.
- After wrapping the elastic bandage, gently compress the end of the bandage with a mosquito clamp. This process will prevent the bandage from loosening due to its structure.
- Then, secure the elastic bandage with at least one wrap of a non-allergenic adhesive bandage (Fig. 39.7).
- Four pieces of dressing material in the form of transparent film are being used. They are cut in the shape of butterflies and then attached to all four sides of the penis to secure the dressing.
- In cases where a large number of stitches are needed on the ventral skin, to prevent maceration and promote better healing, the traction suture on the glans penis can be gently secured to the abdominal skin (Fig. 39.8).

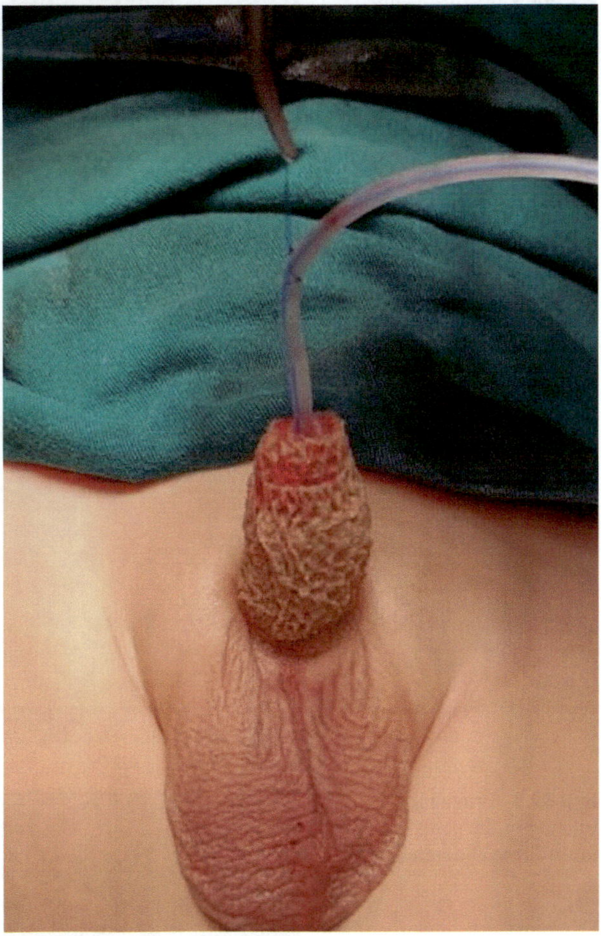

Fig. 39.6 Complete wrapping of the penis with an elastic bandage

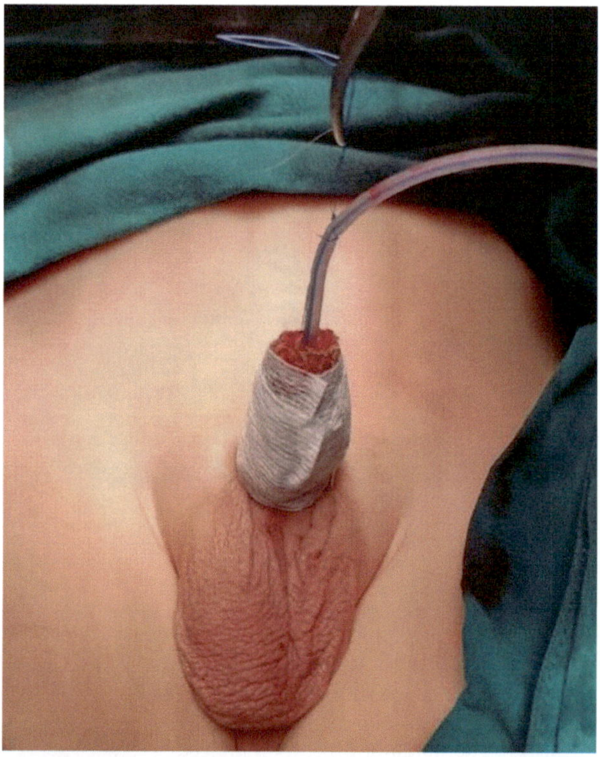

Fig. 39.7 Fixation of the dressing with hypoallergenic adhesive tape

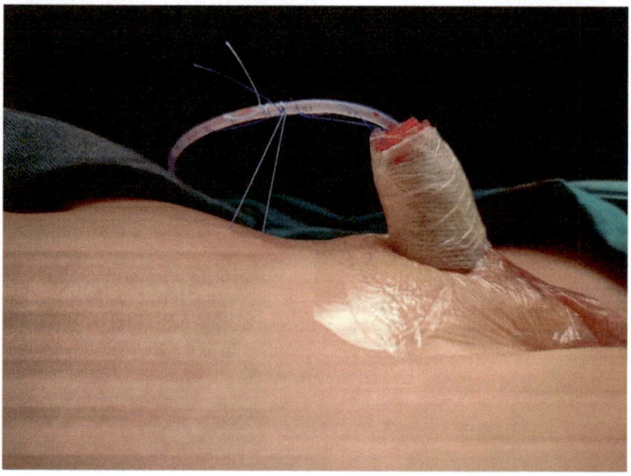

Fig. 39.8 Providing traction of the penis towards the abdominal skin

39.5 Tips and Tricks

- Applying dressings after hypospadias surgery can indeed help reduce swelling and bleeding, and also lower the risk of infection. Post-operative dressings help to keep the surgical area clean and dry, which can facilitate the healing process of the wound.
- Applying dressings too tightly after hypospadias surgery can cause tissue perfusion problems and should be avoided. It can lead to a decrease in blood flow to the surgical site, which may negatively impact the healing process. Therefore, it is important to be cautious of the tightness of the dressings.
- Small rolls of gauze soaked in chlorhexidine can be made to prevent hematoma formation under the graft or flaps that will be used.
- The double diaper method can be applied to patients to make it easier to monitor the hypospadias dressing. This method involves placing a second diaper over the first one to hold the dressing securely in place and prevent it from shifting or coming loose. A catheter is placed between the two diapers. This can help to minimize the risk of infection and make it easier for caregivers to change the dressing as needed.
- During postoperative follow-up, color changes in the glans penis should be monitored, and if there is any suspicion, the dressing should be opened to inspect the surgical site. This is important because changes in the color of the glans penis, such as blueness or purple discoloration, can indicate a potential problem with blood flow to the area. If left untreated, this can lead to tissue damage or even loss of tissue. Therefore, close monitoring and prompt action is necessary to prevent further complications.
- Gently fixing the glans penis to the pubic skin in patients who have undergone reconstruction on the ventral skin and have a large number of sutures can prevent maceration and accelerate tissue healing. This method can help to minimize the risk of infection, promote better wound healing, and prevent complications such as skin breakdown or wound dehiscence. However, it is important to ensure that the fixation is done gently and does not put undue pressure on the surgical site, as this can cause further damage and delay healing.

39.6 Results and Conclusion

There is no definite consensus on postoperative dressing for hypospadias [7]. In fact, some studies have emphasized that dressing may not be necessary for every patient undergoing hypospadias repair [8]. However, we routinely apply it, particularly because it reduces swelling and bleeding, and decreases the likelihood of wound infection. Elastic bandages can be safely used as a dressing technique, but the tightness during application is crucial. It is recommended to monitor the color of the glans after the surgery and intervene if necessary.

References

1. Martins AGS, et al. A wet dressing for hypospadias surgery. Int Braz J Urol. 2013;39:408–13.
2. Sanders C. A review of current practice for boys undergoing hypospadias repair: from pre-operative work up to removal of dressing post-surgery. J Child Health Care. 2002;6(1):60–9. https://doi.org/10.1177/136749350200600104.
3. Gormley A, Fishwick J, Whitnall B. Home dressing removal following hypospadias repair. J Child Health Care. 2007;11(2):158–66. https://doi.org/10.1177/1367493507076779.
4. Whitaker RH, Dennis MJ. Silastic foam dressing in hypospadias surgery. Ann R Coll Surg Engl. 1987;69(2):59–60.
5. Singh RB, Pavithran NM. Elastic and Velcro dressing for penis. Pediatr Surg Int. 2004;20(5):389–90. https://doi.org/10.1007/s00383-004-1206-7.
6. Pfeil M, Lindsay B. Hypospadias repair: an overview. Int J Urol Nurs. 2010;4:4–12.
7. Escolino M, et al. The role of postoperative dressing in hypospadias surgery: a systematic review and meta-analysis of the pediatric literature. Eur J Pediatr Surg. 2023;33:441. https://doi.org/10.1055/a-2048-7486.
8. Van Savage JG, Palanca LG, Slaughenhoupt BL. A prospective randomized trial of dressings versus no dressings for hypospadias repair. J Urol. 2000;164(3 Pt 2):981–3. https://doi.org/10.1097/00005392-200009020-00015.

GPSR Compliance

The European Union's (EU) General Product Safety Regulation (GPSR) is a set of rules that requires consumer products to be safe and our obligations to ensure this.

If you have any concerns about our products, you can contact us on ProductSafety@springernature.com

In case Publisher is established outside the EU, the EU authorized representative is:

Springer Nature Customer Service Center GmbH
Europaplatz 3
69115 Heidelberg, Germany

Batch number: 10726135

Printed by Printforce, the Netherlands